A phrenologist's view of brain organization and
From Johann Kaspar Spurzheim, 1826.

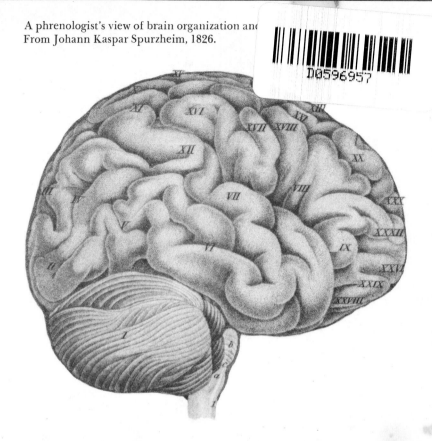

*Guide to the Principal Zones*

I. Organ of Amativeness
II. Organ of Philoprogenitiveness
III. Organ of Inhabitiveness
IV. Organ of Adhesiveness
V. Organ of Combativeness
VI. Organ of Destructiveness
VII. Organ of Secretiveness
VIII. Organ of Acquisitiveness
IX. Organ of Constructiveness
X. Organ of Self-Esteem
XI. Organ of Love of Approbation
XII. Organ of Cautiousness
XIII. Organ of Benevolence
XIV. Organ of Veneration
XV. Organ of Firmness
XVI. Organ of Conscientiousness
XVII. Organ of Hope
XVIII. Organ of Marvellousness

XIX. Organ of Ideality
XX. Organ of Mirthfulness
XXI. Organ of Imitation
XXII. Organ of Individuality
XXIII. Organ of Configuration
XXIV. Organ of Size
XXV. Organ of Weight and Resistance
XXVI. Organ of Colouring
XXVII. Organ of Locality
XXVIII. Organ of Calculation
XXIX. Organ of Order
XXX. Organ of Eventuality
XXXI. Organ of Time
XXXII. Organ of Melody
XXXIII. Organ of Language
XXXIV. Organ of Comparison
XXXV. Organ of Causality

*Also by Howard Gardner*

The Quest for Mind
The Arts and Human Development

# The Shattered Mind

# The Shattered Mind

## The Person After Brain Damage

# Howard Gardner

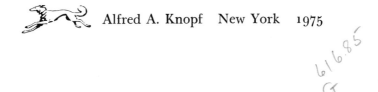

Alfred A. Knopf    New York    1975

Copyright © 1974 by Howard Gardner

All rights reserved under International and Pan-American Copyright Conventions. Published in the United States by Alfred A. Knopf, Inc., New York, and simultaneously in Canada by Random House of Canada Limited, Toronto. Distributed by Random House, Inc., New York.

Library of Congress Cataloging in Publication Data

Gardner, Howard. (date)    The shattered mind.
Includes bibliographical references and index.
1. Brain damage.   2. Cerebrovascular disease—Cases,
clinical reports, statistics.   I. Title.
RC382.2.G28   1975      616.8'5      74-7740
ISBN 0-394-49315-X

Grateful acknowledgment is made to the following for permission to use the material indicated:

Drs. Martin Albert, D. Frank Benson, Norman Geschwind, and Harold Goodglass, colleagues at the Aphasia Research Center, for clinical data on patients treated at the Boston Veterans Administration Hospital.

Basic Books, Inc., for material from *The Man with a Shattered World: A History of a Brain Wound*, by A. R. Luria, © 1972 by Basic Books, Inc., Publishers, New York.

Dr. Arthur Benton, for material from "The Fiction of the Gerstmann Syndrome," which appeared in the *Journal of Neurology, Neurosurgery, and Psychiatry*.

CRM Publications and *Psychology Today* for material from the article "Developmental Dyslexia and the Forgotten Case of Monsieur C.," by Howard Gardner.

Doubleday and Company, Inc., for material from D. Ritchie, *Stroke: A Diary of Recovery*, 1960.

Faber and Faber Ltd., for material from D. Ritchie, *Stroke: A Diary of Recovery*, 1960.

Dr. Roman Jakobson, for material from R. Jakobson and M. Halle, *Fundamentals of Language*, Mouton, 1956.

Thomas Nelson and Sons Ltd., for material from A. B. Carter, *All About Strokes*, London, 1968.

Jonathan Cape Ltd., and Dr. A. R. Luria, for material from *The Man with a Shattered World: A History of a Brain Wound*, by A. R. Luria.

Dr. Richard Jung, for clinical data on patients and artists seen by him.

University of Illinois Press, for material from C. Scott Moss, *Recovery with Aphasia*, Urbana, Illinois, 1972.

F. K. Schattauer Verlag GmbH, Stuttgart, and Richard Jung, for material from the article "Neuropsychologie und Neurophysiologie des Kontur- und Formsehens in Zeichnung und Malerei."

Manufactured in the United States of America

FIRST EDITION

*For my teachers*

Roger Brown
Norman Geschwind
Harold Goodglass
Nelson Goodman

# Contents

# Illustrations

# Preface

Persistent curiosity about human thought processes has prompted me to consult diverse sources. Beginning, like many others, with personal introspection and with literary accounts, I have succumbed to a more "scientific" approach; and I have savored the implications about cognition which can be gained from the examination of children, as in the investigations of Jean Piaget; the description of the "savage mind," as in the writings of Claude Lévi-Strauss; the unraveling of neurotic distortions, as in the case studies of Sigmund Freud. But of the varied mirrors which reflect mentation—which illuminate such fundamental capacities as language, perception, memory, artistry—it is brain damage whose study has seemed to me the most rewarding and fascinating.

Why this should be so, I am not certain. Perhaps it is the bizarre, almost incredible clusters of symptoms which are so commonly encountered on a neurological ward and which virtually clamor for explanation. It may be the excitement of developing a set of hypotheses about a newly observed psychological process, and then having the immediate opportunity to establish its plausibility with the patient in question. Possibly, also, the intrinsically interdisciplinary nature of the salient issues in neuropsychology contributes to its special status: questions of philosophical import lend themselves to empirical investigation even as the physiological substrates of behavior are explored. Prospects for a unified view of the mind may indeed rest upon an understanding of the syndromes produced by injury to the brain.

I suspect, however, that a goodly portion of the excitement surrounding an area of research derives from the circumstances under which one encounters it and the colleagues with whom one collaborates. In this respect I have been most fortunate. The Aphasia Research Center of the Boston University School of Medicine and the Boston Veterans Administration Hospital houses a unique collection of gifted scholars from several disciplines. Together they have made significant progress both in illuminating pivotal issues in the sphere of human language and in charting fresh pathways of study of other higher cortical functions. First as a student, more recently as a co-researcher, I have gained enormously from the opportunity to work with the entire staff of the Center, and to examine several hundred patients seen on its Service. I want to express special thanks to Drs. Martin Albert, Frank Benson, Norman Geschwind, Harold Goodglass, and Edith Kaplan, who introduced me to the techniques of clinical investigation and were always available to discuss puzzling problems.

I was especially fortunate to find myself in this setting, surrounded by knowledgeable clinicians, because I soon discovered the paucity of introductory literature in this field. Notably lacking were materials which describe patients in some detail and then explicate the wider significance of clinical findings. Accordingly, an individual interested in the effects of brain damage, and its implications for normal functioning, has had to wait until the opportunity to interview diverse patients presents itself; read through a widely scattered and often conflicting and disputatious literature; and then strive to collate the disparate data he has gathered with one or other of the major theoretical orientations. The aim of the present work, therefore, is to fill a generally felt need, by aiding students and others who wish to acquire a broad overview of a fascinating field. It is my hope as well that the sometimes controversial conclusions may contribute to useful exchanges among scholars in neuropsychology.

Several friends and colleagues have generously read and commented upon sections of the book. I thank Drs. Russell Butler, Laird Cermak, Judy Gardner, Edith Kaplan, and Edgar Zurif; Kim Ling, Bill Lohman, Jenny Silverman, and Ellen Winner; and my insightful editors, Bob Gottlieb, Dan Okrent, and Melvin Rosenthal. Dr. Richard Strub graciously undertook the unenviable task of reading the entire manuscript in rough draft, saved me from a number of embarrassing slips, made valuable editorial suggestions, and generally encouraged me in completing the project. Thalia Chan and Gladys Bernardinalli assisted ably with the preparation of the manuscript; Ellen Winner skillfully prepared the figures; Bill Lohman kindly offered to prepare the index and performed this task with his customary competence. My work on aphasia and related disorders has been generously supported by the Social Science Research Council, Harvard Project Zero (through grants from the National Science Foundation and the National Institutes of Education), the Milton Fund and the Livingston Fund of Harvard University, and the National Institute of Neurological Disease and Stroke (#NS11408-01). I owe a special debt to my extended family for its constant support.

On the dedication page I name four gifted teachers and valued friends. In their unique and memorable ways,

Professors Roger Brown, Norman Geschwind, Harold Goodglass, and Nelson Goodman have each served as an inspiration to me. I have not attained their scrupulousness of scholarship, their mastery of empirical data, or their telling theoretical sagacity. Yet I hope that in this book I have repaid in some measure their generous encouragement of my work by highlighting the kinds of issues toward which they have directed their students.

HOWARD GARDNER
*Boston, Massachusetts*
*February 1974*

# The Shattered Mind

# 1 Introduction: Brain Injury as an Avenue to the Mind

*To look into our hearts is not enough. . . . one must look into the cerebral cortex.*

—T. S. ELIOT*

It is already commonplace to observe that the brain is the final, most challenging frontier beckoning investigators in the social and biological sciences. Workers in laboratories the world over are probing into the firing of single neural fibers, tracing anatomical connections in the nervous systems of mice and men, placing electrodes in the gray matter of experimental animals and selected surgical cases. While philosophers continue to wrestle with the definition of mind and ponder whether such an entity can ever "know itself," more than one illustrious scientist has declared that the mysteries of the brain may be resolved— or dissolved—in our lifetime.

The excitement attending recent discoveries about the brain should scarcely be minimized. But just what do these discoveries tell us about our "highest," most characteristically human functions? Spectacular as they are, neurophysiological findings at the cellular level seem to me

* All bibliographical references and attributions, as well as explanatory notes and glosses, will be found in the Notes section at the end of the book.

to have but a remote connection to the behaviors and thoughts of individuals like ourselves. Whether research at this microscopic level can eventually bridge the gap between neural synapses and human experience remains to be determined. Equally stunning, yet vexingly problematic, are recent claims that the individual's behavior may be controlled through "bio-feedback" loops, subject to the conscious decision of the individual himself, or to the manipulation of a benevolent (or diabolical) researcher. Although the prospect of voluntary control over bodily processes holds tremendous medical promise, the long-term reliability of these "self-directing" behaviors has not yet been established beyond reasonable doubt. Furthermore, control seems to be exerted primarily over autonomic responses, like blood pressure, rather than over complex learned skills and conscious cognitive processes.

Still another stream of provocative insights has come from "lesion" studies, in which the investigator destroys a certain site in an animal's nervous system and then assesses both the immediate and ultimate effects of this destruction. Application of this highly revealing procedure to human beings, however, is of course prohibited; and inasmuch as the capacities of greatest interest—language, self-awareness, scientific acumen, artistic skill, musical competence—are singularly lacking or hopelessly primitive in most animals, this avenue of understanding also has distinctly constricting limitations.

It may seem then that, however valuable and enlightening these various approaches may prove in their way, they must perforce leave untouched the mysteries of the mind. And yet, through a disturbingly pervasive phenomenon—injury to the brain as the result of accidents, tumors, and above all strokes—it *is* possible to study precisely those "higher cortical functions," those distinctly human competences, which elude investigators probing the performance of individual cells or the "willed" modification of autonomic responses. For every day hundreds of human brains are injured through one or another of these unanticipated twists of fate, and, as a consequence, certain highly complex behaviors and capacities are likely to be impaired; nonetheless, the individual may continue to function at a tolerable or even proficient level, and may be able to tell us, through one or another means, what he can and cannot do.

The variety of brain disorders constitutes a fascinating collection, including capacities altered in so bizarre a fashion as to resemble the vagaries of a science-fiction writer's imagination. Even so, the very cases which, viewed on their own terms, seem so anomalous, may paradoxically have the greatest potential for deepening our understanding of normal functioning.

In the pages that follow, we shall meet many victims of brain injury. Attempting first simply to describe their syndromes, we shall then seek to draw out the implicit lessons concerning our own thought processes, personality characteristics, and sense of self. In the course of this inquiry we shall also consider the history and the present state of neuropsychological research, the methods used by clinical and experimental scientists, the claims and counterclaims about normal (and supra-normal) functioning derived from studies of brain damage. For our purposes the largest and most important cadre of patients are the victims of stroke; and, of these, those whose language capacities have been affected constitute a particularly valuable source of illumination. I came to know one such patient very well during the early months of 1973. Because of the intrinsic interest of his condition, because of the intense humanness of his responses to it, and above all, because his plight exemplifies so many of the themes treated in this book, the case of Peter Franklin will serve as a revealing introduction to the exceedingly complex but perennially intriguing field of neuropsychology.

．　　．　　．

I first met Peter Franklin about two years after he had suffered his stroke. He was a tall, distinguished-looking man in his early sixties, immaculately groomed, with a neat handle-bar mustache, clear hazel eyes, and an infectious grin. Sitting near him in a waiting room, one would have detected no physical infirmities. Yet he displayed a slight limp when walking, he carried himself in a stiff manner, and there was a degree of weakness discernible in his left arm. Mr. Franklin had come to the Aphasia Unit where I work in order to be evaluated and to receive language therapy. He shook my hand firmly, carefully removed his jacket, and crossed his legs as we began to talk.

"How are you today?" I asked.

"Fine, fine," he replied, at first smiling, but then displaying some slight misgiving or discomfort, I was uncertain which.

"Can you tell me what brought you here to the hospital?" I asked.

"What's that?"

"Excuse me," I said (this time speaking more slowly). "How did you get sick? What's wrong?"

"Oh, I see. Now, listen here. Now listen here. Well, I'll tell you. I said, sit down, strewn with clothes, sit, sit down, thank you, thank you. Oh, goodness gracious, goodness gracious. Mrs. Hope, thank God, Mrs. Hope, going to bed. Sleeping. All right, all right. Seconal, seconal [a sleeping pill]. And by the way Victoria Hospital, Maine. I said and, by the way. Dead. Dr. Hope, psychiatrist. Brilliant. All right and two days. Sick. Piss and bewildered. I can't remember. And doctors, doctors. Boys, boys, tip fifty dollars, tip, tip, boys."

"Right," I said. I had reviewed Mr. Franklin's medical charts and so was able to interpret what he had said. I knew that he had spent the summer of 1971 on a small lake in southern Maine, living by himself in a cabin, in close proximity to a long-time friend, Natalie Hope. Both the Franklin and Hope families had vacationed for many years in the Lake Carson area and, even now, after Mrs. Hope's husband had died, and Franklin was estranged from his wife, they returned annually to this spot.

Although the medical charts were not precise on this point, I gathered that Mrs. Hope and Mr. Franklin had dined out together the night of the stroke. Mr. Franklin had complained that he was rather tired and had a slight headache, and so had retired early. Unable to rest, he took some sleeping pills. The next thing he remembered was lying on the floor, with clothing strewn about him; he somehow dragged himself out of the cabin, where Mrs. Hope spotted him walking about, bathrobe half on, drooling saliva, generally disheveled and confused, about nine o'clock the following morning. She had called the local police, who arrived in the company of a doctor about fifteen minutes later. Mr. Franklin had been rushed to the local Victoria Hospital, where he had recuperated for a few weeks before returning to his home in Pennsylvania. In the last sentence quoted above he was apparently alluding to a few youths from a nearby village who had assembled his belongings when he vacated the cabin.

As Mr. Franklin had not referred to the reason for his current hospitalization, I attempted a more direct approach to this sensitive area. "Could you tell me what's bothering you now?" I asked.

Suddenly Mr. Franklin's even demeanor changed and, shaking his fist, he lashed out at me: "Now listen here. Irritate. Irritate. Irritate, irritate, irritate, irritate, irritate, irritate! Questions, questions. Stupid doctors. No good, no good. Irritate. Irritate. Dean, dean, yes sir, yes sir. What's this, what's this. Wall, wall, door." He pointed at various objects around the room and gave vent to several oaths. "That's all, that's all, forget it, forget it." With these last words, Mr. Franklin calmed down somewhat. He then said, as if issuing instructions to himself, "Calm calm down, calm down, it's all right, it's all right." Eyeing me for the first time in several moments, he said, "Sorry, sorry."

I was subsequently to spend much time with Peter Franklin. I learned to be very careful lest I stimulate another such outburst, and yet to insist firmly that he respond to questions, that he avoid darting back and forth among questions, and that he try his best to provide specific information. Although my primary aim was to evaluate certain linguistic capacities, I inevitably touched upon many other aspects of his mental functioning, his personality, his life history. From his own words and from contacts with his friends, I learned that Franklin, a historian by training, had for many years served as dean of a small, prestigious liberal arts college in Pennsylvania. His academic career had been highly successful, and he had been instrumental in maintaining the institution's humanistic orientation against those he perceived as the "philistines" of the natural and social sciences. He had, however, become somewhat embittered in recent years. His wife had left him, he was on poor terms with one of his children, and he had begun drinking quite heavily; he had also been receiving psychotherapy, off and on, for nearly a decade. Nonetheless, even those who disagreed strongly with his views, and resented his arrogant manner, respected the forthrightness and integrity with which he defended his principles and the support which he afforded his faculty and students. Mr. Franklin had been a talented sportsman, an avid amateur musician, and even something of a *bon vivant* in his tastes for food and companionship. Glimmerings of his former eminence and elegance remained apparent; he shaved closely, dressed nattily, received visits and mail from former colleagues; he became visibly annoyed when *The New York Times* and the

Philadelphia *Inquirer* failed to arrive on schedule—even though, as he was surely aware, he was incapable of reading them with any substantial measure of understanding.

One other, seemingly insignificant item from his past turned out to be of salient medical importance. Peter Franklin's parents had discovered, when he was about eighteen months old, that their son was left-handed. As was common in this country at the turn of the century, a strenuous effort had been made to convert him into a right-hander; indeed, Mr. Franklin now wrote and held silverware with his right hand, though he continued to favor his left hand in sports, tool use, and other pursuits of a "less public" nature. The potential significance of this fact was first touched on by the doctor who attended Mr. Franklin outside his cabin in Maine. Noting that Mr. Franklin was unable to speak, and that he was paralyzed on his left side, the physician had asked Mrs. Hope, "Is he by any chance a left-hander? If so, that may affect his chances for recovery." The doctor then briefly explained to her that left-handers have an atypical brain organization and that this sometimes enhances the recovery potential of a stroke victim.

Peter Franklin was (and remains) clearly aphasic—that is, his linguistic abilities were impaired—yet, with some effort, we were able to communicate quite adequately. His speech became easier to understand as I grew accustomed to his habit of repeating words, to the frequent (and seemingly involuntary) imprecation of "irritate," and to his persistent tendency to shift from one topic to another. I found that he would often answer incorrectly when factual questions were posed, such as, What do you put on first, your shoes or your socks? Who is second in command to the President? Can a stone float in water? He would rarely, however, miss the intent of a question which pertained to his own life, and would usually answer appropriately. As an example, when I asked him whether he wished to speak with the president of his college, he replied, "Why sure, President Smith, good friend, good friend, old friend, come right in, sit down sit down, 1954, that's right." Mr. Franklin was unable to set clocks at a stated time, or to read the time aloud; but he always arrived punctually for his appointments and became furious if I (or anyone else) did not. He had difficulties in forming certain sounds—"irritate," for example, came out sometimes as "ear-tate," and even more frequently as a somewhat foreign-sounding "ur-tay"—yet this articulatory problem rarely prevented him from conveying what was on his mind. Outbursts of ill temper remained always a possibility, though they occurred less often as I learned which subjects to avoid and when to terminate a conversation. But there was a rich variety of emotional expression as well: he would laugh heartily at his own jokes and at comical events occurring about the ward; he cried at the mention of Mrs. Hope's late husband, and looked alternately blissful or perplexed, depending on which of his daughters was mentioned.

Although he did not understand complex commands or questions of the sort mentioned above, Mr. Franklin was able to follow what was going on about him and kept close tabs on his own medical treatment and rehabilitation. He could easily hum familiar tunes, and when we sat down at the piano, he surprised me by playing old show tunes excellently with his right hand and even passably with his somewhat weak left hand. He could follow simple conversation and certain commands in French and say a few words, but both his pronunciation and his syntax were even more faulty than in English. He could name most common objects, colors, and body parts, and could read aloud quite well. However, I was unable to determine the extent to which he understood what he read, beyond the names of simple objects or short familiar phrases. Although he had written several books about colonial America, and a collection of essays on education in the humanities, his ability to express himself in writing was now quite poor. And while he could form the letters adequately, he rarely produced a phrase that was error-free, and was totally unable to pen extended discourse. Essentially all his language functions had been reduced to a low level. And yet he frequently displayed an intelligent awareness of what was going on.

This alertness came through most vividly one Saturday afternoon when I came to my office for a few minutes. Mr. Franklin was pacing the halls, as he did for several miles each day, and when he saw me he burst into laughter. He then came over, shook my hand, and exclaimed, "Saturday, Saturday, doctor, golf [he pantomimed a golf swing], tennis [pantomiming a tennis swing], lazy in the sun, enjoy no work, doctors, doctors, Saturday." I joined in the conviviality and he then became somewhat quieter and more serious. He added, "1930, me, Dean Franklin, work, day, night, work, work, work. I understand, I understand, believe me." He then smiled, and walked slowly away, looked back at me and uttered, as if to apologize, a pet phrase of his "Only joking, only joking."

When I saw Mr. Franklin again the following week, he immediately came over to me, winked, and said, "Saturday, Saturday, working hard, working hard. Me, working too." Here was a patient whose ability to communicate had been radically diminished, but whose memory, motivation, and understanding of the world had remained to a considerable extent intact. For certain reasons, such as his ambidextrousness, Mr. Franklin's case does not conform neatly to the diagnostic categories which neurologists have devised over the years. Yet the numerous intriguing issues raised by his case are integral to our major themes, and so we shall return to his story as our development of these themes unfolds.

Peter Franklin was one of the approximately 300,000 Americans in 1971 to suffer a stroke. This meant that his brain had been injured, and brain tissue destroyed, though we were uncertain of the exact cause. Perhaps one of the major vessels leading to the brain had become occluded through the gradual accumulation of fatty materials; an artery may have burst; or a clot lodged in the heart or in a major artery may have broken loose, and was now blocking a smaller artery in the brain. Factors that increase the possibility of such sudden injury to the brain—a stroke of God, it was called in ancient times—include obesity, diabetes, high blood pressure, and inflammation or infection of the blood vessels. Chances for a stroke also rise with age, so that, if other causes do not intervene, it is from this condition that most of us will eventually die. Yet stroke or stroke-like ailments can occur in individuals of any age, including significant numbers of infants and even individuals in their early twenties. Although certain diets and exercise programs appear to reduce the risk, the fact remains that a cerebral vascular accident (the technical term) can strike any individual at any time.

If a stroke is very severe, so that large portions of the brain are destroyed, chances for survival are small. Stroke is, in fact, the third leading killer, just behind heart disease and cancer. Strokes can also be relatively benign, some so mild that they go undetected or unreported, others sufficiently limited that the individual recovers within a few days and displays no discernible aftereffects. Strokes of either extreme severity or extreme mildness comprise a sizeable proportion of the yearly total, but for obvious reasons neither kind is very instructive from a research standpoint. A significant number of strokes each year, however, are of intermediate severity—insufficient to kill the individual or reduce him to a vegetable state, yet serious enough to permanently affect his functioning. Such stroke victims will seldom return to work or resume their "pre-morbid" pace of activity; yet they are likely to get around, to express themselves passably, to interact with other persons, to experience happiness and despair, to share these feelings with others. Many of us know such stroke victims and are frequently torn between a desire to help the individual or to treat him as if nothing has happened, and, on the other hand, a wish to spurn him out of embarrassment, distaste, or fear.

Individuals sustaining moderate strokes receive a great deal of medical attention. They must be followed up by neurologists (much of whose practice, in fact, consists in the treatment of stroke) and not infrequently by neuro-surgeons, cardiologists, and other specialists as well. The more fortunate victims also receive rehabilitation, including speech therapy, physical therapy, corrective therapy, occupational therapy, and, less frequently, family or social therapy.

Many sufferers are examined by psychologists who subject them to batteries of tests. Some of these are primarily for diagnostic purposes: to determine the degree of intellectual impairment, to pinpoint areas of difficulty or of retained proficiency, to detect changes in personality. Other tests aid therapists in devising the optimal program of rehabilitation. But a considerable amount of such testing serves another purpose; for the brain-damaged person is uniquely equipped to provide the psychologist, the neurologist, the philosopher, with clues as to how the brain—or the mind—operates.

It is my purpose in this book to demonstrate that a host of crucial issues in psychology can be illuminated by a thoughtful study of the behavior and testimony of brain-damaged individuals. The basic human capacities that we normally take for granted—language, perception, memory —as well as more intricate or complex skills, such as mathematical reasoning, speed reading, or artistic competence, can be viewed thereby in a new light, and understood in a more profound way. Perhaps most significant, we can achieve a deeper understanding of our sense of self, of the essence of our human consciousness, by study-ing the changes effected in it when things go awry.

A word seems in order here about the attitude of re-searchers such as myself toward such patients. It is a pain-ful paradox, one intrinsic to many aspects of scientific and medical research, that human knowledge and self-under-standing should be advanced through human suffering and misfortune; and it is a paradox of which clinical investi-gators cannot help but be constantly aware. Naturally it is our first duty as clinicians to make the patient as com-fortable as we can and to aid him to the fullest extent possible. Should a conflict arise between the demands of research and those of treatment, there is no question as to how the conflict is to be resolved. And yet, within the limits thus imposed, the opportunity to obtain informa-tion about human functioning must be seized, for the researcher has an obligation to the larger community as well. If there is no denying the interest, often fascination, of the conditions described here, nothing said above or in what follows should be construed as a rejoicing over a state of affairs so tragic for all concerned, and one in which, after all, we (or someone close to us) may one day find ourselves.

Were stroke to reduce each and all of a victim's mental and physical capacities by an equal amount, this outcome would be important to determine, but otherwise not very informative—the brain-damaged individual would emerge as but a slowed-down or imperfect version of the normal. By the same token, if the afflicted person simply regressed to a more childlike state, so that he resembled a teenager, a pre-adolescent, or even a toddler, this finding, again, would be worth noting but not worth pursuing. What happens in brain damage, however, is quite another story. Instead of all parts of the brain, and every human skill, becoming equally impaired, damage is highly selective. One region of the brain may be completely devastated, while the others remain as before; two intact regions of the brain may be isolated from each other because of damage in the connecting tissue; simultaneous or successive injuries at two distinct sites may produce a highly atypical pattern of breakdown.

The brain-damaged patient, then, is a unique experiment in nature. What no researcher may do—make a selective lesion in a human brain—is done every day by inexorable Fate. Indeed, during the last century the psychological effect of nearly every conceivable kind of destruction—and, conversely, of sparing—in the human brain has been noted and its effects studied. Brains are damaged from a variety of causes, and scientific insights can also be obtained from victims of trauma or tumors; but the relative stability and discreteness of a lesion from stroke make it especially revealing to investigators. Sometimes the locus of the stroke is confirmed at autopsy; electroencephalographic, radiological, or isotope studies also provide corroborative evidence about the lesion's site and size. But even if one does not know which region has been destroyed, the effects of brain damage can still be examined. So long as one describes carefully the symptoms found (and not found) in each patient, regularities will eventually emerge, and these patterns constitute a major foundation of psychological knowledge. (For this, among other reasons, we need make only fleeting references to anatomy and physiology in this book; yet these references do deserve explication, and so I have included a brief introduction to the brain and to brain terminology later in this chapter.)

The mission of the neuropsychologist is to interview and then test the brain-damaged patient in a variety of domains, following which he draws up a balance sheet, specifying which skills have been spared, which impaired. Neuropsychological investigations carried out in various countries over many years have yielded totally unexpected insights and tellingly altered our understanding of the human mind.

As an initial example, consider the peculiar condition of *pure alexia*. In this, a patient who has suffered injury in the posterior regions of his brain will suddenly find himself unable to read printed matter. At first, very likely, he thinks he needs new glasses; but his visual perception (of objects, faces, etc.) is normal. The possibility of a general language problem is likewise excluded, for he can speak and understand as well as before. The hypothesis of a difficulty with all "written language" is belied by the fact that he can write—but, amazingly, he cannot even read his own writing! Perhaps even more surprising, the pure alexic can generally read numbers and comprehend symbols related to numerical operations, even while unable to read the words surrounding the numbers. He can read DIX as the roman numeral for 509, but not as "diks." His difficulty is restricted exclusively to the decoding—as distinct from the visual perception or the production—of verbal symbolic materials.

This clinical condition challenges prevalent notions about reading, for it suggests strongly that the decoding of verbal symbols requires more than an ability to perceive and to communicate adequately. And the demonstration that one may be able to decode numbers but not words or letters brings into question any view of symbolic processing as being all of a piece. Is there, then, a specialized reading center in the brain, which has been uniquely injured? Could an alexic unable to read Western languages decode Chinese ideographs? How about letters etched into his hand, musical notation, advertising trademarks? A whole cluster of issues is raised—and can perhaps be solved—by a probing examination of alexic patients.

Here the study of brain damage has helped us dissect a skill into its component parts; a capacity thought to be unitary—the reading of symbols—is shown to be divisible into separate functions. The opposite situation also occurs, when a circumscribed lesion destroys a range of apparently unrelated skills. We find, for example, that a lesion in the parietal lobe of the "dominant" hemisphere causes difficulty in writing, in performing mathematical operations, in telling left from right, in identifying one's fingers. Yet patients with this condition can speak and read adequately, can identify other body parts, and can find their way about. The question arises: have the difficulties cited co-occurred owing to an accident of anatomy, or is there a common psychological thread or underlying structure running through mathematics, writing, and knowledge of one's digits? Such a query is of more than academic interest, for the problems of children who have difficulty in learning arithmetic may reflect a lack of differentiation in their knowledge of their bodies; perhaps the ability to count and to perform mathematical operations could even be enhanced by instruction in distinguishing and manipulating one's fingers.

A somewhat related disorder resulting from injury in the angular gyrus region, again in the "dominant" hemisphere, produces patients unable to calculate, to find their way around complex spatial layouts, or to understand sentences expressing relations such as "on top of," "inside of," "mother's brother," or the passive "A was hit by B." Again a question arises: can an underlying difficulty in handling spatial relations destroy the capacity to orient oneself, to calculate, and to understand certain commands and questions? If so, what is the nature of this potent common operation and how does it arise? Might training in maze-running or object-manipulation help the youngster (or adult) exhibiting difficulty in calculation? Or are the causal relations in the opposite direction, so that training in mathematics will aid the restoration or development of one's linguistic and spatial capacities? And how does the parietal lobe injury relate to the angular gyrus lesion—is arithmetical capacity similarly impaired in both cases?

These examples may be enough to hint at the vast potential of neuropsychological investigations. In each case, preconceptions about how the mind works—often based on the study of normal individuals or on our own casual introspections—are belied by the symptoms and syndromes of brain-injured patients. In one instance, the seemingly unified category of "reading" breaks down into unexpected components; in another, seemingly diverse activities of language, arithmetical calculation, and spatial orientation are related through a common underlying operation which one is challenged to identify. Analogous lessons can be drawn about a slew of psychological topics, ranging from the role played by language in scientific and artistic thinking, to the question of whether each of us possesses a unique and unified mind. The conclusions eventually drawn must come from controlled observations of many patients; but a conclusive consensus can emerge only if each individual patient is carefully and thoroughly investigated. Similarly, while actuarial tables and experimental studies can provide important clues about the rehabilitation potential and the ultimate fate of stroke victims, the different facts of each case preclude authoritative predictions and offer occasional surprises even to the highly experienced neuropsychologist.

By the time Mr. Franklin arrived at our hospital, some two years after his stroke, laboratory tests had already established a number of facts about his condition. We were convinced that he had sustained a fairly large stroke in the central portions of his right cerebral cortex. It seemed likely that the artery which supplies this portion of his brain had been blocked, and a sizeable amount of tissue consequently destroyed. A further indication of the size and severity of his stroke was the persistence of paralysis in his left limbs as well as appreciable loss of sensation on that side of his body. Some further improvement in these motor and sensory functions could be expected if his general health remained otherwise unchanged, but Mr. Franklin would remain perceptibly paralyzed as long as he lived.

The outlook for his "higher mental functions" was not much more encouraging—though, again, some further progress in speaking, understanding, reading, writing, and general alertness might be expected, particularly if he received regular drill and was motivated to practice on his own. A dramatic change in personality and in emotional behavior was highly unlikely, for the stroke seemed only to have accentuated his prior personal traits. Clouding Mr. Franklin's prognosis yet further was the rapid approach of old age, and the possibility that he might sustain further strokes. His frequent depressions were not surprising, particularly in view of his comprehension of the precariousness of his situation. Yet, the fact that he had been "born" left-handed and had been compelled to switch the "dominance" of certain activities raised a lingering hope that there might yet be a significant improvement.

For a person who has been vigorously engaged in many activities, adjustment to the circumscribed life-space of the stroke victim is an especially difficult process. While fundamental aspects of the personality may remain unaffected, the person's entire life-style has been in a single moment radically disrupted. This upheaval takes its toll on the patient's family and friends as well as on himself. Although in rare cases such a misfortune brings a family closer together, a stroke is far more likely to exacerbate family difficulties or to serve as the spur for cutting off a marginal member of the family entirely. Indeed, as the months wore on, and Franklin's disposition remained volatile, the visits from relatives and the letters from friends tapered off.

Many years of careful observation of thousands of stroke victims have enabled neurologists to make rather specific prognoses. Very rarely, a prediction proves wrong: an individual who improves rapidly in the days immediately following his stroke may nonetheless fail to go back to work; a person whose functioning is profoundly impaired for months will be virtually indistinguishable from his non-injured twin five years hence. On the whole, however, prediction of the future course for a patient like Peter Franklin is depressingly accurate.

Advanced as physicians are in their ability to anticipate stroke and to treat its symptoms, a full understanding of its psychological effects—its implications for the person's mental functioning, his emotional status, his special skills, hopes, and fears—is nowhere near at hand. We have only a vague grasp of the extent to which the stroke victim understands the nature of his illness, the degree to which loss of language devastates cognitive processes, the way in which a stroke victim learns new materials. A large portion of this book will be devoted to an exposition of what is known, richly embroidered by speculation about what seems likely but is not as yet satisfactorily documented. Since, however, the challenges confronting neuropsychologists today can be better appreciated if the past development of their discipline is understood, we shall begin with a brief historical review of that development.

The general correlation between the structure of the human brain and the varieties of human behavior (and misbehavior) has been appreciated for many years. Throughout literary and classical writings, one finds allusions to individuals whose behaviors have been grossly affected by injuries to the head. Claims of a general correlation between brain and behavior underwent considerable elaboration and refinement in the early nineteenth century owing to the efforts of the phrenologists, such as Gall and Spurzheim. These investigators of "bumps in the head," who in some cases possessed a profound knowledge of human neuroanatomy, claimed that specific faculties resided or were "localized" in tiny, mosaic-like regions of the brain. Not content to link such relatively broad functions as vision or movement with general brain areas, they purported to uncover discrete centers controlling "attraction to food," "wit," "cautiousness," "thrift," "love of family," and "love of animals," among many others. Their findings took shape in the now-familiar diagram of "mental faculties"—road maps of all human virtues and vices. The evidence for these claims was essentially illusory, but the phrenological movement did, nonetheless, have at least one productive sequel: scientists began a serious search for the relationships (if any) between *particular* structures in the human cortex and *discrete* behaviors.

Two events shortly after the middle of the nineteenth century were instrumental in encouraging this line of investigation. The first was a series of presentations made before the Paris Anthropological Society in April 1861 by Paul Broca, a respected surgeon and anatomist. Broca exhibited to his colleagues the brain of a patient who had sustained a stroke and who had suffered thereafter, until his death, a severe difficulty in speaking. The brain turned out to have a relatively circumscribed lesion in the left hemisphere, specifically in the posterior third of the inferior frontal convolution. After Broca had presented the brain of another, similarly afflicted stroke victim at a later meeting of the Society, he felt justified in "localizing" articulated speech in this area of the brain and in concluding:

No sooner will it be shown that [a given] intellectual function is associated with a localized area of the brain, than the view that intellectual functions are bound up with the brain as a whole will be rejected, and it will become highly probable that each convolution has its own special function.

A phrenologist's view of brain organization and function. *(See page 20.)* From Johann Kaspar Spurzheim, 1826.

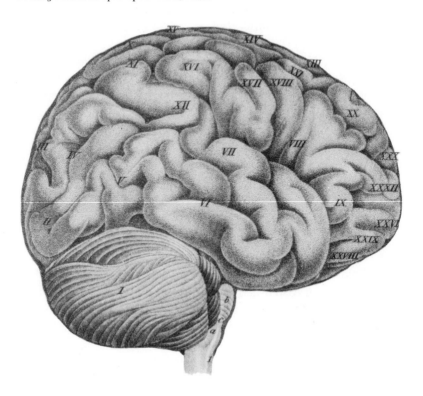

*Guide to the Principal Zones*

I. Organ of Amativeness
II. Organ of Philoprogenitiveness
III. Organ of Inhabitiveness
IV. Organ of Adhesiveness
V. Organ of Combativeness
VI. Organ of Destructiveness
VII. Organ of Secretiveness
VIII. Organ of Acquisitiveness
IX. Organ of Constructiveness
X. Organ of Self-Esteem
XI. Organ of Love of Approbation
XII. Organ of Cautiousness
XIII. Organ of Benevolence
XIV. Organ of Veneration
XV. Organ of Firmness
XVI. Organ of Conscientiousness
XVII. Organ of Hope
XVIII. Organ of Marvellousness

XIX. Organ of Ideality
XX. Organ of Mirthfulness
XXI. Organ of Imitation
XXII. Organ of Individuality
XXIII. Organ of Configuration
XXIV. Organ of Size
XXV. Organ of Weight and Resistance
XXVI. Organ of Colouring
XXVII. Organ of Locality
XXVIII. Organ of Calculation
XXIX. Organ of Order
XXX. Organ of Eventuality
XXXI. Organ of Time
XXXII. Organ of Melody
XXXIII. Organ of Language
XXXIV. Organ of Comparison
XXXV. Organ of Causality

From such a correlation, then, emerged the conviction that each human skill might indeed devolve from a specific locus in the cerebrum.

Just a few years later, G. Fritsch and E. Hitzig, working in Germany, stimulated the cortex of a dog with an electric current. These investigators demonstrated, for the first time, that the stimulation of given areas on the cortex was followed by the contraction of specific muscles. Here was dramatic and indisputable evidence—in living organisms rather than, à la Broca, in excised brains—that particular areas of the brain did indeed control particular muscular movements, and hence particular behaviors.

Physicians in the clinical-anatomical tradition of Broca, and physiologists in the laboratory-experimental tradition of Fritsch and Hitzig, lost little time in building upon these pioneering findings. Clinical practitioners would carefully describe the behaviors of a brain-injured patient and then await the patient's death for decisive confirmation of the site of the patient's deficiency. Case studies accumulated at a great pace, and by 1900 a number of "maps of the brain" presented essentially similar conclusions on the behavioral correlates of each cerebral convolution. In the laboratory, through electrical stimulation of neural centers or excisions of areas of the brain, scientists acquired information about the organization of mental activities in the monkey, the dog, the cat, and the rat. The discovery of certain peculiar clinical pictures, reminiscent of bizarre human syndromes, proved of especial interest. When H. Munk ablated, or destroyed, certain portions of the posterior lobes of the brain of a dog, he found to his amazement that the dog could still "see" but couldn't "recognize." The dog reacted to flashes of light and did not collide with things; yet he no longer behaved appropriately when confronted by once-familiar objects. He would eat soap but not food; he would urinate in a taboo spot; he would fail to act "as usual" when in the vicinity of his bed, his chair, his master. Soon reports appeared of humans who could also "see" in the sense of receiving visual impressions, yet could not "recognize" individuals and objects. The positing of particular forms of agnosia ("lack of recognition") in both animals and humans was the natural outcome; and the anatomical relationships between human and animal brains became an area of growing interest.

One has only to glance through writings of this period to sense the heightened excitement attendant upon these discoveries. After centuries marked by only the vaguest understanding of the relationship between "body" and "mind," and in the wake of the rather ludicrous claims of the phrenologists, it was quickening to contemplate a major breakthrough toward understanding human behavior, human language, and even human thought.

The kinds of studies undertaken during the latter half of the nineteenth century did not instantaneously resolve these questions; but they at least held out hope that clearer appreciation of the nature of language and thought could be obtained from careful study of brain-injured patients. Experiments in nature provided by the bursting of an artery or the blocking of a vessel, along with the interventions possible with animals in the experimental laboratory, could ultimately provide insights into perennial issues in psychology and philosophy.

Yet in the eyes of some, these hopes were perhaps misplaced. The opposing point of view was forcefully propounded by the French neurologist Pierre Marie, who in 1906 electrified the Paris Neurological Society with his bold proclamation that "the third frontal convolution plays no special role in the function of language." Having re-examined the brains originally studied by Broca, Marie concluded that the master's claims were unjustified by the data. Each patient had more extensive lesions than Broca had spoken of: the range of capacities affected had not been thoroughly examined. In opposition to those who described several varieties, Marie argued that there was but one form of aphasia, which could arise from lesions in various cortical areas; and, far from discrete capacities residing in discrete loci, any true disturbance of language would necessarily undermine other intellectual capacities as well.

The implications of Marie's broadsides were profoundly unsettling for the whole enterprise of the previous generation of neurologists. If his argument was valid, there was little justification for linking particular linguistic or specific intellectual functions with given areas of the brain. Marie and his supporters maintained instead that all cognitive functions were widely represented throughout the brain, that any brain injury would result in some diminution of power, and that the degree of impairment depended on the amount of brain injury rather than on its locus. Marie himself, it should be added, did not always endorse these conclusions so strongly and unqualifiedly; but within a few years, successors of his like Henry Head and Kurt Goldstein were making just such uncompromising statements. These neurologists, who came to be known as the "holists" (in contrast to the "diagram-makers" or "localizers"), regarded the brain as a single, highly integrated organ, involved as a whole in any intellectual activity and not susceptible to specific impairments from discrete lesions. The holists took special comfort from the provocative findings of Karl Lashley, an American behavioral psychologist who worked with animals. Lashley found that rats who had been taught to run through a maze retained this ability despite massive lesions in a variety of loci in the brain. From this he concluded that a particular deficit cannot be ascribed to damage at a specific locus in the brain; the degree to which skilled behavior is impaired is dependent instead on the amount of brain tissue extirpated; the different areas of the brain are "equipotential for" or "equally likely to assume control over" any of the diverse functions and behaviors of animals and men.

Both the experimental evidence adduced by the holists

and the philosophical implications of their position held considerable attraction for medical practitioners and experimental scientists during the early years of the twentieth century. Many found it congenial to think of the brain—like the mind—as a unified, indissoluble whole. As a consequence the approach represented by Broca, Fritsch, Hitzig, and other "localizers" fell into disrepute, to such an extent that the legitimate findings they had made and the principles they had discovered were, by and large, either discredited or forgotten. It was said that these individuals did not know how to "examine a case properly," that earlier experiments had not been done correctly, or even that the experimenters had done the wrong studies.

In recent years, however, a more moderate, intermediate position on these issues has been developed. There seems to be a growing consensus that neither the extreme claims of the localizers (to every function its own gyrus, or center) nor those of the holists (all areas of the brain implicated equivalently in all activities) are consonant with the facts. Rather, there is a gradient of neural zones, a cluster of functions, each of which is more likely than not to be associated with a certain brain region; at the same time, there exists considerable variability among individuals and across ages, as well as the strong possibility that a specific kind of impairment may result from a rather wide set of lesions. Increasingly researchers have employed psychological methods—controlled studies using large numbers of patients—together with clinical techniques. It is this more balanced view that may be said, in a general way, to underlie my presentation in this book. I must add at once, nonetheless, the important qualification that many researchers, myself included, often find the localizing approach more fruitful in terms of both clinical usefulness and theoretical suggestiveness; the reasons for this will be discussed—and, it is hoped, successfully exemplified—in succeeding chapters.

Whatever the existing degree of consensus, it is certainly true in any event that numerous legitimate, and some burning, issues continue to agitate the sphere of neuropsychology. Unlike the case with many traditional philosophical and psychological disputes, however, there is a significant possibility of elucidating these issues further, perhaps indeed resolving them. When someone claims that a certain memory impairment is found only with certain materials—e.g., words—there is no need to argue interminably and irresolubly about this hypothesis. A number of sessions with one or two patients over the next few days can provide a decisive answer to the question. If there is controversy among investigators about whether the inability to recognize one's fingers is really associated with difficulty in calculation, this can be resolved by a controlled study with a large number of patients classified and tested according to mutually satisfactory criteria. True, some of the classic issues recur in other guises after tentative conclusions are reached; but they will then increasingly take a more sophisticated form, since the terms in which a given question is posed will have been refined and recast by the earlier findings.

In the pages that follow, we shall examine a large number of neurological syndromes and conditions—both because such conditions are often fascinating in their own right and because these cases may have significant implications for our understanding of how normal individuals function and how children develop. I would like now to touch upon a few of the issues that are presently of central concern—using as illustration the case of Peter Franklin, which speaks to several of these issues. Let us return, therefore, to some of the phenomena cited above.

The central feature of Franklin's illness—a disturbance of language functioning—represents in the view of many investigators the principal problem in neuropsychology.

In all areas of language, and most lamentably in the essential functions of speaking and understanding, he was severely incapacitated; indeed, so pronounced was his difficulty that any conversation with him was fraught with potential for misunderstanding or even non-understanding. Across-the-board difficulties with language following brain damage are not uncommon, and in this respect Franklin resembles most other patients seen on an aphasia service. However, for reasons related to the peculiar organization of his brain (reasons to which we will return later), his aphasia was atypical. Whereas most patients have distinctive profiles of functions spared and functions impaired, with some language capacities much less implicated than others, Franklin's difficulties were of nearly equivalent severity across a range of highly diverse language functions. His case therefore provides an instructive contrast to the classical forms of aphasia examined in detail in Chapter 2.

The varieties of aphasia form a fascinating class of disorders. One group of patients understands reasonably well, yet can only speak in short, elliptical phrases devoid of the "little" parts of speech; a second group has only minimal understanding, yet (perhaps just because of this lack) can talk at great length in a syntactically rich but ofttimes meaningless jargon; still other aphasics can repeat everything while understanding nothing, even as a complementary group is proficient in all language functions save repetition. To those with the linguist's gene, however, there lies, beyond the intrinsic interest of these various conditions, a question of pivotal psychological interest: what is the relation between impairments of language and disorders of thought? In the case of Peter Franklin, as in that of many other victims of brain damage, it becomes crucial to know whether, in the presence of language difficulty, the patient retains the ability to think about the world, his experiences, his present condition. Aphasia thus raises the questions of whether we think in words primarily, in sentence-length units, in images, or perhaps even in imageless entities; and whether words themselves refer to specific objects, to classes of objects, or to the concepts out of which thought is composed. Exploring the lines along which language breaks down tells us whether an impairment of linguistic function necessarily entails a diminution of intellectual powers across the board, or, alternatively, whether the preservation of intellectual status is possible in the face of a severe aphasia. Finally, in the case of individuals with special skills, like the French-speaking, piano-playing Franklin, or with peculiar defects, like the congenitally deaf or the victims of cerebral palsy, lesions in the language area offer a unique glimpse into the ways in which language may develop and the relations among various forms of communication.

In a nonliterate society the effect of aphasia on certain language-related activities is moot. Where reading and writing are so widespread that they have become prerequisites for gaining an education and earning a livelihood, however, the fate of these capacities following brain damage becomes crucial. Had he retained the ability to read and write, Peter Franklin might even have been able to resume his job; once these functions were undermined, his potential for participating meaningfully in the intellectual life of his college was dashed. In Chapter 3 we examine the various kinds of disorders of reading which may accompany brain damage. Undergoing special scrutiny are those occasional strokes which selectively destroy reading capacity, while leaving other language functions essentially intact. First of all, there is the syndrome of pure alexia discussed previously, in which reading of letters is impossible but reading of numbers is spared and writing is also intact; secondly, there is alexia with agraphia, in which both reading and writing are impossible but communication otherwise proceeds without encumbrance.

These disorders not only yield important insights about the relationship of reading to visual perception, linguistic capacity, and overall "symbolic fluency," but also provide vital pedagogical clues about how the normal person learns to read with different writing systems—ideographs, say, as in Chinese, or phoneme-grapheme correspondences, as in English. Through an examination of the alexias, we receive fresh insights about such troublesome problems as "developmental dyslexia," and make an initial acquaintance with the vexed question of the relation between the development and the breakdown of cognitive capacities. Finally, we examine the opposite side of the reading coin —those rare individuals, both children and adults, who possess the mechanics of reading aloud yet are ignorant of the meanings of visual forms when they are translated into sound. The study of alexia, dyslexia, and hyperlexia may eventually alter our approach to language education and rehabilitation: a review of some current pedagogical efforts concludes our third chapter.

Two pervasive human capacities generally taken for granted are the recognition of objects in the world and the memory for events which have transpired. So effortlessly do we engage in these activities from earliest life that the prospect of losing one's memory, or one's recognition power, appears like the stuff of science fiction rather than, as it is, an ever-possible sequel to brain damage. Nonetheless, a brain-injured person like Peter Franklin may fail to acknowledge his own doctors, whom he has known for months; this may reflect a deficit in recognition, a difficulty with memory, or perhaps even some horrid combination of these two disorders.

In Chapters 4 and 5, we dissect two classic neuropsychological syndromes. Taking up visual agnosia, we study those hapless patients who, despite satisfactory visual acuity on standard ophthalmological testing, and in spite of the ability to copy geometrical figures, nonetheless fail to name or otherwise recognize the persons and objects about them. Like the dogs on whom Munk operated one hundred years ago, these persons are "cortically blind"—they know not what they see. Equally pitiable are those individuals who, as a result of excessive drinking, a severe accident, or a surgical excision, can neither learn new material nor recollect events which happened in the recent past. In each case review of these syndromes illustrates anew those recognitive and mnemonic capacities on which we absolutely rely. And, in each case, the notion that recognition and memory are simple, unitary capacities is clearly undermined: failure to recognize under one condition does not necessarily portend failure to recognize under others; memory for nonverbal materials may be quite normal in the very person who cannot remember a list of three words for twenty seconds. Suddenly our own experiences in which we block on a familiar word, or fail to recognize an acquaintance, are thrown into sharp relief.

We have noted in Peter Franklin's case that not all brain damage results in easily recognizable symptomatology. The cases of relatively "pure" disorders described in the early parts of the book are certainly fascinating, in a manner perhaps not unlike a circus sideshow. Such cases, moreover, offer—more, very likely, than those where quite extensive brain damage is involved—a unique perspective on normal functioning. The question arises, however, whether such syndromes as Broca's aphasia or visual agnosia really exist in as clear-cut form as the literature suggests. The issue was highlighted a few years ago by the controversy over the so-called Gerstmann syndrome. For many years it was widely believed among neurologists that a certain lesion simultaneously caused difficulties in writing, calculation, knowledge of left and right, and knowledge of fingers, while sparing related intellective capacities. This occasioned a well-intentioned search for the common psychological or logical thread linking these disparate intellectual functions. Recently, however, more careful studies have seriously challenged the validity of the Gerstmann syndrome, suggesting a far more complex, less formulaic pattern of breakdown in such cases. The entire controversy, while intriguing in its own right, has served as a powerful counterpoise to the pure "case-study" syndrome approach. In addition, the centrality of arithmetical disturbances in the Gerstmann syndrome provides the occasion for a review of disorders of calculation and a glimpse into the functioning of those rare *idiots savants* whose sole capacity is a lightning facility at mental computations.

Throughout the initial six chapters, we will be concerned with lesions of relatively circumscribed size, which lend themselves to the drawing-up of tally sheets listing functions spared, functions broken down. Many forms of brain damage, however, result in deficits far more widespread and much less easily characterized. In the seventh chapter we review four kinds of brain damage which produce effects differing qualitatively from the focal lesions discussed hitherto.

Of particular interest are the various dementias, in which, as a consequence of aging or premature degeneration of brain cells, the individual's entire repertoire of skills is devastated in relatively short order. Also included in this review is the frontal-lobe syndrome most notably associated with lobotomies but in fact a predictable consequence of any sizeable injury to the frontal lobes. In such cases the individual's mental capacities apparently remain unaltered, but his personality and "self-image" undergo a profound transformation which renders him distinctly different from normal human beings (and readily identifiable to the neuropsychologist). We also ponder the rare but fantastic disconnection syndromes, in which one part of the individual's body is left in total ignorance of what the other part is doing, and where, in fact, various facets of the human mind appear ripped asunder.

In examining the aging process, we address directly the

question of how the nervous system deteriorates, which enables us to compare mental dissolution with the developmental processes of early childhood. Unlike strokes or injuries that involve "focal" lesions, the dementias lend themselves to such a comparison, because, to some extent, the stages of development break down in reverse order, with the highest levels collapsing first. Yet dementias do not completely mirror development, since certain highly overlearned skills of later life may prove relatively impervious to brain damage, while other, relatively low-level skills may be mysteriously devastated.

Other issues raised by the case of Peter Franklin are addressed directly in Chapter 7. There is, first of all, the question whether emotional outbursts on the part of patients are a direct consequence of injury to the brain, a psychological reaction to the severe illness, or merely a customary manifestation of the patient's personality before the onset of the disease (his "pre-morbid personality," as it is lugubriously called). In Mr. Franklin's case, there was considerable evidence that he had always been a difficult individual, alternatively charming and arrogant, nasty then apologetic; we therefore felt confident in attributing a healthy proportion of his truculence to his God-given temperament. In many other instances, however, considerable changes in personality are directly attributable to the disease. For instance, disease or injury to the right hemisphere may induce a blithe jocularity in the patient; lesions of the frontal lobes are more likely to engender flat and apathetic responses; while abnormalities in the temporal lobes may yield a bizarre behavioral disorder in which the patient is subject to paroxysms of violent behavior while simultaneously undergoing a strong conversion to religious ideals. Sorting out the factors involved in a patient's emotional state has become a major concern for students of brain disease; helping the patient to control his feelings is a major challenge for all clinicians and therapists.

A second question raised by the case of Peter Franklin

is the relationship between the age at which cerebral injury occurs and the prognosis for recovery. When a young
child suffers a brain injury, even one necessitating the
removal of an entire cerebral hemisphere, he is generally
able to recover all or most of the disrupted functions. This
enviable state of affairs reflects the "plasticity" of the
young, immature brain. Various skills are represented
throughout its bulk, as is shown most dramatically in the
rapid learning of a foreign language: the young brain
seems able to absorb new information at a much quicker
rate, even as it retains this information with greater fidelity.
In a child, therefore, even a circumscribed lesion will
initially cause widespread deficits, but the disrupted functions are far more likely to be recovered. In sharp contrast,
there is much more specialization, and far less duplication,
in the brain of the adult. The older the patient, the more
likely it is that a circumscribed lesion will give rise to
a limited deficit—but the more probable that this deficit
will be permanent. Once a skill has been destroyed in a
mature brain, substantial recovery is unlikely. Here we
confront the main reason why Peter Franklin's prognosis
must remain so guarded.

Franklin is a man reasonably successful in his society: a
scholar, an administrator, a skilled amateur musician,
athlete, and raconteur. Even today he performs at least
moderately well at a few of these activities; nonetheless he
retains but a shade of his former proficiency in them. What
happens, however, to the brain-damaged individual who
has been superlatively skilled at one or another pursuit? In
Chapter 8 we take a detailed look at the fate of various
artists who have suffered brain damage. In particular, we
address the question: Are the artist's skills—his major
means of expression—especially resistant to brain damage,
or, to the contrary, do these exquisitely precise and sensitive capacities crumble easily before its onslaught?

Lamentably for the understanding of cortical functions,

very few brain-injured artists have been accurately examined by neurologists. For this very reason the few case studies of this nature which have surfaced are cherished by researchers, and we shall review these studies in some detail. They are particularly revealing regarding the relationship between language disturbance and artistic effectiveness in the writer, the musician, and the painter; the relative costs of brain damage for the run-of-the-mill practitioner and the extremely skilled individual; the effects of brain damage on both the critical faculties and the creative powers of the artist. Pieced together, the various fragments provide an invaluable picture of how skills are organized in the intact artist, that species of human being which has proved so extraordinarily difficult for psychologists to investigate. In addition, a neuropsychological study of artists highlights the commonalities as well as the differences among the several arts.

We have hinted above that the organization of Peter Franklin's brain was extremely unusual. Recall, for instance, the reaction of the physician who first attended Franklin to his combination of paralysis on the left side of the body and loss of language ability. In Chapter 9 we shall deal more directly with the question of left-right organization in the brain, or laterality; but it seems desirable to provide here at least a brief outline of cerebral organization.

The human brain is an exquisitely sensitive and forbiddingly complex organ whose richness of capacities testifies to, even as it fully justifies, its millions of years of evolution. With its billions of nerve cells, its myriad connecting fibers, its multiple zones, layers, fissures, and gyri, this structure has challenged anatomists, physicians, and other scientists since classical times. Even today, the anatomy of the brain has been only partially mapped out. Medical students find brain study among their most formidable tasks, and even the practicing neurologist must regularly refresh his memory (and buttress his learning) if he is to retain a clear picture of the organ's intricacies, with its countless nuclei, cortical zones, and critical synapses.

Fortunately, a mastery of neuroanatomy is not a prerequisite for understanding of the syndromes which follow upon brain injury. One may even adopt a completely "black box" approach in this field—that is, one may consider the burst blood vessel or bullet as a stimulus, the resultant bizarre behavior as a response, and pointedly spurn any concern with the "wiring" of the black box in which the stimulus-response pattern unfolds. A somewhat less extreme approach is to acknowledge the importance of the locus of injury, and the fact that it determines the kind of subsequent behavior, without getting involved in anatomical details. In this case, one may simply identify the syndromes as numbers (1, 2, 3) which correspond to unspecified but presumably discrete zones or lesions (A, B, C). Such a "blind matching" strategy—reflecting an interest in brain-damage syndromes exclusively as behavioral phenomena rather than as anatomical or physiological problems—is perfectly legitimate, and can be followed by any reader who so desires. Such readers should turn immediately to page 42.

No portion of the discussion in this book calls for a detailed knowledge of anatomy. Nonetheless, I have found it helpful in my own work to carry about a rough "mental map" of the principal regions of the cortex, a sort of poor man's *Gray's Anatomy* of that wrinkled overlay of gray matter which crowns the two cerebral hemispheres. Such a map serves as a convenient collection of pegs on which the various syndromes can be hung. The locations and juxtapositions of parts of the nervous system sometimes offer, moreover, additional guideposts to the relations among (or distances between) various psychological functions.

Each of the two cerebral hemispheres can be viewed

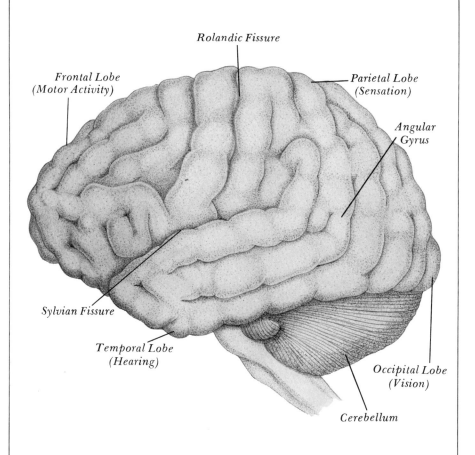

Rolandic Fissure

Frontal Lobe
(Motor Activity)

Parietal Lobe
(Sensation)

Angular
Gyrus

Sylvian Fissure

Temporal Lobe
(Hearing)

Occipital Lobe
(Vision)

Cerebellum

The left cerebral cortex in man. *Illustrated by Virginia Tan.*

along its side, as if the skin and skull which cover it had been mysteriously lifted off. This painless operation reveals the principal lobes of the brain, each of which is associated with a particular kind of sensory or motor function. (Associating a function with a given region of the brain does not mean the function is "housed" there, but only that this region plays a critical role in the operation of that faculty.) At the rear of each hemisphere is an occipital lobe, crucial for visual perception. Along the bottom part of the hemisphere extending toward the rear is the temporal lobe, which figures prominently in auditory functioning and perhaps also in other sensory processes which unfold temporally. Above the temporal lobe (or rather the chasm known as the Sylvian fissure) is the parietal lobe, a massive structure crucial for nonauditory and nonvisual sensory functioning—for example, that involved in the senses of touch, position, and movement. The parietal lobe assumes a crucial role in many complex intellectual functions, such as spatial orientation and calculation; information from this lobe, as well as from the other sensory cortexes, feeds into the pivotal angular gyrus, at the common intersection of the temporal, occipital, and parietal lobes. The interpretation of sensory experience, as well as the relaying of information from one sense domain to another, seems to be critically dependent on an intact angular gyrus.

These three lobes are all concerned primarily with the reception and interpretation of sense data from the external world. In the respective anterior portions of the hemispheres, in front of the Rolandic fissure, are the frontal lobes which constitute approximately one-third of each hemisphere. This region contains the motor strip, from which the action of the different limbs and muscles is governed. The late-maturing frontal lobes also assume a crucial role in the overall planning and regulation of behavior, as well as in the individual's complex judgments and exercise of his will.

Regions of the body ranging from the eye to the toe are involved in reflexes which are mediated by the lower portions of the nervous system. To all intents and purposes, however, voluntary action and sensation are products of the firing of cortical nerve cells. A major lesion in the motor strip of the frontal lobe will cripple the individual as effectively as cutting off or running over his legs; a lesion in the occipital lobe will cause blindness as surely as a nail in the eye. The person may seem intact to the casual observer, but his capacity for various forms of perception, feeling, and action can be destroyed by given lesions in his cortex.

So far, we have considered the brain from one (or the other) of its sides. A brief peek underneath will clarify the curious "crossed nature" of the nervous system.

The schematic diagram of the visual system presented below illustrates a central point about sensory and motor organization in the brain—namely, that neural connections from and to the limbs and organs of the right side of the body feed primarily into the left half of the cerebrum, while those on the left side of the body correspondingly culminate in the right cerebral hemisphere. The historical reasons for this "crossing" will most likely never be conclusively determined; but the pervasiveness of this phenomenon in all higher organisms is clearly established and has important implications.

On a practical level, this crossing has two principal consequences. In the first place, strokes in left-hemisphere motor areas will cause paralysis of the right limbs and right facial area, while strokes of the right hemisphere will have analogous impact on the left limbs and left side of the face. Second, lesions in the right visual (or occipital) lobes and the right auditory (or temporal) lobes will also produce contralateral (or opposite-side) damage.

It is not the case, however, that the right occipital lobe controls the left eye, or the right temporal lobe the left ear.

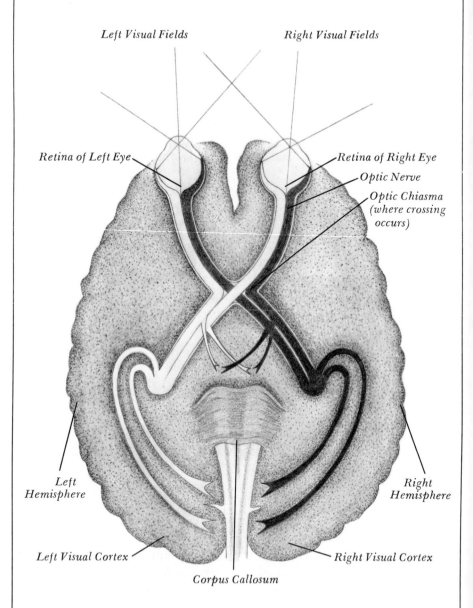

Left Visual Fields

Right Visual Fields

Retina of Left Eye

Retina of Right Eye

Optic Nerve

Optic Chiasma
(where crossing
occurs)

Left
Hemisphere

Right
Hemisphere

Left Visual Cortex

Right Visual Cortex

Corpus Callosum

Contralateral organization of the visual system. Note that the information in the individual's left visual field is received first by the right portion of each retina and then is transmitted to the visual cortex of the right hemisphere. Information in the right visual field is relayed by a similar process to the left visual cortex. Hence the "crossed nature" of the nervous system. (See pages 39–41.) *Illustrated by Virginia Tan.*

Though considerably more complex, the situation can be summarized as follows: An individual's ability to use both his eyes to scan to his left—his so-called left visual field—depends upon an intact right occipital lobe: consequently, injury to that area will "blacken" or obscure, half of the individual's normal visual range, and, correspondingly, injury to the left occipital lobe will block perception in the right half of his visual field. Until and unless compensatory mechanisms develop (which they usually do), the individual will perceive only half of all objects and scenes on which he focuses.

In the case of the auditory system, unilateral damage to the left temporal lobe will not result in any form of deafness—one respect in which the two principal sensory systems differ from one another. Yet significant injury to the left hemisphere will result in a relative inability to monitor the right ear when an individual is presented with information to both ears simultaneously, and, correspondingly, when there is simultaneous input to both auditory channels, right temporal lobe damage will desensitize the person to information entering his left ear. This circumstance allows clinicians to gain valuable information about the locus and extent of brain damage through the technique of dichotic (two-ear) presentation of sound.

Although on gross inspection the two cerebral hemispheres are anatomical twins, a century of study has left no doubt that, in most individuals, each hemisphere controls, or is "dominant for," certain specific functions. The left hemisphere characteristically controls language functioning, so much so that therapeutic removal of the right hemisphere may fail to leave even the smallest detectable effect on linguistic capacity. The left hemisphere also controls the dominant limbs in right-handers, while the right hemisphere seems to be crucial for visual and spatial capacities. Further details on hemispheric asymmetry will be found in Chapter 9; for the nonce, we return to the case of Peter Franklin.

.  .  .

The neuropsychological fascination of Peter Franklin should now be clearer. For he belongs to all of three progressively smaller minorities: those who are predominantly left-handed, hence right-brained-dominant in motor activities—perhaps ten percent of the population; those left-handers whose language functions are represented primarily in their right hemisphere—somewhat less than half of the first group; and finally, those left-handers who have been converted to right-handedness in writing without that transformation materially affecting the organization of language function in their brains. As an individual who wrote with his right hand, performed most other manual functions with his left, and appeared to be right-hemisphere-dominant for speech, Mr. Franklin was an anomaly even for our Aphasia Research Unit. As such, he becomes difficult to draw conclusions about. For instance, he might have had a small stroke in the left hemisphere about which we did not know or he might even have had difficulties in initially acquiring language, about which we were also ignorant. Yet this very anomalousness serves as a challenge to our theoretical notions. If we cannot offer a plausible theoretical account of how functions are organized in Franklin's brain, and how evolution could have yielded such intriguing variations in brain laterality, then our understanding of cognitive processes and the brain remains fragmentary at best.

With the advent of new surgical and other technical developments, it has become finally possible to ferret out the complementary capacities of the two cerebral hemispheres and to determine with some precision the role played by each. In the present inquiry, we shall build on the neuropsychological reports of individuals who have sustained unilateral left- or right-hemisphere brain damage; then we shall assay fresh evidence gleaned from patients whose brains have been bisected for therapeutic reasons, as well as from normal individuals. In the course of this review, we shall encounter an incredibly fascinating pool of data, a set of discoveries which have already captured the popular imagination. At the same time, however, a careful analysis reveals that the data is highly equivocal, with the division of labor between hemispheres susceptible to any number of interpretations, some directly contradicting one another. After propounding some alternative interpretations, I shall indicate my own tentative conclusions about the nature of cerebral lateralization—an issue that clearly raises profound questions about the evolution of the brain and its most effective deployment by contemporary man.

No brain impairment, of course, is greeted with equanimity; but such injuries are particularly painful to behold when they affect a loved one, or a person with whom one has come to empathize. For all the difficulties in our relationship, I grew increasingly fond of Peter Franklin and felt that a bond had developed between us. Yet I had continuously to ponder the individual at the other end of this bond: was I relating to a full person, one whose feelings, emotions, and personality had survived more or less intact despite his severe affliction, or to someone who was a mere fragment of what he had been, capable now only of diminished emotions and perceptions, and a diminished sense of self? Does such a person as Peter Franklin inhabit a strange, exotic country, qualitatively apart, of which we are afforded at most a tantalizing glimpse? Or is there, behind the frequent weariness, the inarticulateness, the inattentiveness, a preserved self and sense of consciousness which, could it but make itself known, would be revealed as one with our own?

In an ultimate sense, of course, the consciousness of an individual thus afflicted, and the central question of how aware he is of himself and his condition, may forever remain a mystery. But as for Peter Franklin, it can be said that he often seemed fully in touch with the realities of his condition and his world—I recall with particular vividness our brief yet significant exchange that Saturday afternoon when I dropped by the office. And yet on so many other days, he did appear, to the contrary, quite oblivious to the world around him. He would sit in front of the television, for example, scarcely noticing that the vertical control was awry, or the picture itself an unintelligible tangle of diagonal lines. A similar oscillation characterized his mood. At times he would harp on his speech difficulty, become increasingly depressed, break down inconsolably into tears; at other moments, he would act as if perfectly fine, devise plans to return to his old job, to go on a round-the-world vacation, even to write more books. He would then break into a frenzy of work on the assignments given him in language therapy; but within a few hours his resolve would be forgotten and there was no further mention of his former style of life. Who could tell if he had simply forgotten momentarily the scope and stimulation of his earlier life, or whether he was so painfully aware of what he had lost that, rather than risk chronic depression, he simply exorcised its memory from his mind?

Because of Mr. Franklin's severe communication problems, I could gain only a rough idea of his thoughts on such questions. Other brain-damaged patients, however, have recovered sufficiently to leave us a record of their recollections of periods in which their functioning was as impaired as his. These reminiscences, though drawn from people scattered in place and time, exhibit striking convergences as to the patients' experiences at the onset of illness, the period of maximum deficit in the early weeks, and the course of their feelings and thoughts along the slow but inexorable road to recovery. Such patients provide profound insights into the topography of their world, and by extension, the life-space of the brain-damaged person.

In the course of our discussion (and especially in the final chapter) we shall touch upon a number of ancillary issues. There is, for one thing, the question of how brain-injured patients should be treated: what kinds of therapy are appropriate, how should family members and others interact with the patient, what are reasonable expectations and demands at various points in the illness, how may the brain-injured person be reintegrated into the society from which he has been so cruelly wrenched? A related question concerns the afflicted person's legal status: Can his decisions and judgments be considered products of a sound mind? Should they be admissible in courts of law or in family councils? Should such an individual be permitted to manage a business, gamble, vote, or alter his will?

Finally, profound philosophical implications flow from the study of brain damage: What are the fundamental natures of cognition, action, and personality? What is the relationship among various mental and physical processes, the definition of consciousness, and the essential nature of the self? These questions, too, will be scrutinized (though scarcely laid to rest) in our concluding discussion.

This, then, is our overall plan: To begin with language and language-related capacities; to look at some of the most common human functions, like perception and memory, through the eyes of the brain-injured person; to consider critically the notion of discrete, isolable syndromes; to examine the process of breakdown in its multifarious forms and to relate it to the course of development in the child; to focus on the effect of brain damage on the most uniquely valuable human capacities, such as artistic skills; to attempt to unravel the mystery of the two hemispheres; and to utilize the shattered and fragmented world of the brain-damaged patient as a means of illuminating—precisely because of its distorted and fragmentary nature—the essential nature of human consciousness, of human identity and selfhood.

A word is in order about the subjects who constitute the basis for our findings. The majority are patients seen on our Aphasia Unit, including some whose case histories I have "worked up" myself; other case descriptions have been taken from the medical literature. Almost without exception, the patients are male, partly because few female veterans have been hospitalized on our Service. (There is, however, no reason to believe that findings obtained with female patients would differ in any significant way from those reported here.) In those instances where the patient's record is public knowledge, I have quoted directly from, and used the pseudonyms contained in, sources acknowledged in the footnotes. In those cases examined on our Unit, I have quoted either from tape recordings or from detailed transcripts made at the time of the interview. Patients' names and other identifying features have of course been altered. Occasionally I have deleted extraneous portions of conversations in order to throw specific features into sharper relief and usually have eliminated my own repetitions and expressed my questions and responses in as brief a fashion as possible. The patients' own words have, however, been faithfully preserved. Regrettably, much is inevitably lost in the transition from aphasic speech to printed text; but I hope that at least some of the experience and feelings of these patients do come through.

One day Peter Franklin said to me, in his usual insistent, somewhat strident tone, "Why, why you do this? Talk, talk, talk, all the time, that's tight, that's right." He then pointed in succession to several other patients with whom I was working, and as his finger ticked off each one, pretended to write in an imaginary notebook. Punctuated with these gestures, the meaning of his question became unmistakable: Mr. Franklin was asking the reasons why I spent my time in extensive conversations and interchanges with the patients housed on our ward.

I gave him a straightforward answer which I believe was truthful and which I hope he understood. "All of us here in the Aphasia Unit," I said (mentioning at this point several other doctors whose names he would recognize), "are trying to find out just what your trouble is. That is why there is so much testing here. Then we meet often, sometimes very often, and put our heads together, and try to understand just what happened to each patient, including you, Mr. Franklin. Sometimes we find out something special about you, for instance, that you were born left-handed" (here I motioned) "but that you now write with your right hand" (another gesture). "That gives us some ideas about how to do your therapy—your speech therapy, your physical therapy, and perhaps other forms of treatment too . . .

"Sometimes what we find out can help you, and even right away. Sometimes, unfortunately, it is of no help to you. But we hope that if we spend a lot of time with many patients over many years" (I pointed to the other patients whom we both knew) "we may understand the brain inside your head—and our heads—a little better. And if we understand the brain a little better, eventually that should help others who come to this unit. So we are very grateful to you for your patience and for your time." Peter Franklin smiled softly and nodded. "That's right, that's right," he said. I think he had understood.

Working with brain-damaged patients is not easy, nor is it always pleasant. Some are quite ill physically, and even a short testing session is uncomfortable for all concerned. A fair number—and the percentage may be particularly high in an older, somewhat indigent population—are not terribly attractive persons: they may have violent tempers, they may scream, swear, or even become physically abusive; perhaps in some measure understandably, they have scant patience for unkempt medical students and button-down psychologists who bombard them with phrases to repeat and cubes to copy. It is not easy to complete a session with such patients and one is tempted to dismiss them or cut short the interview. It would be a mistake and unfair to do so, however, for their behavior may well be beyond their control and they might legitimately benefit from insights reached as a result of testing.

Other patients, and they are clearly in the majority, are kind and generous individuals who have an abiding respect for doctors and who will satisfy any reasonable request. Some of them will sit for hours, executing seemingly inane tasks whose justification they cannot possibly appreciate, and then will, without complaint, proceed immediately to another experimenter or clinician who confronts them with an equally mindless exercise. In the case of such patients, one's misgivings are quite different: Is it really fair to subject them to tests, most of which cannot possibly yield any measurable benefits to the patient in the near future, and many of which are used primarily to satisfy the investigators' (more or less) idle curiosity? Wouldn't it be fairer and more decent simply to cater to the patients' more obvious deficits, supply speech therapy when appropriate, while reducing clinical and especially experimental testing to an absolute minimum? Is it really fair to exploit the goodwill of these people?

Most of us who work with brain-damaged patients in experimental situations have wrestled with this question, only to conclude that there is no simple answer. It is easy to adopt the rhetoric of science (as I did in passing in my explanation to Peter Franklin) and to claim that the future benefits of what one is doing far outweigh any inconvenience or indignity the patient may suffer. Yet one is brought up short by the realization that this rationale is invariably invoked by every medical and scientific practitioner, including those whose work has no conceivable justification and those whose work is downright harmful to those hapless subjects entrapped in the research web. Clearly, obeisance to the gods of "Science" or "Progress" is not enough. On the other hand, it is also tempting to say that these individuals have nothing to do, they are just sitting around anyway, they are bored, and it is good to give them something intellectually engaging. The problem with this argument is that most experimental tasks are anything but intellectually engaging, and that, in any event, it really shouldn't be up to the researcher to decide unilaterally what is (or is not) good for the patient, except in a more circumscribed medical context.

My own tentative solution for this dilemma is as follows: Initially I try to get to know each patient before undertaking any testing. In this way my face becomes familiar to him, and he will, it is hoped, come to regard me as someone concerned with his general welfare, rather than simply as a tester fascinated by his "case" but indifferent to him as a person. When I feel the time has come to begin formal testing, I ask the patient if he would mind spending some time with me. Then, to start off, I try to explain to him as best I can that the testing he is to undergo is part of a general information-gathering program which we hope will benefit him personally and which we believe will eventually benefit other patients. If he has objections, I go over them with him; if he continues to object, I do not proceed further.

During the course of the testing I do not attempt to influence the patient's responses, but I do generally offer him continual encouragement and praise for his efforts. Such praise cannot, it must be acknowledged, be entirely free of ulterior motives; yet it is by no means insincere— for I believe that in nearly all cases the patient *is* doing his best in what are often thankless and trying circumstances, and amply deserves the researcher's gratitude. (These thanks have been edited out in the transcripts for this book, but they could warrantably be inserted in nearly every passage.) If the patient has questions about the task, I answer these after the testing as honestly and thoroughly as I can; if I think he can benefit from being shown errors, I will also share these with him after the testing. I make it a point, however, always to include in the test some items that every patient can pass and also to conclude with items that are easy. This enables the patient to gain or retain some feeling of efficacy, and so may help keep him from feeling completely hopeless about his condition.

It is very important to continue the interaction with the patient after the testing is concluded. To test a patient exhaustively and then avoid further active contact with him is indefensible: To the extent that he remains capable of thinking about the matter, he cannot fail to draw the (correct) conclusion that he has been simply used as an object. And so, inspired by the example of my colleagues, I always attempt to maintain the relationship with the patient while he remains in the hospital and to renew acquaintance when he returns for a visit to the walk-in clinic, or for a more extensive check-up. This includes not only daily greetings (a matter of course), but, more importantly, periodic chats and interchanges in which we attempt to communicate as best we can. These conversations are not always enjoyable for me; but they are, I feel, the very least I can do to thank the patient for his cooperation in exercises which will rarely have had much meaning for him, and to affirm for both of us that he is, despite his affliction, still a worthwhile person with whom another human being desires to maintain contact.

My colleagues and I, of course, know only too well what pitiably small succor we can ultimately hope to offer a person whom the terrible fate of brain damage has befallen. Yet, for the individual locked into such a now-limited world, and increasingly estranged even from his loved ones and friends, such greetings and small talk can make a difference, and for that reason we all undertake it gladly. That it is the intrinsic fascination of these patients' condition that brings us into contact with them is not something we are proud of. For myself, the writing of this book, if not a form of absolution, may perhaps be viewed as at least an effort to share my guilt, as I attempt to portray the intensely interesting cases I have seen and to ponder their implications for normal functioning.

# 2 Aphasia: The Breakdown of Language

*Few things show more beautifully than the history of our knowledge of aphasia how the sagacity and patience of many banded workers are in time certain to analyze the darkest confusion into an orderly display.*

— WILLIAM JAMES

It has sometimes been maintained, by both laymen and scientists, that the study of behavior has in general only confirmed the commonplace, giving superfluous support to what common sense already acknowledges. To dispel this heresy, Professor Samuel Stouffer of the Sociology Department at Harvard used to pass around a list of "social facts" to his introductory class, taking care to gain assent from all that these statements were indeed obviously plausible and true. Stouffer would thereupon triumphantly cite controlled studies which had systematically undermined the validity of each and every one of these "facts."

The condition called *aphasia*—a disturbance in language function following injury to the brain—vividly exemplifies Stouffer's sort of demonstration. Given the information that someone's language function has been impaired, one might plausibly assume that there will be an across-the-board reduction in all of the person's verbal capacities —and that he should experience difficulty in talking, understanding, reading, and writing, and perhaps as well in various other cognitive areas like mathematics or memory. One might also suppose quite reasonably that the most complex linguistic functions—reading technical texts, say, or understanding long sentences—would be the first to disappear, while such relatively "primitive" capacities as repetition or the following of commands might be spared.

What actually happens in aphasia, however, is far more complicated. And the facts of aphasia, moreover, illuminate not only the process of breakdown in the afflicted individual but also aspects of cognition and language in the intact person. The relationship between such capacities as reading, writing, naming, repeating, understanding sentences, understanding commands, spelling, and calculating is exceedingly intricate: almost any of them can be destroyed or spared in relative isolation from the others, or various pairs may appear or disappear together. Some combinations, on the other hand, just do not happen—even though from a common-sense standpoint they might appear inextricably linked—and such non-occurrences are equally revealing.

The issues raised by aphasia are mysterious and fascinating. There is the effect of brain lesions upon the capacities of deaf persons, of users of sign language, of those who can communicate via Morse code or musical notation. There is the fate of language capacities in children who have strokes or tumors or are involved in accidents. Individuals with special skills—among them musicians, painters, those who speak a multitude of languages—also undergo respectively characteristic transformations when their language areas are injured. In each of these various cases, special questions arise: Are all tongues of the polyglot equally affected? Can the musician still compose? Is the child's language function altered like the adult's? Are deficiencies in ordinary language paralleled by communication difficulties in Morse code or sign language? There is, moreover, the possibility of radical personality change in the aphasic individual. And, finally, there is the most vexing and debated issue of all: the relationship between language and thought, the question of whether a person deprived of his ability to communicate via language can still retain his capacity to think. As yet, research has not provided clear-cut answers to this raft of questions. But promising leads have already emerged, and there is every reason to believe that further accumulation of case materials, in combination with judicious experimental studies, should eventually provide the solution to these intriguing puzzles.

When an aphasic patient like Peter Franklin enters a neurology service, he undergoes an intensive examination, aimed at pinpointing which of his faculties has been affected, and in what way. The attending physician evaluates his state of awareness: Is he alert, attentive? Does he know where he is, what the date is, what's wrong with him? His general behavior and his physical appearance are analyzed: Is he neat? Does he respond appropriately to questions? Is he generally depressed or ebullient? Are his emotional responses in keeping with his condition—concern about his linguistic and physical problems without excessive despair or unwarranted glee? Are his senses intact—can he see and hear adequately, can he distinguish odors, does he react when pricked by a pin? What of his memory—can he relate his past history, can he nod appropriately when asked questions about recent events, does he remember where various objects have been hidden by the examiner?

Some patients will be deficient in one or more of these areas; a separate evaluation will then have to be undertaken to ascertain whether the given deficit(s)—say, loss of memory, change in personality, or inability to attend—could have caused the linguistic impairment. Most aphasic patients, however, in particular those who have sustained limited lesions in the left hemisphere from a stroke or a bullet, will pass muster nicely on these nonlinguistic measures. Indeed, they may achieve a creditable score on the nonverbal portion of an intelligence test, a series of exercises in which they have to copy block designs, assemble jigsaw puzzles, point out errors in line drawings, arrange a series of pictures into a coherent story, and the like. They can be expected, however, to perform quite poorly on the verbal portion of the test—if the results were normal, they would not be deemed aphasics.

If, as in most cases, performance on the above-described "mental status examination" is adequate, then a direct evaluation of linguistic capacities is undertaken. Language testing is done in numerous ways, depending on the amount of time available to the examiner, the major purpose of the testing (medical evaluation, therapy, research, teaching), the degree of impairment, and the endurance of the patient. A plethora of tests having varied advantages and drawbacks can be administered. In my own work, I rely heavily on an excellent test developed at the Boston Veterans Administration Hospital by my colleagues Harold Goodglass and Edith Kaplan.

Our testing of aphasic patients usually involves four steps. First, we take note of the patient's ability to express himself, both in spontaneous conversation and under more controlled conditions, for instance, when he is required to name specific objects, to repeat a phrase, or to utter familiar sequences, such as the days of the week or the letters of the alphabet. Next, we evaluate the patient's capacity to understand verbal communications addressed to him: general conversation, comprehension of isolated words, ability to carry out commands, and mastery of progressively more complex utterances, until we reach the limits of his understanding. Third, we proceed beyond spoken language to other aspects of linguistic functioning:

the patient's ability to read aloud and to understand what he reads; to write out various kinds of messages; to spell aloud and to comprehend spelled words; to sing a song with and without lyrics. If he is known to have some unusual or specialized linguistic skill, such as knowledge of a foreign language, ability to read music, or familiarity with a code or some other nonverbal communication system, we attempt to evaluate his performance in any such area. Finally, we monitor other areas of cognition ostensibly less closely related to language: his ability to execute or imitate various kinds of actions (e.g., lighting a cigarette or pretending to brush his teeth); to recognize elements in the environment, without having to name them; to calculate, to distinguish right from left, to draw free-hand and to copy, to set clocks, to remember events, and to locate objects which have been hidden. At the conclusion of this examination, which can take anywhere from an hour at one sitting to several hours over a number of days, we are usually able to place the patient into a diagnostic category and to indicate which features of his condition are common, which unexpected or even unique.

When Peter Franklin was examined, he presented a clinical picture typical of aphasics in that he exhibited some deficits in each of the four major categories outlined above. As his test profile (see below) indicates, there was significant impairment on nearly all language functions, yet on none was he grossly deficient. His reading and writing were perhaps somewhat better than that of the average aphasic in our hospital; this could be due to the fact that he was partially left-handed, but also to the scientifically less interesting fact that he had been a college professor. Reading and writing were, after all, his major activities before he entered the hospital, while most patients on whom the test has been "standardized" have been laborers or tradespeople. Mr. Franklin had also undergone a detectable alteration in personality, being apparently more variable emotionally, more volatile than before; and he had unquestionably suffered some diminution in his intellectual capacities. Thus considered, his case lends powerful support to the claim that language function is of a piece, with aphasia necessarily implicating the full range of language capacities.

Mr. Franklin's case was extraordinary, however, precisely by virtue of the extreme averageness of the findings. Just as there are few genuinely average or "mean" Americans, it is the rare aphasic who has so undistinguished a profile as his. After my work with nearly two hundred aphasics, bolstered by discussions with colleagues who have together seen several thousand, I can safely affirm that the various language capacities can be, and usually are, differentially affected in aphasia. It is far more common, that is, to see patients whose ability to speak is significantly more, or notably less, impaired than their ability to comprehend; or whose repetition capacity is significantly superior or inferior to their spontaneous speech; or whose writing is far worse or whose reading is far better than could have been expected in a random distribution of these capacities.

How, then, to account for the lack of zigs and zags in Franklin's profile, his remarkably unremarkable pattern of abilities and defects? Certainly his ambidextrousness, which may be correlated with a more diffuse cortical representation of language functions than is found in the normal right-hander, could well be the key factor here. It is also possible that, in the two years since his accident, he had evolved many compensatory mechanisms; we cannot, of course, re-create the more distinctive and differentiated clinical picture which may conceivably have existed shortly after his stroke.

In the pages that follow, we shall meet three aphasics who have more distinctive profiles, with clear areas of spared and impaired functions. Although such cases are (as indicated) far more common, what makes these three

PETER FRANKLIN

| | 1 | 2 | 3 | 4 | 5 | 6 | 7 | |
|---|---|---|---|---|---|---|---|---|
| No melodic line | 1 | 2 | 3 | 4 | (5) | 6 | 7 | Melodic line runs through entire sentence |
| Longer phrases in conversation average 1 word | 1 | 2 | 3 | (4) | 5 | 6 | 7 | Longer phrases in conversation average 7 words |
| Articulation always impaired | 1 | 2 | 3 | 4 | (5) | 6 | 7 | Articulation unimpaired |
| Absence of varied grammatical forms | 1 | 2 | 3 | (4) | 5 | 6 | 7 | Normal range of grammatical forms |
| Frequent paraphasias* | 1 | 2 | (3) | 4 | 5 | 6 | 7 | No paraphasias* |
| Speech filled with content words: few grammatical particles | 1 | 2 | (3) | 4 | 5 | 6 | 7 | Speech filled with grammatical particles: few content words |
| Auditory comprehension grossly impaired | 1 | 2 | 3 | (4) | 5 | 6 | 7 | Auditory comprehension normal |

DAVID FORD

| | 1 | 2 | 3 | 4 | 5 | 6 | 7 | |
|---|---|---|---|---|---|---|---|---|
| No melodic line | 1 | (2) | 3 | 4 | 5 | 6 | 7 | Melodic line runs through entire sentence |
| Longer phrases in conversation average 1 word | 1 | (2) | 3 | 4 | 5 | 6 | 7 | Longer phrases in conversation average 7 words |
| Articulation always impaired | 1 | (2) | 3 | 4 | 5 | 6 | 7 | Articulation unimpaired |
| Absence of varied grammatical forms | 1 | (2) | 3 | 4 | 5 | 6 | 7 | Normal range of grammatical forms |
| Frequent paraphasias* | 1 | 2 | (3) | 4 | 5 | 6 | 7 | No paraphasias* |
| Speech filled with content words: few grammatical particles | 1 | (2) | 3 | 4 | 5 | 6 | 7 | Speech filled with grammatical particles: few content words |
| Auditory comprehension grossly impaired | 1 | 2 | 3 | 4 | 5 | (6) | 7 | Auditory comprehension normal |

* Paraphasias are distortions resulting from substitution of a word or neologism related in sound or meaning to the intended word.

### PHILIP GORGAN

| | 1 | 2 | 3 | 4 | 5 | 6 | 7 | |
|---|---|---|---|---|---|---|---|---|
| No melodic line | 1 | 2 | 3 | 4 | 5 | 6 | ⑦ | Melodic line runs through entire sentence |
| Longer phrases in conversation average 1 word | 1 | 2 | 3 | 4 | 5 | 6 | ⑦ | Longer phrases in conversation average 7 words |
| Articulation always impaired | 1 | 2 | 3 | 4 | 5 | 6 | ⑦ | Articulation unimpaired |
| Absence of varied grammatical forms | 1 | 2 | 3 | 4 | 5 | 6 | ⑦ | Normal range of grammatical forms |
| Frequent paraphasias* | 1 | 2 | ③ | 4 | 5 | 6 | 7 | No paraphasias* |
| Speech filled with content words: few grammatical particles | 1 | 2 | 3 | 4 | 5 | ⑥ | 7 | Speech filled with grammatical particles: few content words |
| Auditory comprehension grossly impaired | 1 | ② | 3 | 4 | 5 | 6 | 7 | Auditory comprehension normal |

### RICHARD MACARTHUR

| | 1 | 2 | 3 | 4 | 5 | 6 | 7 | |
|---|---|---|---|---|---|---|---|---|
| No melodic line | 1 | 2 | 3 | 4 | 5 | 6 | ⑦ | Melodic line runs through entire sentence |
| Longer phrases in conversation average 1 word | 1 | 2 | 3 | 4 | 5 | 6 | ⑦ | Longer phrases in conversation average 7 words |
| Articulation always impaired | 1 | 2 | 3 | 4 | 5 | 6 | ⑦ | Articulation unimpaired |
| Absence of varied grammatical forms | 1 | 2 | 3 | 4 | 5 | 6 | ⑦ | Normal range of grammatical forms |
| Frequent paraphasias* | 1 | 2 | 3 | 4 | 5 | 6 | ⑦ | No paraphasias* |
| Speech filled with content words: few grammatical particles | 1 | 2 | 3 | 4 | ⑤ | 6 | 7 | Speech filled with grammatical particles: few content words |
| Auditory comprehension grossly impaired | 1 | 2 | 3 | 4 | 5 | ⑥ | 7 | Auditory comprehension normal |

* Paraphasias are distortions resulting from substitution of a word or neologism related in sound or meaning to the intended word.

unusual is the exceptional purity and prominence of their symptoms—which is the reason I have selected them. Even as Peter Franklin's case tends to support those who regard aphasia as an undifferentiated phenomenon, the cases of David Ford, Philip Gorgan, and Richard Mac-Arthur substantiate my own contention that aphasia takes a variety of forms involving very different patterns of assault on language function.

David Ford was a thirty-nine-year-old Coast Guard radio operator, who had enjoyed good health (except for diabetes) until he suffered a stroke in March 1972. The cerebral vascular accident initially left him confused, without language, and with a marked weakness in his right arm and leg. At the time of his admission to our Unit, three months later, Ford's confusion had cleared and he was able to walk with a cane; but he still had little use of his right arm and hand. He was a pleasant and intelligent individual, who displayed appropriate frustration when he failed at various tasks, but was otherwise not overly depressed. He was alert, attentive, and fully aware of where he was and why he was there. Intellectual functions not closely tied to language, such as knowledge of right and left, ability to draw with the left (unpracticed) hand, to calculate, read maps, set clocks, make constructions, or carry out commands, were all preserved. His intelligence quotient in nonverbal areas was in the high average range.

I asked Mr. Ford about his work before he entered the hospital.

"I'm a sig . . . no . . . man . . . uh, well, . . . again." These words were emitted slowly, and with great effort. The sounds were not clearly articulated; each syllable was uttered harshly, explosively, in a throaty voice. With practice, it was possible to understand him, but at first I encountered considerable difficulty in this.

"Let me help you," I interjected. "You were a signal . . ."

"A sig-nal man . . . right," Ford completed my phrase triumphantly.

"Were you in the Coast Guard?"

"No, er, yes, yes . . . ship . . . Massachu . . . chusetts . . . Coastguard . . . years." He raised his hands twice, indicating the number "nineteen."

"Oh, you were in the Coast Guard for nineteen years."

"Oh . . . boy . . . right . . . right," he replied.

"Why are you in the hospital, Mr. Ford?"

Ford looked at me a bit strangely, as if to say, Isn't it patently obvious? He pointed to his paralyzed arm and said, "Arm no good," then to his mouth and said "Speech . . . can't say . . . talk, you see."

"What happened to make you lose your speech?"

"Head, fall, Jesus Christ, me no good, str, str . . . oh Jesus . . . stroke."

"I see. Could you tell me, Mr. Ford, what you've been doing in the hospital?"

"Yes, sure. Me go, er, uh, P.T. nine o'cot, speech . . . two times . . . read . . . wr . . . ripe, er, rike, er, write . . . practice . . . get-ting better."

"And have you been going home on weekends?"

"Why, yes . . . Thursday, er, er, er, no, er, Friday . . . Bar-ba-ra . . . wife . . . and, oh, car . . . drive . . . purnpike . . . you know . . . rest and . . . tee-vee."

"Are you able to understand everything on television?"

"Oh, yes, yes . . . well . . . al-most." Ford grinned a bit.

As can be seen, Mr. Ford's output in this brief exchange was extremely slow and effortful. Nearly every sound required a "fresh start," and many were imperfectly pronounced. For example, the "s" in "speech" was sometimes slurred so that the word sounded more like "peech" with a sharp breath before the beginning of "p." There were errors in the choice and ordering of sounds; for example, *turnpike* became "purnpike," *write* came out as "ripe" and "rike," *o'clock* sounded like "o'cot." Mr. Ford more easily pronounced letters made with the front of his mouth, particularly with the lips, words beginning with *m, p,* or *b:* like a baby, he found it easiest to say "pa-pa," "ma-ma," or "ba-ba." Often the emission of a word would be spread out over several seconds, as each syllable struggled to his lips before entering into the world. Each word emerged separately, and most seemed directly dependent on the presence of an environmental stimulus, like an object, a person, or a word provided by someone else. There were occasional ejaculations which came out much more rapidly and effortlessly, almost unconsciously, such as "you know" or "Jesus Christ." It was difficult to avoid the impression that these fluent words were coming from some other part of his brain; the suspicion that some speech was effortlessly produced was strengthened when I asked him to name the days of the week.

"Mon, er, Sun-day."

"That's right, Sunday. And then Mon . . ."

The remaining days came out so quickly and accurately that even Mr. Ford was surprised. Similarly, he was able to count to twenty and to recite the Pledge of Allegiance with little hesitation. Once when asked the letters of the alphabet, he began promisingly with "A, B, C," but then abruptly continued with "four, five, six": one "over-learned" series was apparently interfering with another. Counting to twenty by twos was also more difficult, apparently because this sequence had not been overlearned or overrehearsed to the same extent as the numbers in consecutive order or the days of the week. Mr. Ford could sing well, issuing a bell-clear melody: the words to "Home on the Range" were somewhat less than perfectly enunciated, but still sounded qualitatively better than the same words emitted in spontaneous conversation. Asked to repeat phrases which I modeled, Mr. Ford returned to his halting, imprecise manner of articulation, except occasionally when the phrase was very familiar, such as "all right." He had an easier time repeating words that denote familiar concrete objects (*book, boat, candle, nose*) than those that express grammatical relations (*but, or, if, where*) even though the latter were words that appear much more frequently in the language. Again, different mechanisms seemed involved in producing the different categories of words.

This disparity between the naming of objects and the use of grammatical terms has been considered the hallmark of the kind of aphasia Mr. Ford was suffering from. Usually named *Broca's aphasia*—after Paul Broca, the man generally regarded as the first to identify and describe it— it features a speech pattern reduced almost entirely to "content" words, as if the person were constrained by ignorance or economic considerations to speak at a very slow rate in "telegramese." Verbs almost always appear in their simplest, non-inflected form. Thus, all forms of *go (go, goes, went, will go, have been going)* are likely to be reduced to either the infinitive ("Me go") or a participle ("Doctor going now"). Nouns tend to be expressed only in the singular, except when the plurals have a distinct, separately stressed ending, as in *hors-es* or *church-es.* On the rare occasions when complete sentences are used, they are almost exclusively declaratives, except for an occasional (and perhaps inappropriate) command. The patient has little "melody" in his speech and particular difficulty in initiating an utterance. He therefore searches for a stressed word which can catapult him into speaking, sometimes borrowing it from his interlocutor, often overusing a single "pivot" like "This guy" or "Boy." Parts of speech that are more abstract or "grammatical" in function—conjunctions, prepositions, articles, adverbs—are exceedingly uncommon; if they appear at all, it is likely to be in the context of an overused phrase such as "and so on" or "this or that." In sum, the patient is restricted for the most part to the key words most crucial for communication.

No definitive explanation for Broca's aphasia as yet exists. It seems most plausible, however, to assume that the mechanism for producing the motor patterns of speech has been injured, and that the patient therefore gravitates to those words most easily accessible within his damaged system. These are likely to be the names of either prominent objects or basic actions, for whose use strong environmental support exists at the time of speaking. If one is trying to come up with the name of a person or object, there are various actions and sensory associations which can serve as cues. "Grammatical" words, on the other hand, while very common in speech, cannot be aroused by external stimuli —there are no *if*'s, *and*'s, or *but*'s in the world, and it is difficult even to imagine how one might cue the words *nor* or *by*. Normally, once a given sequence of speech has been launched, these "filler" words can be aroused by intra-word associations; it is just such an initiating sequence, however, that eludes the Broca's aphasic, except in the case of highly overlearned patterns or phrases.

Our conversation indicated that Mr. Ford's comprehension was relatively intact. At no point did he misinterpret my queries about topics of a general sort. His ability to understand and answer correctly such relatively difficult questions as "Does a stone float on water?" or "Do you use a hammer for cutting?" was also good. He sometimes erred in pointing to a sequence of four items named in succession—a task that may have overloaded his capacity to "rehearse" items. I also found a difficulty with more subtle questions in which attention to the precise meaning and order of grammatical components was crucial—for example, with such instructions or questions as "With the pencil, touch the paper"; "Put the cup on top of the fork and place the knife inside the cup"; and "If I say, 'The lion was killed by the tiger,' which animal is dead?" Correct answers here required precise understanding of the grammatical terms *on top of* and *with* and of the passive construction *was . . . by*. Since it is just such elements that were absent from Ford's speech, it was not surprising that he was maladroit in applying them.

Mr. Ford's ability to name objects was surprisingly good.

He correctly, though slowly, identified his elbow, wrist, and lips; he also named the floor, the sink, a tape recorder, and a desk. He sometimes missed on words that were relatively unfamiliar, such as *tile, shin,* and *stem* (of a watch); yet when asked to point to these items, he instantly gave the correct response each time.

I also probed the patient's ability to handle language-related tasks. He read aloud very slowly, in a manner strongly reminiscent of his spontaneous conversation; grammatical terms were frequently omitted or slurred. (It was fascinating to find that he could read the words *bee* and *oar* aloud but failed on the far more common, but less nounlike, *be* and *or.*) Silent reading was carried on somewhat more rapidly, and he was able to answer simple yes/no questions about the material. It took him several minutes, however, to read a paragraph, and he hardly ever read on his own, either for pleasure or for information. When asked why, he indicated that reading was just too wearing and time-consuming; also, that he sometimes lost his place, unaccountably shifting from one line to the next. We secured for him a *Reader's Digest* with large print; he acknowledged that reading was then easier, but he still spent very little time with literary materials. Mr. Ford's writing was as slow, effortful, and grammar-free as his spontaneous speech. However, he could copy written materials quite well with his left hand and was even able to point out spelling errors.

Since he had been accomplished in Morse code, Mr. Ford was seen by a "bilingual" colleague. He performed as well in producing and identifying single letters as in ordinary English, making occasional errors but invariably indicating his understanding of these symbols. However, his ability to recognize and produce words was poorer in Morse than in English. Presumably he had not mastered this language of his adulthood to the level of his native tongue.

Finally, I explored the patient's ability to recognize objects and to carry out sequences of actions. His recognition (through pantomime) of objects presented exclusively to his eyes, his ears, or his fingers was instantaneous; his ability to name such objects was consistent across sensory modalities. His execution of commands and his imitation of various gestures were also fine. Indeed, his only difficulties came in carrying out actions which involved the area of his mouth. Asked to pretend to blow out a match, he made a rather loud, sputtering sound. When I actually held a lit match in front of his mouth, however, his performance improved markedly; he emitted a soft, steady stream of air, which smoothly terminated as the light was extinguished. There was a similar disparity involved in his difficulty in coughing on command and his ability to clear his throat when it was deliberately irritated.

These last performances were considered mild signs of *apraxia*. In this condition, a person who understands what is required, and whose motor apparatus is sufficiently intact, nonetheless fails to carry out a desired action. Mr. Ford met both stipulations, for comprehension was sufficient, and his ability to carry out the requisite motor sequences was demonstrated by his superior performance with the lit match and the tickled throat.

Such dramatic differences between demonstrated skill when an action is elicited and supported by multiple cues in the environment, and when it is arbitrarily requested by the experimenter, are crucial to an understanding of all breakdowns of higher cognitive functions. What is involved in the patient with Broca's aphasia is a difficulty in utilizing and programming the (more or less) intact motor apparatus of speech when a relatively non-evident and demanding task is posed. Mr. Ford had great difficulty in producing words when he had to find and articulate them on his own; he improved somewhat with familiar words and with a model for repetition; he was qualitatively superior when simply required to complete a fa-

miliar and overlearned sequence. And other such impairments of "higher" functions—agnosia, apraxia, etc.—can
similarly be diagnosed only if the patient's physical apparatus, his sensory and motor systems, are reasonably
intact; only under such circumstances can disorders in
understanding and in expression be attributed to a breakdown in a "higher-level" skill, such as willed behavior,
interpretation of meaning, or comprehension of a situation.

The next aphasic patient exemplifies the second major
type of the disorder to be discovered. Following Broca's
epoch-making demonstrations in the early 1860's, there
was a heightened interest in all kinds of language disorders. Just ten years later, a young German neurologist
named Carl Wernicke suggested that there were two broad
varieties of aphasia: the first described by Broca, in which
comprehension was relatively intact but production of
spontaneous speech was severely impaired; and a second
form, resulting from a lesion in the posterior portion of
the left temporal lobe, in which exactly the opposite clinical picture obtained—such a picture as can be clearly
elucidated through a comparison of Mr. Ford with Philip
Gorgan.

There was no difficulty in conversing with Mr. Gorgan.
Except during the first few days after his admission to the
hospital, when he was too weak to do or say much, Mr.
Gorgan emitted a steady stream of clearly articulated,
richly intonated speech patterns. His command of syntax
was excellent, and he employed a variety of grammatical
forms, including adjectives, adverbs, conjunctions, and
prepositional phrases. Anyone completely ignorant of the
English language would have thought him speaking fluently—a conclusion no one would reach after auditing
Mr. Ford's tortured output. For someone knowing English, however, the difficulty with Mr. Gorgan was the

impossibility of understanding just what he was talking about.

"What brings you to the hospital?" I asked the 72-year-old retired butcher four weeks after his admission to the hospital.

"Boy, I'm sweating, I'm awful nervous, you know, once in a while I get caught up, I can't mention the tarripoi, a month ago, quite a little, I've done a lot well, I impose a lot, while, on the other hand, you know what I mean, I have to run around, look it over, trebbin and all that sort of stuff."

I attempted several times to break in, but was unable to do so against this relentlessly steady and rapid outflow. Finally, I put up my hand, rested it on Gorgan's shoulder, and was able to gain a moment's reprieve.

"Thank you, Mr. Gorgan. I want to ask you a few—"

"Oh sure, go ahead, any old think you want. If I could I would. Oh, I'm taking the word the wrong way to say, all of the barbers here whenever they stop you it's going around and around, if you know what I mean, that is tying and tying for repucer, repuceration, well, we were trying the best that we could while another time it was with the beds over there the same thing . . ."

At first, Mr. Gorgan appears to be a rather amateurish double-talk artist who has picked up a few pointers, but who so consistently overdoes things that hardly a semblance of the coherence vital for the effect is created. More extended observation suggests a psychotic monologue, the sort of "word salad" found on the most disturbed wards of mental hospitals. Indeed, there may well be certain parallels in the respective mechanisms giving rise to the babbled jargon of Wernicke's aphasia and to "schizophrenic salad." However, if the distinction between psychosis and organic brain disease ever means anything, it must be invoked here. The schizophrenic talks as he does because, presumably as a result of extreme interpersonal conflicts, he has undergone radical changes in personality. The Wernicke's aphasic, on the other hand, has suffered a lesion in a specific region of his brain. If the region has not been completely destroyed, his output may gradually improve; if it has, he will probably never talk normally again, despite the efforts of the greatest therapists or the most efficacious drug treatments. This pessimistic prognosis need not apply to the youthful schizophrenic.

According to classical aphasiological theory, Broca's area is responsible for the conversion of ideas, perceptions, and intended messages into smoothly articulated patterns of speech, structured by the appropriate syntactical forms. Lesions there will produce the paucity of speech found in Mr. Ford. In the other major type of aphasia, Broca's area is still intact, but appears to be largely dissociated from direction by the patient's conscious ideas and intentions. Present is the outward *form* of normal speech, its flow, its connective and adjunctive words interspersed among the more crucial substantives; largely absent is direct and accurate reference to specific elements in the environment, as well as the capacity for coherently interweaving particles and substantives into a meaningful whole. Wernicke's area appears crucial in two functions: relating incoming sounds to the representations (or "meanings") which allow understanding of discourse; selecting and arranging meaningful units for eventual conversion into comprehensible, coherent speech. These functions are obviously essential for understanding and emitting language. According to this traditional model, reading and writing depend upon a preserved ability to extract meanings from linguistic materials and to encode ideas into meaningful units. Therefore the functions should be impaired in Wernicke's aphasia, except perhaps in the case of certain highly skilled persons who might be able to read some materials without translating the images into sounds, or to produce certain written messages without first mentally expressing their content in spoken form.

This model is obviously very simple, and begs many

questions. For example, such crucial terms as *meanings,
meaningful units,* and *sound patterns* are in need of scrupulous definition. Nonetheless, even as it stands, it does
help to clarify the clinical picture found in Mr. Gorgan
and other Wernicke's aphasics. Asked to name objects in
his vicinity, Mr. Gorgan succeeded fully only with the
most familiar ones (e.g., *book, ear*). His responses were
hardly ever wholly wrong, however. He would often produce a word which came at least from the same category
as the desired one, saying, for instance, "chair" for *table,*
"knee" for *elbow,* "hair" for *comb;* likewise he would
sometimes get the correct sounds, but produce them in the
wrong order; "plick" came out for *clip, butter* was renamed "tubber," and *ceiling* became "leasing." Even more
frequently, Gorgan would make a series of stabs at the
correct target. For *ankle* he said, "ankley, no mankle, no
kankle"; *comb* elicited the sequence "close, saw it, cit it,
cut, the comb, the came"; *paper* was called "piece of handerchief, pauper, hand pepper, piece of hand paper"; *fork*
was called "tonsil, teller, tongue, fung." Sometimes, as
these examples show, he would manage to hit, or at least
circle in upon, the sought-for-target; sometimes not.

Mr. Gorgan clearly has some notion of what the designated objects are. He does not try to comb his hair with
his fork, nor does he sit on the table. This "functional"
understanding makes it more likely that the word produced will come from the same category as the desired
target. He also has in many cases a partially preserved
image of the specific sounds that constitute a given word.
But he has largely lost control of his word-finding or -naming mechanism. Like a soldier in a strange country, who
knows there is an enemy somewhere but is unfamiliar with
the terrain and type of warfare, he searches about, periodically lunging in various directions, sometimes coming close
to, or even to grips with, the enemy; but he is just as likely
to shoot completely wide of the mark or get caught in a

booby-trap. Much the same may be said of the patient's spontaneous speech—occasionally accurate, but evincing a basic lack of precision. Glimmerings of a guiding idea are present, but each new word engenders its own associations which are difficult to stifle, these associations being both meaningful (what objects or action go with this word) and syntactical (which forms of speech are likely to appear in this linguistic environment). As a result, his spontaneous production is rife with semantic links and syntactic expeditions that all lead him away from the desired target and make it exceedingly difficult for the listener to figure out what is going on. Nonetheless, if the interlocutor is sufficiently tenacious (and resourceful), posing questions until enough of the relevant fragments have been marshaled, he can eventually secure useful information from the patient. It is by this laborious procedure that case histories of Wernicke's aphasics are usually obtained.

Because of the hazy relationship between general understanding of the situation through nonverbal cues—which is usually good—and specific control of linguistic resources —which is not—the patient's difficulties are reflected in all functions which draw upon language. Mr. Gorgan's writing was a replica of his spontaneous speech; without paralysis, he readily took the pencil and, before he was even asked to write anything, briskly produced the following specimen: "Philip Gorgan. This is a very good beautifyl day is a good day, when the wether has been for a very long time in this part of the companing. Then we want on a ride and over to for it culd be first time . . ."

Mr. Gorgan was able to read single words aloud quite well and usually succeeded in the oral reading of single numbers and letters. But when he was given passages of any length, "paraphasic" errors occurred like those above; there was little evidence, furthermore, of comprehension. Presented with cards with commands written on them, he would read the words more or less correctly yet fail to initiate the slightest attempt to carry out the command. Even swear words failed to produce a blush, though he sometimes issued them on his own in an appropriate context.

Ability to handle more difficult questions, of the sort that only occasionally stumped Mr. Ford, was nil. Mr. Gorgan was never able to carry out "Put A on top of B" commands, and performed at a level no better than chance when queried about "floating stones" or "lions killed by tigers." However, there was, strangely, one island of preserved comprehension: Mr. Gorgan consistently carried out "whole body" commands like "stand up," "stand at attention," "turn around three times and sit down," or "assume the position of a boxer"; yet he failed to execute commands of comparable difficulty when these required the movement of specific limbs—"raise your hand," "make a fist," "touch your chair," etc. This remarkable preservation of capacity in a single category of commands is quite common in Wernicke's aphasics, but is not as yet understood. Perhaps, as Norman Geschwind has proposed, the ability to move the body as-a-whole involves different neural pathways (the so-called "extra-pyramidal tract"), and possibly also a different facet of auditory comprehension.

For an individual with such excellent melody and articulation, Mr. Gorgan's repetition was rather poor, peppered with the paraphasic errors encountered in his ordinary speech; the only exception was with highly familiar phrases like *on the other hand,* which were usually repeated accurately. Yet despite his difficulty in reading and writing, he could often detect spelling errors in written materials; apparently these words just did not look right as visual patterns and he was able to indicate the locus of error, just as he could point out that a cow was missing a tail. Similarly, though unable to produce an acceptable sentence on his own, he could often arrange cards bearing individual words to form a syntactically appropriate sentence. The key substantives, unfortunately, were apt to turn up in the wrong places: "The book put the man down" or "The dog was bitten by the man." This performance suggested that he was more sensitive to grammatical construction than to meaning—a pattern opposite to that often exhibited by patients with a Broca-type aphasia.

Mr. Gorgan had spoken some French as a young boy, and, during the first days of his illness, he would often switch in and out of French, giving his name, approximate age, and a few other facts in French as well as English. As he recovered his ability to speak English, however, he was increasingly reluctant to talk in French. He seemed annoyed when French words intruded into his spontaneous speech and rejected efforts to test his French with "Non, non merci, none of that française stuff, thing, if you don't mind." Mr. Gorgan sometimes exhibited understanding when a more complex, in contrast to a simple, form was employed: thus he erred in designating a "chair," but succeeded with "a piece of furniture on which one sits." The greater redundancy in the longer phrase—if one picks up either the word "furniture" or the word "sit," one may get the correct answer—may aid the patient; in the first instance, either one catches the word on the fly or it disappears forever.

Unlike the case with Mr. Ford, Philip Gorgan's nonlinguistic skills were generally diminished. He recognized familiar objects in different sensory modalities but often produced paraphasic names for them. Asked to "pretend to brush your teeth" to "wave goodbye," or to "sip through a straw," he often failed to understand the command altogether. Even when it was understood, he did not carry it out appropriately, but instead would behave in a primitive, highly concrete way. For instance, he would press his index fingers physically upon his teeth, as if the fingers were the toothbrush. Or he would run his hands through his hair, as if they constituted the comb. Even when a model for imitation was supplied, he would continue to defy the experimenter and utilize some portion of his body as if it were the required implement. Only when the actual physical object was given him could he execute the act properly. Mr. Gorgan thus exhibited the same pattern for the full range of motor activities that characterized Mr. Ford's performances in the area of the mouth: apraxic responses, except in the presence of the physical object. Unlike Mr. Ford, however, Mr. Gorgan was unaware of his errors and made no attempts to correct his apraxic responses. The mimed act and the action with the physical object would be performed as if they were two entirely unrelated tasks.

On other tests of intellectual capacity, such as calculation or drawing, Mr. Gorgan performed at a level substantially poorer than would have been expected from a man of his age and education. Although the possibility that he would have been equally impaired before his stroke cannot be excluded, it is far more likely that this depression in intellectual functioning was in fact a sequel to his brain injury. Often he would seem to have at least a general idea of the task, but his errors betrayed an inability to get beyond an imperfect, vague understanding. For example, a pair of numbers to be added would be multiplied; an object that was hidden would be remembered but its locus would be designated incorrectly; a set of blocks would be copied correctly in outline, but the red and white blocks within the configuration would be interchanged. Related tendencies were discernible in Mr. Gorgan's efforts to play the piano or sing a song: the overall scheme of the tune would be preserved and individual fragments would be discernible, but there would be irrelevant cacaphonous intrusions (an extra phrase, say) or reversals of passages (one part incorrectly placed before another). And, as with his spoken speech, the patient would have difficulty in bringing a musical performance to a close. His monitoring mechanisms—his ability to examine and criticize and terminate segments of his performance —seemed to have been lost along with his language ability. The fragments of music and speech continued to be produced, but the end for which they were being emitted remained only dimly discernible.

Messrs. Ford and Gorgan, in sum, presented complementary clinical patterns: Mr. Ford's strengths—comprehension and general intellectual capacity—were the weak points of Mr. Gorgan's profile; Mr. Gorgan's preserved capacities—the motor components of speech and writing, the ability to articulate easily, the inclusion of grammatical particles in speech, and the appreciation of these features in written discourse—were all salient lacks in Mr. Ford's clinical picture.

On a first meeting, our third patient, Richard MacArthur, seemed to display neither set of defects. His ability to speak was certainly adequate; there were occasional pauses, but not more than in many a slow and thoughtful individual with an uninjured brain. Questions were responded to appropriately; sometimes a word was not understood, or a question had to be repeated, but no more so than in an individual who was slightly hard of hearing or who had learned English as an adult. Yet a serious automobile accident had in fact left Mr. MacArthur, previously a foreman in a large industrial factory, with a disabling aphasia.

When we engaged in small talk, his responses were entirely appropriate—not especially rich in information, perhaps, but certainly adequate. He told me his name, his residence, his family's history, the events leading up to his illness, the kind of work he used to do. For example, asked about his work, he replied, "Well, let me tell you, Dr. Gardner. It's like this. I've been a supervisor for the Telephone Company up in Lawrence for all these years. About twenty years in fact. I was in charge of twenty-five men, the finest group of men you'll ever want to meet, I can assure you."

"What specifically did you do, Mr. MacArthur?"

"Oh, specifically, why sure. Well, I would come in every morning about eight o'clock, check in, you know they have those big new time-clocks, and then I'd make the rounds, checking up on all the fellows, like at the electric lathes, and all that. Is that what you mean?"

It is possible to detect Mr. MacArthur's difficulty even in these short responses. There is, for instance, a tendency to produce overlearned, not entirely apposite phrases; to be extremely concrete in responding; to get lost in minutiae without, on the other hand, providing relevant details. Yet the vacuousness of the conversation was not excessive, even in longer discussions.

It was when we shifted to more circumscribed tasks and questions, however, that a striking impairment became apparent. I asked Mr. MacArthur to name some common objects around the room. When I pointed to a clock, he responded, "Of course, I know that. It's the thing you use, for counting, for telling the time, you know, one of those, it's a . . ."

"But doesn't it have a specific name?"

"Why, of course it does. I just can't think of it. Let me look in my notebook."

A similar kind of response greeted other familiar objects, such as parts of the body. When I indicated his elbow and asked him to name it, he responded, "That's the part of my body where, my hands and shoulders, no, that's not it." At this point he grasped his elbow and rubbed it back and forth as if to evoke the name by some kind of magic. "No, Doctor, I just can't get it, isn't that terrible?" When presented with a wallet, he said, "This is a kind of bag you use to hold something; you may hold materials in it and keep it in your pocket."

If asked to pick the correct name from among a group of words, Mr. MacArthur would generally make the appropriate selection. Even then, however, he was uncertain about his choice, and remained so even when directly given the answer. Told that one sat in a *chair,* he spelled the word out: "C-H-A-I-R, C-H-A-I-R, that could be right, but I'm not sure. A chair. A chair. I'll have to double-check that word." When I told him that the part of his body in question was an elbow, he repeated the word over and over again, saying, "It could be an elbow, I've heard that word before, but I just don't know."

In aphasiological terms, Mr. MacArthur was suffering from a severe *anomia,* a difficulty with the names of objects and elements. This problem was manifested in two ways: shown the object, the patient had extreme difficulty in producing its name; told its name, he was subject to considerable uncertainty about what the name referred to, and whether it was in fact correct.

In one sense, of course, every aphasic can be considered anomic, in that every aphasic has difficulty in producing and combining names in the appropriate fashion. In practice, however, the term *anomia* is applied chiefly to cases like Mr. MacArthur's, in which the naming difficulty exists in the face both of relatively intact spontaneous speech and of comprehension of written and spoken language. According to the classical description of aphasic disorders, anomia results from damage to that region of the brain in which elements from the various sensory systems come together and are associated with one another—the area known as the angular gyrus. In order to know the name for a chair, the auditory configuration *châr* must be linked to knowledge gained from looking at and sitting upon chairs; in other words, auditory, visual, and tactile information must merge in this specific region. A lesion within this area of rich intersensory associations may spare the patient's speech and understanding, but impair his ability to come up with the name of a specific object at a given moment in time.

As in other kinds of aphasia, there is no trouble in perceiving the sound of the name: Mr. MacArthur effortlessly heard and repeated the word *chair*. Nor is there any indication that the patient cannot produce the name in an appropriate context. Thus, looking for a place to sit, MacArthur might well say, "Hey, would you mind handing me a chair?" The nub of his problem inheres, rather, in this: for a person to be able to produce a word in isolation from any given context, he must possess a certain mental flexibility; he must be able to take himself mentally out of the here and now and, at least implicitly, enter into a situation where he would normally use the term— such as "I'm going to sit on a chair," or "You sit down in a chair," or "This room has a table, a desk, and some chairs." It is this flexibility that the anomic has substantially or wholly lost. (The classic, paradoxical example of this condition is the patient who is unable to say "no" upon request. He finally throws up his hands in despair, shouting, "No, no, I told you I can't say 'no' "—an outburst that in no way allows him to succeed the next time he is asked to produce the term of negation.)

The more familiar the object, and the richer the sensory associations aroused by it, the greater the likelihood it will be named. Thus a small, fragrant, and manipulable object like a flower proves easier to name than a large object which is known only visually, like the sky or the ceiling. Conscious of their embarrassing deficiency, patients sometimes attempt to cue themselves. Mr. MacArthur, for example, kept a notebook in which he jotted down helpful hints. If the patient's condition is relatively mild (or he begins to recover), such ploys as touching the object in question or retrieving a well-learned phrase may successfully elicit the name. In severe cases like MacArthur's, however, these *ad hoc* procedures seldom work.

Most of Mr. MacArthur's other cortical functions, such as his praxis, knowledge of directions and spatial layout, ability to sing, and to copy stick and block designs, were remarkably intact. Yet his naming difficulty did extend beyond mere word-finding to other aspects of his intellectual functioning. For example, asked to interpret a proverb, he seemed unable to get away from the literal sense of its specific component words, unable to rephrase it so as to bring out its latent essential meaning. The saying *Too many cooks spoil the broth* evoked the reply, "Too many cooks, you know, cooks standing around the broth, they are talking and cooking." Cautioned not to mention cooks or broth in his response, he was completely stymied for a while, and finally conjured up an overly generalized answer: "If you want things to work out in the right way, you've got to be careful about that sort of thing."

Such a difficulty in interpretation is usually attributed to an excessive tendency toward "concrete thinking." The patient is deemed unable to divorce himself from the immediate situation, to abstract its essential underlying elements, and so provide a summary which highlights the main point while also generalizing to participants other than cooks and cook's helpers. This apparent loss in "abstract attitude" could certainly be detected in Mr. MacArthur's conversation, for he hardly ever pitched a response at the appropriate level of generality: he either hovered over particulars, or retreated into such broad and sweeping generalizations as could be applicable to everything or to nothing. Furthermore, he had difficulty in some seemingly trivial tasks, such as indicating "What date appears on the first page of a brand new desk calendar?" This question at first elicited no comprehension whatsoever, and then a series of hackneyed phrases, like "You mean the two months, a month has thirty days, and one has thirty-one, is that what you mean?" Only when a calendar was physically brought to him, and each page was turned over one by one, did Mr. MacArthur begin to catch on.

Such responses may in fact reflect a general loss of the

capacity for abstract thought, or perhaps instead only an extreme difficulty in finding words to express the precise ideas in one's mind. Kurt Goldstein, who deemed naming to be central to all forms of aphasia, strongly argued that an anomic patient had lost the capacity for abstraction *per se.* These aphasics were, in his view, incapable of assuming a new mental set, of mentally transporting themselves to the situation where a name would be forthcoming, of grasping common properties among diverse objects, of shifting their attention voluntarily from one aspect of the situation to another. Required to sort a group of blocks, they would home in on one feature—say, size or color— and then prove unable to shift to another means of classification, even when encouraged to do so. Once having taken a word in one way—the word *cape,* say, as a geographical landform—they would experience grave difficulties in appreciating its other meaning (a garment). Goldstein claimed that failure at various nonlinguistic tasks of abstraction such as sorting elements, colors, or shapes correlated highly with the naming disorder evinced by patients with lesions in the angular gyrus region.

In the case of Mr. MacArthur, however, as well as of other anomic aphasics I have examined, the apparent loss of "abstract attitude" seemed intricately and peculiarly tied to language. On sorting tasks of the kind devised by Goldstein and his associates, Mr. MacArthur performed adequately. He was also able to separate out line drawings which were superimposed upon one another, thereby demonstrating a capacity for "figure-ground" discrimination supposedly absent in this form of aphasia. His quotients on both the verbal and the nonverbal parts of a standard intelligence test were within normal limits, though probably depressed to some extent from their levels prior to his accident.

As previously noted, Mr. MacArthur was highly conscious of his problem, and kept a notebook in which he jotted down troublesome words together with a capsule definition of each. This notebook grew to be quite large, and he could be observed poring over it frequently, adding to or revising definitions, which he "double-checked" whenever he encountered a difficulty. A specimen page contained the following entries:

> *chair:* to sit on [Here appeared a simple sketch.]
> *ceiling* (top)
> *tile floor* (bottom)
> *wheel chair:* for people who can't walk by their self
> *cane, caine:* to help people walk
> *cabinet* (new bed)
> *matress* [sic]: for sleeping on
> *wall:* used from floor to ceiling—wall is from bottom to
>      top. [Here appeared a diagram of the whole room.]
> *wrist-band:* for watch
> *foot:* below leg than knee and last thigh [with a sketch
>      of a leg]

Either because of his scrupulous study of his notebook, or through a natural process of recovery, or both, Mr. MacArthur improved significantly in the months following his admission to our hospital. On a return visit some months later, he was able to name familiar items with little difficulty and did not exhibit the strange dissociation of word-sound and meaning which had plagued him during the early part of his hospitalization. Some of the old symptoms surfaced, however, when relatively uncommon words were introduced in spontaneous conversation, or when he was required to name less familiar elements (e.g., a *magnifying glass,* an *archaeologist*). There was also a lingering inability to shift mental set from one question to another, and a persisting tendency to be extremely concrete in his responses. Yet the patient had developed means for alleviating these various difficulties or at least rendering them less visible. He would whisper to himself or would silently mouth a doubtful word until he had arrived at a meaning, then come forth with his response clearly and with confidence. Thus, the casual observer might be even less aware of Mr. MacArthur's difficulty than I had been on the day of our opening interview.

While there is widespread agreement on the symptoms and the lesions involved respectively in Wernicke's and Broca's aphasias, the condition of anomic (or nominal, semantic, or amnesic) aphasia has evoked more controversy. In part, the diversity of opinions reflects the fact that, as noted, some sort of naming difficulty marks every form of aphasia. As a result, many different syndromes of naming difficulty, stemming from disparate causes, are often lumped together under a single name. A second reason for the controversy is disagreement over the extent to which the disorder is limited to the linguistic sphere. As we have seen, Kurt Goldstein attributed a difficulty in naming to a loss of abstract (or "distanced") attitude, irrespective of the realm of functioning. However, a reasonable percentage of anomic aphasics, including Mr. MacArthur, do not display notable difficulty on nonlinguistic tasks of abstraction. There are also disputes about other aspects—for example, whether there is necessarily a difficulty in reading or in calculation, and, if so, whether it is the language difficulty that causes these associated disorders, or whether some more fundamental factor underlies both the linguistic and nonlinguistic lapses. Anomia is thus seen as a cause by some, an effect by others.

Yet, whatever their disagreements, few aphasiologists would deny the existence of a distinct group of patients whose spontaneous speech and comprehension seem reasonably normal, except with regard to the definition of terms and the appropriate uses of specific lexical items. And since this form of aphasia is clearly milder and less debilitating than the other forms we have examined, it often happens that the recovering Wernicke's aphasic comes to resemble an anomic aphasic, in that his syntax remains superior to his ability to use substantives and he resorts frequently to circumlocution. Unlike the Wernicke's aphasic, however, the anomic emits very few paraphasias: faced with uncertainty, he knows enough to say nothing, while the Wernicke's aphasic, who displays less uncertainty in any case, is likely to continue talking. The recovering Broca's aphasic may also have difficulty in producing names. He is more likely, however, to know what he wants to say, yet find himself unable to arrange his articulatory apparatus appropriately for producing the desired word.

When an aphasic patient is grossly impaired in both expression and comprehension, he exhibits an amalgam of these various forms of aphasia. This happens initially to many stroke victims who nonetheless go on to recover in a matter of days. Those who do not recover usually have a large lesion involving much of the cortex of the left hemisphere. This latter group are called "mixed" or "global" aphasics; they have all the defects, and none of the preserved capacities, of Wernicke, Broca, or anomic aphasics. Global aphasia is quite common, particularly among elderly people. Unless there is rapid remission, the prognosis for such patients is very dim, because so much of the language area has been destroyed. They are often confined to wheel-chairs, devoid of functional communication; until someone figures out how to tap the uninjured right hemisphere, or to exploit the remainder of the left hemisphere, these individuals are unlikely ever to communicate effectively again. They may still display normal emotional reactions, becoming appropriately sad or happy if nonverbal cues are strong; but one cannot escape the conclusion that much of the "whole person" is lost forever.

Broca's, Wernicke's, anomic, and global aphasia together account for perhaps two-thirds to three-quarters of all aphasics. Other syndromes are much less frequent and, as a result, the subject of much greater dispute. (See the discussion of the Gerstmann syndrome in Chapter 6 for a particularly controversial example.) Yet the contribution of these syndromes to our overall picture of language function is sufficiently substantial to justify at least a thumbnail sketch of a few of them.

The capacity to repeat what has been said may seem unimportant, until it is realized that much of language learning presupposes the intactness of this function. But is repetition a merely elementary function—one which even a parrot can perform—or a high-level cognitive operation, presupposing an intact intellectual and perceptual system? Two curious syndromes encountered with some frequency speak to this question.

Like the anomic aphasic, the individual with *conduction aphasia* has good comprehension; his spontaneous speech is fluent, though somewhat more halting and dotted with paraphasias. The unique disturbance of such a patient consists in a special difficulty with repetition. He will respond appropriately to words or statements, demonstrating full comprehension, but at the same time be unable to repeat what he has heard, instead muttering, stuttering, often giving up in despair. The reasons for this peculiar disturbance are not understood, and may well differ across patients. Yet it is generally conceded that something must be happening to the message after it has been heard and processed, so that, while remaining in the mind and the memory of the patient, its particular phonological pattern eludes the articulatory system.

Exactly the opposite set of features is present in *transcortical aphasia*. In one variety, transcortical motor aphasia, the patient has good comprehension and little spontaneous speech; in a second variety, transcortical sensory aphasia, the patient has fairly fluent spontaneous speech but little comprehension. Both groups of patients, however, can repeat excellently—sometimes better, in fact, than a normal person. Indeed, the transcortical sensory aphasic can even mimic messages composed in foreign tongues or in nonsense syllables, apparently oblivious to the meaninglessness of what he is saying. (It is somewhat unsettling to witness a patient repeating "What a bajoom day in the borogroves" without the slightest trace of a smile.) The transcortical motor aphasic will resist such "silly" repetition but will echo faithfully in his native tongue; his own output is much enhanced if he latches on to the terms introduced by the examiner. And, perhaps because a written message also provides a model of sorts, he finds it much easier to read aloud than to speak on his own. In both varieties, a diminution in repetition ability seems to correlate with improvement in the patient's general condition: an indication that repetition may be an automatic as well as (or instead of) a voluntary behavior. The lesion responsible for transcortical aphasia spares most of the language-producing area *per se,* but cuts it off from other parts of the brain—in the case of the sensory variety, from the areas of comprehension; in the case of the motor variety, from the messages that the patient spontaneously desires to convey.

The most extreme and bizarre form of transcortical aphasia has been called "isolation of the speech area." In this rare but fascinating disorder, the patient can neither speak spontaneously nor comprehend what he hears. He appears to be mute, wholly ignorant of what is going on about him—until he hears a message, whereupon, like the sensory transcortical patient, he will parrot back verbatim what he has heard. The message has been perceived, a phonetic analysis has been made, the articulatory muscles proceed to repeat exactly what has been heard; then, deprived of environmental or ideational support for communicating further, the person ceases to produce any sound until the next message is intercepted.

Careful study of such patients, however, indicates that the parroting is not completely faithful. First of all, the patient is capable of some new learning. If he repeatedly hears a song on the radio, he will eventually be able to reproduce the melody, even including the words some of the time. He will also make subtle but revealing changes in messages directed to him. Told to "say hello," he will reply with "hello," indicating that, at some point in transmission, the extraneous instruction "say" has been deleted. Grammatical changes may also be made when appropriate. Asked to repeat "I am a doctor," the patient may surprise listeners by responding "You are a doctor." In one classic exchange, a German patient was asked to complete the sentence "Der Leben ist . . ." This would place the normal speaker in a quandary, for the question appears to seek completion of the sentence "Life is . . . ," yet *Leben* is neuter in gender and so ordinarily takes the article *das,* rather than the masculine *der.* One patient with isolation of the speech area, however, neatly solved the problem as follows: "Der Leben ist ein guter Mann" ("The man named Leben is a good man"). By converting the word *life* into the proper name *Mr. Life,* he was faithful to the syntactic requirements (a masculine form) while also producing a meaningful phrase. One does well not to overinterpret such isolated anecdotes; all the same, it seems possible that built into the language system is a Chomskyan sensitivity to certain of the syntactic and semantic requirements of ordinary language, and that these constraints will not be totally violated even by a patient completely cut off from the world, so long as his system for repeating has not been totally disrupted.

Taken together, conduction aphasia and the transcortical aphasias dramatize the complexity of a single aspect of language functioning. In one variety of aphasia, repetition is impaired while other functions remain relatively intact; in the other, only repetition is spared. It follows that repetition is neither highly complex nor trivially elementary, but constitutes a separate, distinctive capacity, which must be considered in terms of its own psychological and linguistic mechanisms. (It has sometimes been suggested that there may even be two repetition mechanisms: one fairly automatic and "nonsemantic," the other presupposing an initial processing of the message for meaning.) Certainly, in any event, repetition cannot be ignored. For if one cannot repeat, one will be unable to acquire the building blocks of new words or new languages; while so long as one can repeat, the phonetic and syntactic components of language will still be at some level functional. Indeed, examination of this little-studied capacity underscores the extent to which overall linguistic skill represents the sum of a large number of relatively separable functions, and reveals at the same time the subtle and hitherto unforeseen interrelations of these functions.

There is not space to summarize the other varieties of aphasia here, though some will come under scrutiny in later chapters. Other, equally bizarre combinations of symptoms are possible—for example, in the pure alexic patient, who is able to write while being unable to read; the pure alexic with agraphia, who can neither read nor write yet who retains intact his other language faculties; the acalculic person, who has a selective difficulty in dealing with numbers; and the apractic patient, who can comprehend and speak perfectly yet is unable to execute acts which have been requested verbally. While the details of this or that syndrome continue to be disputed, the incredible variety of possible aphasic disorders certainly constitutes an effective refutation of the simple hypothetical models of language disturbance which were outlined at the start of this chapter. The findings show, moreover, that by no means do language disorders necessarily involve an across-the-board reduction in skills—else the existence of complementary syndromes like Broca's and Wernicke's aphasias would be impossible. Nor is there an immutable hierarchy of difficulty or ease; were that the case, then repetition, say, would be, as it is not, invariably the best-preserved or invariably the worst-damaged capacity.

It might be tempting to conclude here, as the eminent English neurologist Henry Head did fifty years ago, that the realm of aphasia is a vast chaos; that every possible breakdown of any system can occur in any conceivable combination. Indeed, many aphasiologists would protest that the catalogue of syndromes presented above represents an oversimplification; they would rightly point out the numerous patients who elude the neat categories taught to neurological residents. Yet, true chaos is *not* the case. The breakdowns we have examined correlate reliably with the lesions indicated; existence of a circumscribed difficulty, for example in production of speech, co-occurs with a relative paucity of syntactic forms and a superabundance of concrete nouns. Furthermore, certain syndromes conceivable in the abstract have never, to my knowledge, arisen in fact. Thus, there are no reported cases in which either language expression or language comprehension is significantly impaired and yet naming is unaffected. Nor are there instances where such disruptions exist in the face of a preserved ability to write. In other words, writing and naming disorders are part and parcel of all aphasic difficulties, whereas, say, reading and repetition deficits are not. The study of aphasia is indeed complex, and the extent and types of impairments astonishing; but given enough thought about the nature of language and sufficient study of its disorders, some sense can be made of the aphasic cosmos. In this connection, we should note that all major present-day students of aphasia—as well as such supposed antagonists of past generations as Henry Head and Carl Wernicke—have each put forth diagnostic categories consistent with those described above: a variety of Broca's (or motor) aphasia, a type of Wernicke's (or sensory) aphasia, and disorders which highlight, respectively, difficulties in providing names, repeating messages, and reading texts, as well as disorders featuring a relative preservation of repetition in the face of severe impairment of other linguistic mechanisms.

Accounts of aphasic disturbances go back to classical times. As early as 400 B.C., Hippocrates described a loss of speech capacity that he called *aphonia*. Valerius Maximus reported a selective difficulty in reading in 30 A.D., and his countryman Sextus Empiricus was the first to use the term *aphasia,* though not in its present sense but referring, rather, to a "condition of mind, according to which we say that we neither affirm nor deny anything." By the time of the Renaissance, clinical descriptions of aphasic disorders abounded from such euphoniously named commentators as Antonio Guaineria (c. 1440) and Baverius de Baveriis (c. 1480). In later centuries, such nonmedical observers as Goethe and the Duc de St. Simon described individuals who had suffered apoplectic strokes and were left with language impairments. Dr. Samuel Johnson had the misfortune to suffer a stroke in 1783, but the good fortune to recover his capacities almost immediately thereafter. He drew up a graphic account of his condition, and even performed what may have been the first aphasia testing, requiring himself to compose verses in Latin in order to confirm that his mind was still sound. (It was.)

Two very careful students of aphasiological history, Arthur Benton and Robert Joynt, assure us that by 1800 every major kind of aphasic disorder which has subsequently found its way into the medical literature had been reported somewhere by somebody. Why, then, was there so little systematic knowledge about aphasia as late as 1860? For one thing, no one had yet publicly confirmed that language loss followed lesions in the brain's left hemisphere. True, an obscure French physician, Marc Dax, had realized early in the nineteenth century that a "loss of the memory for words" follows "alterations of the left cerebral hemisphere and not of the right hemisphere." But, perhaps fearing that this counterintuitive observation was insufficiently documented and would therefore be disapproved of or disproved, he shared his conclusion only with a few close colleagues in a "private communication." At the time, after all, there seemed no reason in the world to expect language to favor one side of the brain. It was left to Dax's more self-confident successor, Paul Broca (see Chapter 1), to make a public proclamation of the anatomical bases of aphasia at a meeting of the French Anthropological Society in 1861.

The tremendous upsurge of interest which followed upon Broca's historic revelation led, within ten years, to the positing of Wernicke's aphasia (though the disorder was not actually named after Wernicke until some time later). Faithful to the localizing passion of those days, Wernicke and his followers pinpointed regions of the brain which in their view subserved such functions as comprehension (auditory verbal images), reading (visual word images), writing (kinesthetic or tactile word images), repetition (connecting the comprehension and speech areas), and so on. Such leading researchers as Joseph Jules Déjerine, Charles Bastian, and, later, Karl Kleist clung to the notion that each narrowly specific aspect of language function was localized in some discrete portion of the brain and so could be separately damaged or separately spared. Kleist, indeed, claimed to have found the loci for word-sound deafness, word-meaning deafness, name deafness, and even sentence deafness.

For about fifty years, these individuals represented the mainstream of neurological analysis. However, working in quiet obscurity in Great Britain during the latter part of the nineteenth century was a thoughtful neurologist who took a markedly different view of language disorders. For

Hughlings Jackson, all parts of the brain were found to participate in every cognitive activity. Comprehension was not represented only in the posterior portion of the first temporal gyrus of the dominant hemisphere; instead, the perception and interpretation of acoustic signals took place all over the brain, but to a relatively greater extent in the left temporal lobe, and to a relatively lesser degree in the frontal lobes or in the right hemisphere. The different aspects of language functions were not, then, wholly discrete. Rather, the higher-level aspects—such as the ability to formulate and to utter a complex proposition, or to read or write a lengthy text—were more extensively organized, and implicated larger brain areas; conversely, similar and more automatic functions—the ability to utter an oath, say, or to read and write one's name—were controlled by much smaller, localized brain areas. It was for this reason, therefore, that brain damage typically disrupted higher, more organized and developed functions, while commonly sparing less-developed ones. Even severely aphasic patients could read and write and speak, if you required only names or oaths; but an aphasic patient only slightly impaired would still exhibit difficulties in reading, writing, and naming, if one looked carefully enough.

The tension between the Continental and the Jacksonian positions has persisted until this day. Broca, Wernicke, and their successors found it more useful to focus on particular loci within the brain and to characterize the function subserved by each. Jackson, objecting to such a "parceling out" of human abilities, preferred to view the brain in a more "organismic" way, as a network of related tissues, all of which were implicated to some degree in every psychological function; all functions, in his view, were interconnected, there being no expression apart from understanding, no repetition apart from naming, no thought apart from language. The Englishman never tired of reminding the "localizers" that "localization of symptom is not the same as localization of function"; establishing that a lesion in the angular gyrus results in an impaired capacity for naming in no way proves that naming specifically "takes place" there—indeed, since dead tissue cannot mediate behavior, symptoms are *by definition* a manifestation of whatever tissue has been spared and *not* directly of that which has been destroyed or disconnected.

The simmering dispute between the "localizing" and "holistic" approaches erupted into open conflict in 1906 when, in a series of three papers published in the journal *Semaine medicale,* the French neurologist Pierre Marie proposed "Revisions on the Question of Aphasia." Marie challenged the whole line of research initiated by Broca, claiming that "the third frontal convolution does not play any special role in the function of language." According to Marie, a lesion purely in Broca's area would produce merely a difficulty in articulation: no problems with language *per se,* and hence, no intellectual disorder, would be anticipated. On the other hand, once Wernicke's area was implicated, there *was* a true language disturbance, one that would be reflected in speech, reading, writing, understanding, indeed in all communicative functions. There is only one aphasia, therefore—Wernicke's aphasia: if an individual has difficulty with his motor functioning as well, he has Wernicke's aphasia with a superimposed articulatory disturbance. Either language is impaired or it is not; if impaired, there is inevitably a disturbance of all intellective activity, most particularly the "inner speech" on which thought depends.

Marie's attack created an uproar, but met vigorous resistance from the French neurological establishment, in particular from M. and Mme. Déjerine. After several fiercely polemical exchanges, during which Marie retracted some of his more intemperate claims and the Déjerines in turn conceded that Broca's own cases had been somewhat equivocal, the dispute between the two sides receded from public view. But Marie had effectively undermined the solidity of the localizing position, and from many different quarters there now came a more differentiated and flexible view of the aphasias. This reorientation coincided, moreover, with a similar widespread shift in psychological analysis, from a strict concern with elements toward a greater concentration upon the wholes that the elements comprised. At the same time, neurologists like Anton Pick began to develop psychological models of aphasia, in which the steps from "conception" to "speech" were outlined and hypotheses formed regarding the various kinds of possible disruption of this sequence. Perhaps such trends in the study of aphasia were simply symptomatic of a more general shift in the *Zeitgeist*.

Two individuals in more recent years who espoused the organismic, antilocalizing approach were the English neurologist Henry Head and the German-American neurologist Kurt Goldstein. Each issued large compendia on aphasia, full of controversy, strongly and uncompromisingly assertive. In *Aphasia and Kindred Disorders of Speech,* a work in two massive volumes, Head was critical of most previous workers in the field, with the exception of Marie and Head's own venerated mentor, Hughlings Jackson. Rejecting Wernicke and his followers as simplistic theorists and clumsy observers, he claimed that:

> This school of thought . . . enabled teachers of medicine to assume an easy dogmaticism at the bedside and candidates for examination rejoiced in so perceptive a clue to all their difficulties. But serious students could not fit these conceptions of aphasia to the clinical phenomena.

In his view, "Marie's criticisms passed like a harrow over a weed-choked field." Despite a very complete review of earlier aphasiological research, however, Head's own contributions to the field were scanty, except for a series of useful bedside tests. Without much amplification or critical incisiveness, he outlined Hughlings Jackson's approach and then presented an extensive series of cases. These latter were often interesting, but Head was ensnared in his own trap: having cautioned against undue theorizing, he produced far too much sheer description and failed to place his cases within a meaningful systematic framework, save for a prosaic classificatory system which simply recapitulated earlier attempts. As a consequence, aside from his somewhat biased historical account and his polemical philosophical position, Head has made little impression on active workers in aphasia.

Goldstein's contribution is much more substantive. Not only was his critique of the localizing school more temperate, but he discovered and documented numerous important neurological phenomena. Goldstein assimilated his own findings to the theoretical perspective of Gestalt psychology; he directed neurologists' attention to general changes in patients' behavior, such as loss of an abstract attitude, insensitivity to figure-ground relations, and the explosive ("catastrophic") desire of certain patients to escape the examining situation. Curiously, however, as Norman Geschwind has pointed out, there is a schism running through Goldstein's writings: his theoretical views are strongly organismic, yet his recitation of case studies conforms in most particulars to the classical localizing approach. Indeed, Goldstein sometimes went beyond this school in the precision of his localizing—for example, attributing conduction (or central) aphasia to a lesion in the insula of the brain.

Nonetheless, because he was a keen observer, a tireless theoretician, and a prolific writer in German and English during most of his ninety years, Goldstein's works are very widely known. The present generation of neurologists, and in some measure psychologists, was raised on Goldstein (or on translations or summaries of him); in both their substance and their general manner and tone, his studies have been highly influential—a fact by no means to be regretted, for Goldstein's work in aphasia has stood the test of time and some of his case studies are incomparable in the plenitude of their clinical descriptions and detailed testing. Of the currently most influential schools of aphasiological analysis, each bears an active relation to Goldstein's position.

The point of view developed by Norman Geschwind draws upon the classical localizing tradition (which constituted Goldstein's own education) while avoiding its extremes. No claims about centers for word-meaning, word-image, or word-sound are put forth, and investigation focuses on a careful examination of the anatomical correlates of specific disorders. The schools headed by Henri Hécaen in France and Harold Goodglass in Boston stress teamwork between psychologists, linguists, and neurological workers and specialize in experimental investigations with groups of patients. The tradition launched by Alexander Luria in Russia embraces the localizing approach as a means of understanding the more elementary forms of disorders, while adopting an at least partly holistic stance in regard to lesions in areas governing the more highly developed functions. And, like Goldstein, Luria is deeply concerned with the biological properties of the organism and the dynamic interactions of neural fields. Each of these schools understandably seeks to go beyond Goldstein and to correct his excesses—Geschwind, by criticizing Goldstein's sweeping philosophical assertions and by sponsoring empirical investigations of anatomical connections in primates; Hécaen and Goodglass, by employing sizeable subject pools and gathering data under controlled experimental (as opposed to bedside-testing) conditions; Luria, by studying different levels of development and breakdown in diverse subject populations and by taking into account the capacities of "analyzers" in each sensory system. From these various streams of research are emerging, I believe, the most important present-day contributions to our knowledge of aphasia.

How do these various schools stand on the central question posed earlier: the nature of language and thought, and the relationship between these crucial psychological functions? Contemporary observers are less bold in directly confronting the question than such early polemicists as Marie or Kleist. Almost no one would make the bald statement that linguistic and thought processes are identical, or, on the other hand, that language can be completely divorced from thought. Nonetheless, significant differences still exist among the most informed aphasiologists. Those who, like Geschwind, retain a localizing bent caution against the positing of generalized functions like "cognition" or "thought." In their view, the intelligent thinking person possesses a whole range of skills representing diverse cortical systems, many operating at a high level of competence. While a dementing process may impair a large number of these abilities, aphasia clearly does not: an individual can be severely aphasic and yet solve problems which do not involve language, draw with accuracy, and retain his pre-morbid attitudes, personality, and intersocial relationships. Alternatively, an individual can have intact speech mechanisms, as in the isolation syndromes, or even excellent language, as in right-hemisphere disease, and yet be wholly deficient on a gamut of cognitive tasks, such as in drawing, mathematics, spatial orientation, or perceptual-motor skills. It is better, according to this view, to speak of a range of linguistic and a range of cognitive skills, some of which overlap, but many of which do not, functioning instead in comfortable independence of one another.

This orientation differs significantly from that of the Head-Jackson-Goldstein school, whose descendants include a large number of contemporary aphasiologists, among them Eberhard Bay, Eric Lenneberg, Macdonald Critchley, and J. de Ajuriaguerra. While conceding the existence of a few freakish syndromes which implicate only a few linguistic functions, this latter group stresses the pervasive coevality between linguistic and cognitive functions. Emphasis is placed on a presumed regression to a more primitive developmental level—e.g., the adoption of a "concrete" attitude; such a regression, it is alleged, will be found in any individual with significant brain damage, particularly one with destruction in his language zone. If a Broca's aphasic copes successfully in the area of nonverbal intelligence, this engenders the claim that he is not *really* aphasic—the disorder is considered to be one of articulation and not of language. A severely aphasic artist who continues to draw, to play an instrument, perhaps even to compose, elicits a variety of reactions from members of this camp. Either it will be asserted that these are not cognitive skills, but rather overlearned habits no longer requiring voluntary control; or the diagnosis of aphasia may itself be challenged; or the critic may throw up his hands and simply say that here is an aberration, an abnormal individual with a bizarre arrangement of capacities in his skull— perhaps he is playing the piano with his cerebellum!

On a more serious note, such commentators highlight a concept which is also heavily emphasized by the Russian school, notably Luria. This is the notion of *inner speech* —a type of internalized language function believed to be close to, if not identical with, the processes of thought. In the young child, it has been noted, much of thought is externalized—the child thinks aloud; as he matures, however, these processes apparently move inward (into the inner "associative" regions of the cortex, as it were), becoming increasingly elliptical, and, it is believed, eventually collapsing into the actual operation of thought. In an aphasic, the capacity to employ this inner speech is assumed to be destroyed, resulting not only in severe incapacity in the linguistic realm, but also in an inability to carry on the cognitive processes involved in other forms of thinking. For words, in this view, are not mere tokens associated with objects; rather, they *are* our concepts of the world, the very "stuff" of cognition.

Proving the existence (or nonexistence) of inner speech is most difficult: Heated arguments rage over its optimal definition, and one's own conclusion on the necessity for "inner speech" in thought seems to depend on whether one equates inner speech with all symbolic activity, or adopts a more restricted definition, entailing for instance the deployment of certain syntactic relations. Despite terminological disputes and theoretical misgivings, however, the general notion that thought processes involve a considerable amount of "talking to oneself" convinces many on introspective or psychological grounds. Indeed, Luria himself is sympathetic to the idea that learned language eventually comes to play a controlling role in thought; but he shrinks from asserting that all thought processes must involve language in some sense. This caution is probably wise, in view of demonstrations that many aphasics are able to solve intricate problems, providing only that no distinctively linguistic capacities are required. The psychologist Jean Piaget, moreover, has documented young children's cognitive sophistication in the absence of linguistic capacities. Piaget has argued strenuously that an individual's linguistic maturity simply reflects his general cognitive (or operative) capacity rather than, as the "language-thought" school tends to hold, somehow determining it.

Even though the relationship between language and thought remains perplexing, our brief survey justifies some conclusions. First of all, it is clear that not all cognitive activity is dependent upon language, else severely aphasic patients would fail the full range of problem-solving tasks. By the same token, however, linguistic and cognitive processes cannot be entirely divorced, for a high correlation has been demonstrated between specific language disorders—for example, difficulty in carrying out logical commands—and specific nonlinguistic deficits, such as performing calculations, or finding one's way about a maze. Whether an aphasic individual can perform the highest-level, most demanding intellectual tasks is debatable; yet, except when these tasks are explicitly dependent upon language functions (such as the verbal portion of intelligence tests), it may be difficult to demonstrate significant deficits. In short, many aphasic individuals can think at a high level (even as many talkative individuals cannot), but their performance at a specific task seems to depend on the kind or severity of aphasia sustained, on the degree to which that task requires some kind of explicit or implicit use of language, and on the extent to which the patients themselves have previously conducted the activity without the mediation of language. Naturally, tasks which by their nature depend upon language (for example, the writing of criticism or poetry) completely elude aphasic patients. Thus, an answer can be given to our central puzzle, but this answer is less complete, and more complex, than we would like.

These descriptions of aphasia are neither simple nor devoid of controversy. As is probably apparent, my own bias is in the direction of the "localizing" Geschwind-Luria school, rather than the "organismic" Jackson-Head-Bay school. However, this bias reflects less my conviction that one or another school is correct in its assertions about the physiology and anatomy of the brain (an area about which I know little) than my belief that at present the localizing approach is more useful for psychological and pedagogical purposes. As a psychologist, I find it relatively immaterial which area of the brain has been affected by a lesion; what is crucial is that certain functions have been impaired, others spared, and that this symptom picture clarifies my own thinking about behavioral and cognitive processes. To the extent that everything is related to everything else, as the Jackson school argues, differentiation and analysis become much more difficult. By the same token, I find it pedagogically unsatisfying and unproductive to blur distinctions wherever they may exist and to stress, or perhaps overstress, the interrelatedness of all capacities. Unless one can make comparisons, unless one can set up categories which can be distinguished, compared, and used as a basis for further study and subsequent modification, there is little possibility of effective instruction. Moreover, there seems to be scant hope for scientific progress; once one has declared the irreducible connections between diverse functions, few meaningful empirical investigations suggest themselves. Thus, I come to the following admittedly extreme judgment: even if, in the last analysis, the Jacksonian view of brain functioning proves more accurate, the "localizing" approach is more likely to extend our knowledge at the present time. Nonetheless, I have made, in Chapter 6, an attempt to present the opposing point of view; between that discussion and the indication of my bias presented above, the reader should be able to avoid any serious misunderstanding.

It must be admitted that the typology of aphasia attempted here, even if completely accurate, is based on only a small sample of the population: middle-aged right-handed adults in Western society who have suffered from focal lesions, usually produced by a sudden stroke in the central portions of the surface of the left hemisphere. Each time this select circle is broken to allow in additional groups, the picture becomes more complex. For example, young (preadolescent) children do become aphasic when they suffer head injuries, but the cause and effects are distinctly different. Injury in almost any area of the young child's brain will produce at least some aphasia, since the lines of language (and nonlanguage) are by no means clearly demarcated. The resulting patterns are also different. There are no fluent, Wernicke-type aphasics among children: nearly every child aphasic either is entirely mute (in which case it cannot be proved that he is aphasic) or displays the slow, effortful and limited output of the Broca's aphasic. Why there is no Wernicke's aphasia in children is not known. Perhaps this condition requires a Broca's area which has "overlearned" language to such an extent that it can continue to spew words forth even in the absence of stimuli provoking the outflow. No child has spoken enough language to allow such an outflow and, as a result, there are no youthful aphasics who chatter away like Mr. Gorgan or even Mr. MacArthur.

Although the initial verbal output is limited in childhood aphasia, prospects for eventual recovery are much greater. Despite extensive brain damage in the young child, including removal of the entire left hemisphere, the child is likely to speak normally again and in the near future. This reflects the well-known flexibility and widespread representation of skills in the brain of the growing child; perhaps the child has learned to speak using both hemispheres and whichever is spared merely takes over the helm of language. Indeed, at least some of the dispute between localizers and antilocalizers can be attributed to their interest in different subject groups: localizers tend to focus on older subjects, where fixed lesions produce permanent impairments; antilocalizers look to young subjects who can recover impressively, independently of the locus, and even the size, of the lesion. Such an optimistic view may not apply, however, to children with congenital aphasia. Such individuals may lack normal structures crucial for the learning of speech; and substitute mechanisms will not easily be evolved or adapted.

All generalizations falter when it comes to left-handed persons. In many cases, this condition is due to genetic factors: in others it is a consequence of early brain damage, or, possibly, a grossly abnormal environment. At any rate, perhaps ten percent of the population is wholly or largely left-handed, which means that this hand is favored for most activities. Anywhere between thirty to fifty percent of this left-handed group, and especially those with family histories of left-handedness, are likely to have representation of language functions wholly or in large part in the right hemisphere; even more commonly, left-handers are characterized by bilateral representation of speech. These estimates are based on several indices: the incidence of aphasia among left-handed individuals with localized lesions in the left or right hemisphere; the use of "dichotic" listening tests, in which the language skills of each cerebral hemisphere are pitted against the other; and the results of sodium amytal tests in which one or the other hemisphere is put to sleep so that the effects of this barbiturate on the individual's language capacities can be ascertained.

Like young children, left-handers have speech more widely represented in their brains. As a result lesions in a variety of loci are likely to produce aphasia, yet, by the same token, recovery from it is more probable. In certain cases, unfortunately—that of Peter Franklin, for example —injury is sufficiently pervasive, or language representation sufficiently localized, that the pattern of recovery resembles that among right-handers.

Because of a dearth of studies the anatomical representation of language in individuals from alien cultures and backgrounds is not known. Although there is every reason to believe that the same general principles are universally applicable, it remains to be determined whether individuals whose language places a greater emphasis on pitch may be significantly impaired by damage to the "musical" right hemisphere. And it also is not known to what extent the possession of an ideographic written language (as in China and Japan) may spare reading in cases of left-hemisphere lesions or whether lesions to the "pictorial" right hemisphere will destroy the capacity to read. We shall dwell on these issues in subsequent chapters, but it is worth hypothesizing that the particular constituents of each language, as well as the genetic traits of different ethnic groups, may influence the type and severity of aphasia.

The more atypical an individual and the less common his arsenal of skills, the poorer our success at predicting the effects of lesions in his left hemisphere. Just as the young and the left-handed often defy considered judgments, the highly skilled musician, painter, athlete, or chess player may, in some cases, perform at an extremely high level after aphasia, while, in other instances, he is reduced to but a shadow of his former capacity. The outcome appears to depend on a number of factors: the age at which the skill was learned, how well it was mastered, which neurological structures were implicated. For example, if an individual relies wholly upon written music, his musical capacity is likely to be affected in a more severe way by aphasia than the individual who has learned to play by ear. Similarly, the individual whose artworks are representational or who has previously depicted narrative sequences in his paintings will find his performance far more affected than the artist who has worked with purely formal patterns, such as arrangements of lines, colors, shapes, and textures. Language is so crucial that in the course of evolution powerful pressures have caused it to develop in roughly analogous ways in most individuals. Such strong biological constraints have generally not, by contrast, served to predetermine the acquisition of less pervasive skills like playing the violin, becoming a gourmet cook, or mastering the game of bridge; as a consequence, individuals acquire such skills in idiosyncratic ways. When the brain is injured, the particular way in which one of such skills has been acquired becomes crucial in determining whether it will be destroyed or spared.

The degree to which the individual's personality and emotional state are affected by aphasia is also variable. Some individuals indomitable before being stricken remain so, while others, who appeared equally indomitable, may change radically, lose all motivation, and remain contentedly (or discontentedly) in their wheel-chairs. Yet, there are recurrent patterns. Broca's aphasics tend to retain their previous personalities, and their emotional responses are appropriate as a rule. They evince an understandable frustration at tasks failed, and may well become depressed if they show no progress. Wernicke's aphasics are generally found in a convivial frame of mind, perhaps because they are less aware of what is wrong with them. However, a sizable minority eventually develop a paranoid streak. They observe that others are not reacting to them in the usual way, and may detect the astonished looks and embarrassed grins which often greet the nonsense they are spewing forth. Incapable of appreciating the reasons for this derision, they may conclude that others are harboring a secret or making fun of them; the result is a barrage of accusations or secretive maneuvers. Fortunately, as comprehension improves, this tendency is apt to disappear. A little paranoia, in fact, is sometimes a hopeful prognostic sign. Overall, aphasia does not usually alter an individual's basic personality and emotional makeup; in most cases, there is an awareness of the difficulty, appropriate depression over its debilitating effects, moments of elation when signs of improvement appear. Yet there is clearly an interaction between one's pre-morbid personality and his reaction to such a traumatic experience, so that those inclined toward pessimism or melancholy will exhibit far more despair than those with blithe spirits or sunny dispositions.

Still a fascinating mystery is the kind of aphasia found in individuals whose customary language is in some way extraordinary. When an individual has known more than one language, the result is not always uniform. As a general rule, the language that has been better known, or the language that has been known earlier in life, is better preserved. When the language that was known earlier is also better known, prediction is relatively easy. When, however, the individual spoke one tongue as a youth, yet has favored the other in his adult years, the pattern of breakdown, or of sparing, is difficult to foretell. Sometimes a language learned during a brief period in life—for example, one of the classical tongues—may be mysteriously preserved. In such circumstances, it is tempting to speculate that this language is "located" or was "learned" in a part of the brain which has been spared by the injury. Equally bizarre results have occurred in relation to unusual social circumstances. For example, during wartime, individuals who have become aphasic have found themselves entirely unable to speak a tongue they had formerly known well, if that one happens to be the language (say, German) of the enemy. Naturally it is quite embarrassing when the tongue that is spared happens to be, or appears to be, that spoken by the enemy. One Norwegian woman ignorant of German was extremely chagrined when, after becoming aphasic during the Second World War, she suddenly acquired a prosody which sounded like German to the untutored ear!

Particularly when the person is a compound bilingual —when he knows both languages equally well and has used them interchangeably—his output, syntax, and comprehension after being stricken will be roughly equivalent in both. On the other hand, if he is a coordinate bilingual —if he learned the two languages at different times and has hardly ever used them together during any given period of time—it is more likely that the languages will be differentially affected. When the individual receives sustained practice in the language in which he is less proficient—for example, if Mr. Gorgan had been drilled in the French that he once spoke fluently—the less-preserved language may rather rapidly attain the level of the better-preserved one. At that point, the general process of language recovery, rather than the person's particular facility in each tongue, determines the level of proficiency eventually regained by the aphasic polyglot.

What happens following injury to the language zone in individuals who are blind, deaf and dumb, or mute, or to persons who have mastered a special symbol system such as Morse code or American Sign language? All too often, unfortunately, the examinations of such unique patterns have been undertaken by people whose enthusiasm about their unusual case has far surpassed their knowledge of the proper techniques. If this caveat is borne in mind, some representative findings can be cited.

One individual who had been born with the capacity to hear, but whose parents had been deaf, had learned both sign and ordinary language. When he suffered a lesion in the language area, he became globally aphasic; his ability to use sign language, however, was better spared than his capacity in ordinary language. Natural signs were much better preserved than finger spelling, presumably because the latter function required knowledge of standard English, while the former was subserved by those areas of the brain which govern motor action and a general "knowledge of the world." Eventually all of the language functions in this patient improved to equivalent levels, thus suggesting that each function is dependent to some extent on the language area but that sign language is perhaps somewhat more robust in the presence of a lesion.

While a lesion in the language area seems more disruptive to ordinary language, a lesion outside this zone may be more destructive of paralinguistic capacities. For instance, an individual who suffered disease in the frontal areas of his left hemisphere did not become aphasic but lost the ability to execute Morse code signals. His disorder apparently produced an apraxia which selectively impaired the fine-finger movements required in this semilinguistic system. Another person with a lesion in his right hemisphere remained able to read Morse flashlight signals perfectly but lost the ability to decode the same signals when these were presented by flags oriented in space. The spatial abilities for which the right hemisphere is dominant were apparently crucial for decoding in one medium of Morse code signaling.

In deaf-mute individuals, the ability to decode sign language is, in general, somewhat better preserved than the ability to decode natural language which has been written out; similarly, in those cases where some oral language or lip-reading has been acquired, sign language is usually better preserved than these ordinary language functions. Although finger spelling is usually fragile, in at least one case it seems to have been better preserved than other sign-language forms. Despite such intriguing discrepancies between the various systems, however, injury to one language system does generally implicate all other ones; an individual who becomes aphasic in ordinary language also becomes so in lip-reading and various forms of sign language. Indeed, in the most carefully studied case of aphasia in a congenitally deaf person, the authors conclude that "aphasia in the congenitally deaf is entirely equivalent to that in normal hearing people. . . . The congenitally deaf encode and decode language by the same fundamental processes as those with normal hearing."

In view of the limited number of cases (hardly over a dozen) in the literature, firm or sharply defined conclusions about aphasia in individuals with atypical language systems are ill advised. What is heartening, from the point of view of research, however, is the virtual certainty that further case studies and additional data on such persons promise to illuminate the most general properties of all communication systems. When only a handful of deaf-mute individuals has been studied, each case will necessarily seem unique. But the same was true for Broca when he examined *his* first patients. Now, however, the broad lines of aphasic disorders in normal right-handed adults are already quite well established; the same should eventually come to pass with reference to language disorders in polyglots, musicians, deaf-mutes, and young children. Such knowledge may prove of more than academic interest: armed with knowledge about the range of communication systems, we will be in a superior position to design ones suited to all aphasics' needs and capacities.

If asked to summarize on one leg the multiple points introduced in this chapter, I would probably stress the finding that the crazy-quilt amalgam of aphasic disorders can be viewed coherently if the population is restricted to a relatively typical group of adult right-handers, and if performances on the principal language tasks—reading, writing, repetition, naming, spontaneous speech, and understanding—are carefully evaluated. Most aphasiologists —localizers as well as holists—have described the same major syndromes; no factor analysis or computer program is needed to discover when an individual is a Broca's, Wernicke's, or anomic aphasic.

When it comes to the theoretical questions underlying the fascination of aphasia—and in particular, the most tantalizing of all, the relationship between language and thought—there is less widespread agreement. Yet, I have tried to suggest that even this dispute has been somewhat overblown: no one holds the most extreme views any longer, and most would concede that certain language disorders, such as Broca's aphasia, leave reasoning processes relatively intact, while other language impairments, such as Wernicke's aphasia, take their toll from a variety of (though by no means all) domains of cognition. Whether or not one stresses the identity between cognitive and linguistic processes seems to depend on several factors—the kinds of aphasia being talked about, the cognitive functions at issue, how one sees the relationship between "inner speech" and "thought," and whether one is talking about the mature adult (where it is easier to separate these functions) or the young child (where the overlap is far more notable). If one's definition of inner speech is closely tied to spoken language, then stressing the identity of cognitive and linguistic processes is untenable; if however, one holds a subtler view of inner speech, as a kind of mental manipulation of symbolic elements, then the close relationship between thought and language is much more plausible. Those who disagree with this conclusion—and it is by no means the only possible one—are encouraged to clarify what they mean by "inner speech" or by "basic thought processes," so that an empirical test of their position can be undertaken.

To the casual visitor to the aphasic clinic, its denizens are bizarre indeed. Some, like Mr. Ford, seem to understand exactly what is going on, yet can hardly emit a clear sentence. Others, like Mr. Gorgan, talk a blue streak, but render the average double-talk artist into a paradigm of clear thinking and precision in speech. Some, like Mr. Mac-Arthur, suddenly become bizarrely tongue-tied. And rare individuals can either parrot everything that is said, while understanding nothing; communicate quite well, yet mysteriously clam up when asked to repeat two numbers; or display such curious combinations as writing without reading, or hearing speech while failing to understand it as a language.

Entering the mind of the brain-damaged is, as must have already become abundantly clear, a most difficult assignment. Empathy can come in some measure from talking and listening to aphasics, or from reading descriptions of their behavior, particularly ones lengthier and more comprehensive than those offered here. Yet it may also be helpful if we realize that in our everyday experience we have all, at least superficially and momentarily, entered their world. For example, as young children once, and as observers of young children now, we see individuals whose understanding of their world is quite adequate but who issue only short predications, rich in substantives, devoid of conjunctions, prepositions, or other grammatical building blocks. True, the speech is not labored, and the child quickly advances to utterances of notable length and complexity, but at least for a few months his telegrammatic utterances bear strong similarities to those of the Broca's aphasic. By the same token, our attempts to communicate our wishes and needs in a poorly mastered foreign tongue are often biased in favor of substantives and action verbs, while deficient in adjectives, adverbs, and other "little" words which tend to elude us.

Analogies to the output and comprehension of the Wernicke's aphasic are somewhat less compelling. When we are in a foreign country, hearing a language we but dimly comprehend, we probably share some of the recovering Wernicke's aphasic's confusion at utterances addressed to him. We search for the recognizable word amidst the rapid-fire babble of the foreigner. When we have been working too hard, when we are under the influence of liquor or drugs, when we are falling asleep, the control of our language resources becomes much less firm. We may take off in long flights of fancy, appropriate in grammar but skimpy in meaning, somewhat reminiscent of the free associations of the Wernicke's aphasic. Our latent capacity to produce the jargon which sometimes intrudes into the latter's speech is evident when we try to accompany a song whose lyrics we do not know, or mimic a nursery rhyme or a foreign tongue. Another "Wernicke's aphasic" is the young child (a year older than the Broca-like toddler described above) who allows his language-producing apparatus (his Broca's area) to run on freely, as when he is creating nighttime monologues before falling asleep. Finally, there is the sleep-talker, a transcription of whose speech might easily be confused with that of some of the patients seen on our Service. In each of these instances, though presumably for diverse reasons, our language output is proceeding in a relatively unmonitored way; our mastery of the phonological component, the rhythm, the prosody of our language is manifest, but the communication of specific information is attenuated.

The anomic aphasic, perhaps closest to the normal individual, is easiest to simulate. Indeed, whenever a word is on the tip of one's tongue, or perhaps just shy of that locus, many of the anomic's feelings and behaviors are likely to be manifest. His state may be simulated further when we are overtired, or when we are trying to talk about a subject on which we are poorly informed, or which is "over our heads." Suppose, for instance, that you had to discuss the Japanese economy or the tools used by a geologist. You will find yourself (unless, of course, you do happen to be expert in these areas) constantly searching for words, unsure even when suitable candidates are supplied, engaged in considerable circumlocution, embracing whatever concrete exemplars you can think of, and hovering about them, just like Mr. MacArthur and his cooks about the broth.

Even more frustrating, and equally reminiscent of anomic aphasia, is the inability to name an object that one has clearly recognized. As one casts about, often in vain, for the correct label, producing guesses related in sound or meaning, one may truly feel as if the language area were inexplicably dissociated from the various sensory associations to the object. There is, finally, the frequent experience of encountering an individual or an object one has not seen in some time, or which one associates with an entirely different milieu. The correct word often fails at this point, and yet, when that person or object is introduced into his usual surroundings (or when one is able to do this by a leap of the mind), then the name readily emerges. How similar this is to the plight of the anomic aphasic, whose best hope for access to the missing word is somehow to re-create the circumstances under which that word is customarily issued.

Similar analogues can even be found to the more bizarre forms of aphasia or aphasia-like disturbances. When shutting one's eyes, one is reduced to the condition of the individual who can write but not read; if one is illiterate or has even known an illiterate, he can share the state of mind of the person who can neither read nor write but whose language capacities are otherwise impeccable. Someone who is tone-deaf or color-blind is somewhat like the individual who is word-deaf—an entire realm of sensory stimulation is closed to him. In learning a new language, one may be able to understand pretty well and utter stock phrases, yet experience particular difficulty in repeating directly what is heard; one then resembles the conduction aphasic. On the other hand, when one fails to attend to what has been said, the meaning may not get through, even though the acoustic echo of the message lingers on; in such cases repetition without understanding can occur, as with the transcortical sensory aphasic. Finally, if one is totally ignorant in a foreign language and yet has learned some poems or songs, he can proceed like a transcortical patient, able to repeat or finish up the song, perhaps even to make a few appropriate grammatical adjustments, but otherwise speechless and uncomprehending in that tongue. And so on.

None of these analogies is perfect, and the imaginative observer may well conceive more apt ones. My only point here is to emphasize that the processes affected in aphasia are the very ones which serve us without fanfare during normal communication. Fortunately, we can usually take these for granted, and, fortunately, only a few of us will ever become aphasic. Nonetheless, if we are to understand the person who finds himself in this strange and pathetic condition, it is most helpful to realize that he is an individual like us, with a brain constructed like ours, and that some of the neurons left in his brain are analogous to those servicing us at the present time. Understanding his predicament, and perhaps even helping him recuperate, may depend upon our appreciation of whatever common linguistic links he shares with us. Introspective analysis of the highly complex activities involved in comprehending an utterance, saying a few well-chosen words, or even mind-lessly repeating ourselves, may be a prerequisite for speci-fying what the aphasic has lost; such self-examination may also enable us to appreciate which aspects of thinking, speaking, understanding, and feeling he still retains.

Understanding of the common links between normal and pathological functioning is a major dividend of neuro-psychological research. In addition, critical examination of the breakdown of a process may yield unexpected insights into its acquisition. Both of these lessons are amply real-ized in the study of disorders closely related to aphasia, such as those which undermine the capacity to read. It is to such "alexic" difficulties that we now turn.

# 3 Reading Difficulties: Lessons from Alexia

*It was a very long time before it dawned upon men that all the words which men utter are expressed by a few sounds and all that was needed was to select from the big and confused mass of ideograms, phonograms, and all their kind, a certain number of signs to denote, unvaryingly, certain sounds.*

—EDMUND BURKE HUEY

In October 1887, Monsieur C., a French businessman in his late sixties who had amassed a fortune selling woven goods, experienced several attacks of numbness in his right leg, some feebleness in his arms, and a slight difficulty in speaking. These symptoms soon disappeared, and C. went back to work and thought little more about it, until he discovered that, while able to distinguish objects and persons without any difficulty, he could not read a single word. C. made an appointment with his ophthalmologist in order to be fitted with an adequate pair of glasses.

Much to C.'s surprise, the ophthalmologist, the world-renowned Edward Landolt, did not prescribe glasses. Instead, after a careful examination, he referred C. to an equally eminent colleague, Joseph Déjerine, neurologist at the Bicêtre Hospital in Paris, and one of the pioneers in the emerging field of neuropsychology. C.'s reading difficulty, the two men agreed, could not be rectified by glasses, for it had nothing to do with visual acuity. C. had suffered a relatively rare yet fascinating type of stroke which, while having little effect on his general perceptual capacity, had made it impossible for him to see objects in one-half of his visual field, and had destroyed his capacity to read. For the next few years Déjerine followed C.'s course very closely, noting the details of his condition and performing crucial experiments which have contributed to a better understanding of the process of reading in normal and in brain-injured persons.

The neurological examination began with a presentation of letters of the alphabet. C. was unable to identify any of the letters yet had no trouble in copying them. His way of copying was instructive, for he treated a letter as a design and carefully traced each stroke, rather than as a single graphic unit to be re-created in his own style of handwriting. Indeed, he described the letters as if they were line drawings; *Z* was a serpent, *P* a buckle, *A* a trestle or stand. C. protested that he was losing his mind, for he understood perfectly well that the signs were letters, yet was totally at a loss in identifying them. Shown words, the results were much the same: copying was faithful to a fault, but the identity and the meaning of the words were totally lost. A man of intelligence who had been knowledgeable about political and cultural affairs, C. was now blinded to print and, medically speaking, *alexic*.

Surprisingly, however, C. was able to express himself without difficulty, to recognize and name instantaneously obscure technical and scientific instruments, to understand everything said to him, to recall the most minute details of past events. Even more astonishing, he could still write without difficulty, both expressing his thoughts spontaneously and transcribing what was dictated to him; yet he was quite unable to decipher his own handwriting, unless he could independently remember what he had written or had been dictated to him. In fact, he preferred to write with his eyes shut, for he got "tangled" when he monitored his own writing. When letters were etched on his hand, or when his fingers were guided through the air in the form of a word, he could instantly identify these verbal materials. In short, all his language functions, including writing, were preserved with the exception of the decoding of words and letters presented to his eyes.

Yet there were certain written materials which did make sense to C. To be sure, when shown the French newspaper *L'intransigeant* he was unable to read its title in a fifteen-minute trial; but when shown the newspaper *Le Matin,* he immediately called out its name. He could not identify the individual letters *R* and *F;* but when a circle was drawn around "RF," he instantly reported "République Française." C. himself explained that these recognitions were due to an appreciation of the "form" or "picture" which these symbols assumed. Identifying *Le Matin* was not a matter of deciphering seven letters or three syllables, but rather the recognition of a familiar shape; (RF) was like a traffic signal or a cattle brand, not a group of letters enclosed in a circle. C. was "reading" these "signs" in the same way that a Westerner might learn to recognize a Russian signature despite ignorance of the Cyrillic alphabet, or a child the name of a restaurant by the appearance of its billboard or marquee.

Too energetic and active a man to be felled by his misfortune, C. continued his favorite activities during the years following the onset of his alexia. No longer able to read music, he had his wife perform opera parts which he learned by ear and later sang. He continued to play cards, for he recognized the different numbers and suits; furthermore, he was able to read numbers, to perform elaborate calculations, to follow his business and stock market investments. Why the particular lesion in his brain should destroy recognition of verbal and musical symbols, while sparing numerical ones, remains nearly as mysterious to neurologists today as it was to C., but at any rate his capacities in the numerical realm were not in the least impaired. Indeed, until ten days before his death, C. led a normal existence—at least one as normal as imaginable for an individual who has been selectively blinded.

In early 1892, C. suffered a second, more serious stroke, which still spared his intelligence but left him unable to write—*agraphic,* as well as alexic. Within ten days he died, and Déjerine was permitted to come to the deceased man's home to remove and examine his brain. While cases of alexia had been reported previously, there had been no adequate anatomical evidence about its cause. Study of C.'s brain left little doubt, however, as to the reasons for his original difficulty. The left half of C.'s visual field was completely intact—therefore he would see lines and objects on that side; his language area was also intact—therefore he could speak, understand, and write. But because of the accidents (or design) of the human nervous system, C. was not able to transmit information from the preserved part of his visual system in the right hemisphere to the areas in the left cerebral hemisphere where (in right-handed people) lexical names and concepts are housed. C. could see forms and could copy them adequately; but, because of an interruption of a crucial pathway, this visual information could not travel to the language area. C. could thus name letters aloud, could write spontaneously to dictation, and could even recognize *by touch* letters written in his hand, for the necessary pathways within the language and tactile systems had been preserved; what he could not do was recognize and name a visually perceived letter or word.

But why, if part of the visual center was disconnected from the language center, was C. still able to recognize and name persons, objects, playing cards, even numbers? Déjerine could not provide a satisfactory answer for this question, but some recent studies, which we shall discuss later, do provide clues to this intriguing phenomenon.

The two syndromes exhibited by C.—pure alexia and subsequently alexia with agraphia—are paradigmatic examples of the kind of "isolated" disorders which occasionally surface in the neurologist's office or ward. Owing to a bizarre injury to the nervous system, an individual may find his linguistic and perceptual capacities unimpaired, while suddenly and mysteriously deprived of a capacity fundamental in our society. In many cases of alexia the capacity to read simple materials eventually returns, and sometimes complete recovery ensues. On other occasions, however, injury to the nervous system is sufficiently pervasive so the individual is never again able to decipher written text. In the case of pure alexia, the patient must communicate through speech and writing; in the case of alexia with agraphia, the patient is restricted entirely to oral language.

Many patients, of course, suffer reading disability as part of a more widespread disorder. Sometimes the reading difficulty is secondary to visual problems, in which case the patient can no longer perceive the visual world and becomes more or less "blind"; in many other cases, the patient's linguistic competence has been impaired and, while he can copy written text, he can no longer understand it. The patients described in the previous chapters —indeed, nearly all aphasics—suffer a significant impairment of reading capacity. In global and Wernicke's aphasia, reading for comprehension is largely destroyed, although some oral decoding of graphemes (elements of writing) may still be possible: the patient may read and bellow aloud "Stand up," yet he won't make the connection to, or perform, the action. In Broca's and anomic aphasia, reading for meaning is usually possible but the patient may experience severe difficulties in reading aloud; he cannot find or articulate the sought-after sounds. Even where reading is relatively well preserved (as in cases of conduction and transcortical motor aphasia), the patient's writing is almost always seriously impaired. Indeed, so pervasive and predictable are agraphic difficulties that they provide virtually no clues for the diagnostician. Presumably this is because writing, a supremely complex and multifaceted activity, requires intactness of a whole range of perceptual, motor, linguistic, and cognitive systems— even as the weakest link breaks the chain, a significant difficulty in any of these cortical functions will undermine the patient's ability to express himself in written language.

The reading deficits that accompany aphasia are instructive, and we shall consider them at the conclusion of this chapter. However, the "pure" disorders of reading are of special interest, for they illuminate one of the most troublesome problems in our society: the inability of perhaps ten percent of our children and adults to read with skill. A consideration of the parallels between alexia (acquired reading disability as a result of brain injury) and developmental dyslexia (reading difficulty which emerges in early life) also provides the opportunity to consider more generally the relationship between processes of development and processes of breakdown in human cognition and to examine methods for ameliorating both conditions. Finally, the curious sequel of events which led to the discovery, dismissal, and recent rediscovery of the neurological underpinning of various reading difficulties offers an intriguing glimpse into the manner in which medical research, with occasional stumbles and detours, makes its way.

The inability to read is surely one of the most serious handicaps which can burden an individual growing up in our society. Not only does access to decent jobs or higher education demand a certain facility in reading, but even finding one's way around a city or avoiding dangerous locations becomes a tremendous problem unless verbal

signs are understood. Imagine driving a car or riding a
subway in a strange city if one cannot interpret a map,
or read a sign; consider handling one's own business or
legal affairs if one has always to ask someone else what has
been written; imagine missing the crucial information
"½ PRICE SALE—TODAY ONLY" or "DANGER—LIVE WIRE";
contemplate keeping up with what's happening in the
world, in the community, or in the classroom, if the
printed word is "Greek" to you. Ever since reading became an essential skill in Western society, however, it has
been noted that a significant proportion of individuals
had extraordinary difficulty learning it, and a somewhat
smaller number—perhaps three percent of the population
—seemed unable to read at all.

How the community handles such problems provides a
clue to its prevailing scientific and ideological climate.
For many years the nonreader was regarded as simply
retarded or dull, and banished from school, if not from
the working community—a point of view that has by no
means disappeared. But after repeated documentation that
many nonreaders were as bright as, perhaps even brighter
than, their peers, more enlightened authorities allowed
that reading problems might be a selective disability. Children who had such difficulties were then labeled and
treated in a variety of ways. Often it was assumed that they
were "perceptually handicapped," that they could not see
as well as they should. Much time was then spent with the
eye doctor or with a teacher who would drill the child on
discrimination of signs of similar size, shape, and orientation. Sometimes children who could not read were called
minimally brain-damaged, and efforts were made to correct
their difficulties through medical intervention. Very frequently, such reading deficiencies were tied to emotional
or psychological problems; children and their families
were encouraged to undergo counseling or therapy, with
the expectation that clearing an "emotional block" or

"anxiety attack" would translate into dramatic progress on standardized reading tests.

The ineffectiveness of these methods for most dyslexic children, however, led investigators to search for alternative approaches. One particularly insightful researcher was the Scottish ophthalmologist James Hinshelwood.

Summarizing the accumulated knowledge on alexia in 1917, Hinshelwood pointed out that reading disorders secondary to brain damage were of two principal sorts. The first, epitomized by C.'s condition when he was initially followed by Déjerine, might be called *pure alexia,* or word-blindness. In this condition, the individual is entirely normal in his language functions except for a selective blindness to written verbal materials. The second variety, represented by C.'s condition during the last ten days of his life, could be termed *alexia with agraphia.* Here the individual can still speak and understand perfectly, but is able neither to read, to write, nor to spell— he has been reduced to the status of an illiterate. The individual with pure alexia still understands letters and words as "graphic entities"; he has simply lost the capacity to relate their appearance to their sound and meaning. In contrast, the individual affected by alexia with agraphia no longer understands words or letters as graphic entities; his knowledge of the relation between the alphabet and spoken language has been destroyed. While Déjerine had been among the first to distinguish these varieties, by the time of Hinshelwood's summary they were established clinical phenomena, with well-documented anatomical localizations.

Still, some cases seen by Hinshelwood seem to have been as amazing as Déjerine's original patient. One polyglot, for example, found himself totally unable to read the words of his native tongue, English. Yet he could read some French, even more Latin, and Greek perfectly. Another patient was totally unable to read or name any letters but could effortlessly read such difficult words as *stetho-scope, electricity,* and *infirmary.*

Hinshelwood's consuming interest, however, lay in another group of patients, whom he described as "congenitally word-blind." These were children who had a glaring deficiency in one area: the capacity to read verbal materials. They had no trouble seeing lines and forms, nor did they experience any difficulty in talking, recognizing numbers, or performing other school tasks. Like C. in the last days of his life, they were selectively impaired in decoding visually presented verbal materials and, necessarily therefore, in writing and spelling. Hinshelwood was perhaps the first to make this connection explicit in his insistence that "without an adequate knowledge of [acquired word-blindness] congenital word-blindness cannot be properly understood." In his view, these children lacked certain connections between their visual and speech centers and therefore presented the same difficulty as adults whose left hemispheres had been injured from one or another cause.

It might be thought that discovery of this parallel between acquired and congenital defects would have resulted in revised theoretical notions about the brain, as well as practical applications in training those with reading problems of whatever origin. (Hinshelwood himself worked intensively with one of his first patients, a fifty-eight-year-old teacher of foreign languages who had become alexic, and helped him relearn the alphabet through six months of daily practice. He then acquired a children's primer for this patient and taught him some simple words.) As we have seen, however, a concatenation of circumstances caused the localizing approach, which related specific cognitive defects to discrete brain lesions, to fall into disrepute during these early decades of the century. Indeed, the kinds of cases which Hinshelwood, and Déjerine before him, had seen were alleged to be nonexistent. These early investigators, the argument went, did not examine patients properly, nor did they have acceptable histological methods for studying brain tissue. What they had regarded as isolated disorders were actually more widespread difficulties, affecting language and perception generally, resulting from injury to larger portions of neural tissue. For perhaps thirty years, the notions of alexia, alexia with agraphia, and the relation between congenital and acquired disorders of reading were either forgotten or discredited, particularly in the English-speaking world.

While those who worked with dyslexic children were floundering among the disparate methods concocted by theorists of different camps, some understanding of the reading process in normal children was beginning to emerge. In getting to know their world, children seem to pass through a number of stages reminiscent of the order in which written communication appears to have evolved historically. They first gain knowledge of the world of objects through a variety of actions and sense modalities; for example they see, touch, smell, bounce, and bite a rubber ball. Similarly, they see, hear, and feel a dog, learn to call it by name, and, soon enough, refer to it in its absence. Most children have never seen a kangaroo or a whale, and none have seen a unicorn or Mickey Mouse, yet with little effort they learn to recognize and name these creatures from pictures. This form of recognition and naming resembles pictographic communication, the type of writing system which was devised first: drawing of the entire animal is associated both with a range of potential sensory impressions and actions (you could pet, smell, or hear a kangaroo) and with a sound cluster (kăng′gà rōō′).

By the time he is three or four, the child, though not yet a reader, will recognize certain written words. He will be able to identify his name, perhaps his address, the words *Coke* or *Coca-Cola, Sesame Street, Howard Johnson's,* or *Spic and Span.* By and large, these graphic configurations function as pictures for him. He perceives the name and

sound of the whole entity rather than its constituents; seeing the word *Coke,* he may call out *"Pepsi"* or *"Tab"*; and
if *Coca-Cola* appears in another font, in capitals, or in
different-sized letters, he will probably fail to recognize it.
He is like the individual who recognizes signatures on a
Japanese print without knowing how to read Japanese; or
like Monsieur C., who identified *Le Matin* and  Ⓡ𝔽
from their visual configuration rather than from their
constituent sounds.

This approach to verbal materials has been called the
"look-say" method and has sometimes been regarded as an
effective way to introduce reading. Yet teachers have soon
made a transition from the "look-say" to the "letter-sound,"
or "phonics," method; for only the latter provides a
strategy for reading words not encountered before. At
best, the looker-and-sayer can decipher the word *knock-
out* by combining the sounds "knock" and "out" whose
visual appearance he has memorized; he is helpless when
faced with a term like *lunar module,* a name like *Bonaparte,*
or a nonsense syllable like *mimsey,* whose constituent
parts he has not seen heretofore.

One group of youngsters seem unable to make this
transition to "phonics." As Macdonald Critchley, one of
the world's most renowned authorities on reading problems, has pointed out, "the dyslexic child has no problem
at all in identifying and distinguishing straightforward
signs and signals even though they may be used in communication. He can understand traffic signs, pick out, sort
and name various makes of automobiles, aircrafts, birds,
or clouds, indeed anything except verbal symbols." Most
such children can learn, with effort, that the configuration
BOOK stands for the sound *book;* what they cannot learn
is that the initial sound of the word comes from the
grapheme *B,* the closing sound from the grapheme *K,* and
so on. Unable to make these associations between a single
sound and an arbitrary sign, they are necessarily impaired

in writing and spelling, although their accomplishment in other fields such as mathematics, painting, or music, may reach the "high superior" level. Indeed, some apparently dyslexic children, among them Thomas Edison, George Patton, the surgeon Harvey Cushing, and the sculptor Auguste Rodin, have gone on to make substantial contributions in their chosen fields, and one—Hans Christian Andersen (though he never learned to spell)—became a masterful writer.

For too many years, children who could not relate single letters to single sounds were erroneously but regularly classified as mental defectives. Neurologists who saw adult patients with acquired reading problems were among the first to realize that children with reading difficulties might well be perfectly normal in all other respects. What these children apparently either lacked completely or were slow to develop were the kinds of connections between the visual and language areas which could also be interrupted in later life by a stroke or tumor. Such an anomaly might go completely undetected in an illiterate society, but because of the way in which many modern societies happened to evolve, this variation in brain structure created tremendous difficulties for a select group of children.

Gradually, recognition of developmental dyslexia became widespread; yet this awareness did not lead immediately to effective methods of treatment. The most promising source of insight—studies of isolated acquired alexia— was either unknown to or systematically ignored by reading authorities. Rather, as we have seen, a variety of *ad hoc* and often questionable techniques were employed in a vain effort to make these children readers. Some of the methods were imaginative but inappropriate gimmicks— letters of different colors, typewriters which spoke. Others, such as the effort to teach such children to crawl and walk again, enjoyed a considerable vogue, only to be discredited when controlled studies supporting their claims were not forthcoming. In recent years some developments have given new hope that at least some aspects of acquired alexia and developmental dyslexia are remediable. It is instructive, and somewhat disquieting, to realize that these developments followed closely from a careful consideration of the case of C. and others described at the turn of the century.

One of the most potent impetuses to more effective treatment of dyslexics came from the work of Dr. Samuel T. Orton, who, at the very time in the 1920's and 30's when the work of Déjerine and Hinshelwood was in disrepute, was carefully examining children with congenital word-blindness in Iowa City, Iowa. Like Hinshelwood before him, Orton concluded that there was nothing wrong with the perceptual or linguistic capacities of his patients, but that they had special difficulties in associating written symbols to the sounds they made and the objects they represented. One of his crucial contributions lay in his systematic outline of the irregularities and errors common in the reading and writing of dyslexic children. Such children exhibited a strong tendency to read a word from right to left, confusing words like *was* and *saw;* they had particular difficulties with letters whose orientation is significant in their identification (for example, *p, q, d,* and *b*); they often "mirror-wrote" and read as efficiently, or inefficiently, upside down as right side up; in fact, some could write equally well, or poorly, with either hand.

In Orton's view, this apparent facility provided a key to the riddle of dyslexia. By the time that reading is usually taught, cerebral lateralization has already occurred in most individuals. This means that one hemisphere of the brain, in most cases the left one (which, you will recall, controls activity on the right side of the body and is essential for all language functions), has already established ascendancy over the right hemisphere (which controls activity on the left side of the body but plays a negligible role in ordinary language). In dyslexic children, however, the two hemispheres are apparently still "competing" for dominance and there is no clear division of labor between them. Rather than the left hemisphere guiding perceptions and activities in one direction only, any activity may proceed equally well in either direction. This is why, in such children, writing is as likely to go from right to left as from left to right, reading can similarly proceed in either direction, and letters are read and written without the necessary attention to the placement of strokes or the angle of contours. Before normal reading and writing may occur, hemispheric dominance will have to be established, thereby eliminating the "confusing memory images" of the nondominant hemisphere and the tendency to go from right to left, while bringing to the fore correct visual images and appropriate directionality.

To the condition he described, Orton gave the name *strephosymbolia,* or "twisted symbol." Because of the child's confused images and orientation, his efforts to read and write evoked sounds and pictures that had at best an approximate relationship to what was wanted. Orton had no ready-made solution to this difficulty, but felt that repetitive drill would eventually result in the association of the correct letter-form with its appropriate sound and "the permanent elision of the reversed images and reversals in directions." He strongly favored strengthening those capacities which were undeveloped in the child, rather than exploiting (as in the "look-say" method) those which were normal. Some of his followers have focused on treatments which would encourage the more rapid establishment of cerebral dominance, such as favoring one hand, foot, or eye; while superficially appealing, there is little evidence that this approach succeeds; nor is it known whether, if dominance could be facilitated, this would be healthy or damaging for the child. In many cases dyslexia seems due chiefly to a developmental lag, and as the child grows older, the condition spontaneously disappears. It is at best a guess whether such children would have been better or worse off had hemispheric dominance been accelerated in them through clinical intervention.

Orton's approach signaled a healthy return of interest in the relationship between reading and the organization of the brain. Although a causal relationship between incomplete lateralization and dyslexia has yet to be conclusively demonstrated, a correlation between a developmental lag in the attainment of dominance and a cluster of language problems *has* been well documented. Another approach, inspired by the work of Norman Geschwind at Harvard Medical School, involves an explicit return to concern with patients having acquired disorders in reading, in an effort to determine the range of reading difficulties and the possibilities for remedial training. A number of instructive phenomena have been uncovered in the course of this research.

First of all, it has been shown that there is a strong association between acquired reading disability and acquired inability to name (though not to match) colors; at the same time, preservation of the ability to read numbers and name objects is typical with the lesion which produces pure alexia. In attempting to account for these perplexing findings, Geschwind has suggested that both colors and letters involve arbitrary links between a purely visual configuration and a name. Neither letters nor colors exist in the world as separate entities (though of course there are many letter-like shapes in the world, and many objects with hues). In contrast, objects do exist in the world and any individual has multiple sensory associations to them, including tactile, auditory, kinesthetic, and often olfactory impressions. While numbers *per se* do not exist in the world either, the learning of numbers by using one's fingers involves strong tactile and kinesthetic associations; furthermore, any activity in the realm of numbers entails an active manipulative process involving counting, ordering, transforming, and coordinating. The differences between the relatively static and unisensory domains of letters and colors, and the relatively active, multisensory domains of objects and numbers, is naturally reflected in brain organization. To recognize and name a letter or color, the individual must proceed from the purely visual configuration to a name; even a fairly discrete lesion in the brain may destroy the connection between these domains. On the other hand, the person confronted by an object or number will have a larger number of associations aroused—even if the purely visual-language connections have been destroyed, there are enough associations between visual and other modalities (such as the fingers involved with counting, or the actions involved in throwing a ball) to enable the individual to recognize and name the target by means of an alternate anatomical route. For instance, the message 2 (but not the message $D$) might go from the visual to the tactile area, and thence to the region where naming takes place.

Striking support for this line of reasoning comes from scattered reports of individuals who could once read two kinds of written languages—one using a phonetic alphabet like English, and one employing ideographs like Chinese. Certain lesions which will impair ability to read the phonetic language will apparently spare the ability to read the ideographic language (and vice versa). Presumably this is because writing in the ideographic language, involving as it does symbols similar to objects or pictures of objects, arouses a range of sensory and motor associations that make it more resistant to brain damage than that in the purely visual-phonetic language. Systematic studies of alexic patients have also confirmed the clinical impression that these patients have less difficulty identifying objects and symbols which have been learned in an active way and which arouse many kinds of associations than they do in identifying objects and symbols which are known only from their visual configuration and with which the individual has had less active contact. Numbers are easier to read than words, number-related signs offer less difficulty than punctuation marks, and objects like telephones, fingers, or clocks are easier to name than equally familiar objects like the sun, the clouds, or the ceiling, which a person knows from their visual forms but with which he has had little direct physical experience.

Careful examinations of patients afflicted with alexia and agraphia have shown that, when materials are presented to them in certain ways, they are able to read much more than had been hitherto supposed. For example, one patient recently seen at the Boston Veterans Administration Hospital could initially neither read words aloud nor respond to written commands. Nonetheless, when shown a group of words and a picture, he could easily point out which word went with the picture; when shown a group of pictures and a word, he could make a similar association; when shown a group of words all but one of which belonged to the same category, he could pick out the exception; when given a category name, he could easily point out an exemplar; finally, when shown a word and asked qualitative questions about the object to which it referred (e.g., shown *tarantula,* the patient is asked, is it *large* or *small, harmful* or *harmless*), his answers were generally appropriate. We concluded that while his ability to "sound out" a word had been destroyed, his "semantic reading"— i.e., his understanding of the penumbra of meaning surrounding a word—had largely been preserved. Various other patients have displayed a similar pattern, which often took the form of revealing misreadings of words. One patient, for example, read *tape* as "reel," *tallow* as "candle," *learn* as "book," and *elbow* as "macaroni"! Others could easily read advertisements for items whose names they could not recognize in isolation. One patient with pure alexia was totally unable to read individual letters, yet could effortlessly identify symbols which were simply concatenations of letters, like IBM, NBC, USMC, or WPA. Another could not name letters, yet volunteered words beginning with those letters, and proceeded to spell these words!

Such findings suggest that, among at least some alexics —and in contrast to most developmental dyslexics—there is considerable sparing of reading capacity, of both the comprehension of meaning and the ability to identify individual words and symbols. The key lies in presenting the target item in the right context, or asking the appropriate question. From this, certain remedial implications follow: To make it easier for such patients to read, one must determine which verbal materials they were familiar with earlier, which words and abbreviations they could previously identify. In written communications to them, it is important to use words with rich semantic content and to offer the patient different means of recognition, such as matching or elimination. Most difficult for such individuals, as for Broca's aphasics in spoken language, is the recognition of the "little" words of language like *and, but, if,* or *in.* While common as flies, these words lack strong semantic associations. Perhaps an optimal rehabilitation program would include reactivation of the comprehension of familiar nouns and verbs, use of known trademarks and abbreviations, plus intensive drill and memorization of those few highly important little words which seem to become most inaccessible in cases of acquired alexia. Some of the alternate connections between visual recognition of the written message and comprehension of meaning might also be utilized in the treatment of developmental dyslexia.

Findings obtained with alexic patients also have application to aphasic patients with reading difficulties. This latter group can also benefit from exercises which open auxiliary channels or exploit the context in which verbal materials are presented. We have seen, however, that the pattern of language disorders varies significantly depending on the type of aphasia; so, too, methods for aiding reading must be adapted to the attendant alexia.

Patients with lesions in the anterior portion of the left hemisphere, in particular Broca's aphasics, are usually able to understand the meaning of substantive nouns, verbs, and adjectives, particularly those rich in sensory associations. The extent to which the meanings of these words can be pictured, felt, touched, or smelled seems a critical determinant of their readability. The difficulties faced by this patient group come in deciphering small, "grammatical" particles; in reading aloud; and in absorbing lengthy texts. (This latter problem may reflect a tendency toward fatigue, a difficulty in making the proper eye movements, or a tendency to neglect the right half of space.) Accordingly, in the preparation of a text for such patients, it is advisable to keep it short and to stock it chiefly with the kinds of lexical items which populate telegrammatic communications. A plethora of prepositions, adverbs, and conjunctions complicates the task; a diet of concrete nouns and verbs simplifies it considerably. We might say that these patients read in the manner of the "look-say" method, deriving a global meaning from a familiar visual gestalt. Consistent with this hypothesis, patients with anterior aphasia hardly ever fail to match a concrete noun with its appropriate picture, while they will frequently produce or accept a misspelled version of the concrete noun.

Virtually the opposite clinical picture obtains among posterior aphasics, especially those afflicted with Wernicke's aphasia. These patients have retained the mechanics of reading, and in some cases can read a text aloud with few errors or omissions; yet they will largely fail to comprehend its meaning. (Sometimes, as in the case of transcortical sensory aphasia, they will read nonsense words and foreign phrases without even blinking.) Unlike anterior aphasics, such patients are relatively sensitive to elements of syntax, and as a result, they are more likely to comprehend a longer passage replete with redundant elements. Where the anterior aphasic more readily decodes the agrammatical phrase "boy drinking," the posterior aphasic is more likely to succeed with the more long-winded "the little boy is drinking his cool white milk." The ability of many posterior aphasics to read texts aloud demonstrates that they are using a phonetic rather than a "look-say" method: their frequent disregard of the meaning of the given message suggests an inability to proceed from visual gestalt to intended sense. However, the stability of the gestalt is demonstrated by the typical ability of posterior aphasics to detect a spelling error even while remaining ignorant of the word's meaning.

For all their differences, both anterior and posterior aphasics are more likely to succeed in reading aloud than silently and in comprehending words which designate concrete, manipulable objects. Presumably this is because such objects, and by cortical osmosis the words which designate them, arouse far more sensory associations in the brain. Even in the face of extensive brain damage, such elements are likely to have retained enough of their customary associations to allow partial decoding of their meaning.

In this sense, most aphasics resemble the patient suffering from alexia with agraphia more than the patient who is purely alexic. Irrespective of the form of aphasia, the word *telephone* is more easily enunciated and understood than the word *tell* or *sky* or *ceiling,* apparently because the latter words, less tangible and concrete, arouse fewer sensory associations. (It is perhaps such highly concrete words which best lend themselves to the type of subliminal perception which purportedly seduces movie-goers to the canteen.) Only among pure alexics is ability to read a word correlated directly with its length: *be* is easier than *bee, phone* or *tell* simpler than *telephone.* Such patients are painfully piecing together words letter by letter, and thus they benefit from brevity of words rather than from accessibility of word meaning. Alone among the many varieties of brain-damaged individuals, they appear to have a reading difficulty which stands apart from their overall linguistic competence.

Examination of reading in aphasia confirms, then, that reading is far more than the simple decoding of graphic symbols. Even when this capacity is intact, the patient may remain oblivious to meaning; the pivotal ability to relate sound or sight to meaning has been impaired. And in those patients whose comprehension of spoken language is relatively spared, significant deficits in reading are still likely. Such difficulties may arise because of the greater difficulty of scanning connected text, the necessity for decoding the more elusive grammatical components and inflections, and the absence of assorted gestures, props, and intonations which aid the comprehension of spoken language.

Analogies to each of these disorders exist among children. Some have difficulty in eye movements, resulting in problems with line scanning; some are lost without the situational cues of ordinary spoken language; a few can grasp "telegrammatic" writing, while encountering marked difficulties with endings, inflections, and other "low-meaning verbal components." But perhaps the most interesting analogue to aphasic reading occurs in a small group of abnormal children who master the mechanics of reading at an exceptionally early age. While the average dyslexic child performs normally in most cognitive areas, only to experience a severe and crippling difficulty in reading, the hyperlexic child performs poorly in virtually every area with the striking exception of reading.

The history of such children usually resembles the account of an individual with "minimal brain damage." The typical hyperlexic youngster is characterized by developmental lags: milestones of sitting, walking, saying the first word, and talking in full sentences have usually been delayed. In addition, they may be gawky, clumsy, or "funny-looking"; and they may exhibit certain signs of autism, such as avoidance of eye contact or spurning of peers. What distinguishes these youngsters from other learning-disabled children is this: by the age of three or four, and usually without appreciable aid from parents or siblings, these children have mastered oral reading.

This precocity is best conveyed by citing the highlights of a few case histories. A boy aged four years and ten months, studied by Peter and Janellen Huttenlocher, could read a third-grade-level passage fluently despite woefully inadequate speech and understanding and an IQ in the mentally defective range; so much did he enjoy this activity that he sought to read all materials in sight. A three-year-old youngster seen by these investigators could read newspapers aloud and also recited everything in sight, including dictionaries and telephone books. Two other investigators, Charles Mehegan and Fritz Dreifuss, describe a six-year-old who could not desist from reading:

> Reading had the features of a compulsive ritual: he could not be distracted or easily deterred. If he were given a book, he had to start at the beginning, reading the entire title page, including the publishing house, date of publication, Library of Congress number, etc. He showed great resistance to interruption and would return later to this point and carry on the exercise. While reading, he stood slightly back from the exercise as though to gain perspective, moving to and fro in a rhythmic fashion with arms flexed at the elbows and palms turned inward in a somewhat oratorical attitude.

In each of these cases, as well as others reported in the burgeoning literature on hyperlexia, the youngster gives no evidence that he comprehends what he has read aloud. Reading for him consists strictly in the oral decoding of visual graphemes: his prosody and accentuation do not vary with the sense, nonsense words are read as effortlessly and as emphatically as meaningful ones, jokes are not laughed at, commands not honored, and even references to the present situation may be missed. Like the youngster who has learned to pronounce Hebrew vowels and consonants, but has never acquired any word meanings, the child spews forth, in machinelike fashion, the assorted sounds which characteristically accompany the particular written symbols. Not surprisingly, some of these children also habitually "echo" words and phrases spoken in their hearing; in this, as in their reading, they manifest a "purely linguistic" function that seems to have matured on its own, without the customary ties to meaning which convert verbal sounds and sights into communication. As the Huttenlochers summarize: "The children all repeated speech sounds rather than formulating verbal messages about their own experiences as normal children do." It may well be that the language areas in these children's brains have matured at a normal or even precocious rate while those regions which organize nonverbal meaning are abnormally slow in maturing, physiologically impaired, or disconnected from the areas of speech and sight.

Given, for whatever reason, the existence of isolated oral reading in certain children, a question arises about such capacities in brain-damaged adults. In my own research, I have indeed encountered a number of patients who can read aloud with consummate skill, yet without the slightest sign that they know whereof they speak. It seems clear that these patients have retained the rules of English orthography: given a visual configuration, they can sound it out; and, in some cases, given a word, they are even able to spell it aloud! Yet, like hyperlexic children or the unschooled Hebrew chanter, theirs is a written world without meaning, their reading capacity as "isolated" as the analogous ability of certain brain-damaged patients to repeat without comprehension whatever oral messages happen to be intercepted. Such capacities, of course, do not do the patient much good; they are at best curiosities, which may embarrass relatives or entertain onlookers. But they serve as a powerful reminder that the reading process is scarcely unitary, and that its "mechanics" may well be selectively spared in the anomalous child or the injured adult. Nor should one forget the converse: the retained ability in certain alexic and dyslexic patients to decode familiar visual configurations for meaning, while failing to attach the correct sound sequence to it. Such a limited skill may also embarrass and/or entertain, but with a crucial difference: the world of such patients can generally be entered by spoken messages, and if written messages are perceived at all, the all-important meaning will be grasped.

Between the aphasics who exhibit diverse reading disorders and the hyperlexic children in whom reading is the outstanding capacity, the complex of factors which contribute to skilled reading is effectively illuminated. Yet, in general, the condition of dyslexic children most closely resembles the experiences of acquired alexics like Monsieur C. The most effective treatments for developmental dyslexia, therefore, employ methods which might easily have been designed by Déjerine or Hinshelwood. In 1915, Bishop Harmon, reviewing the evidence on dyslexia, suggested that such children must be taught on the plan of the Chinese, with each word having its own ideographic symbol. Wittingly or not, Paul Rozin and his associates at the University of Pennsylvania have recently devised just such a method, which has proved effective in teaching visual language to severely dyslexic inner-city children. These investigators have assigned an English meaning to thirty different Chinese characters. The ideograms can be read from left to right and combined to form a variety of English sentences. After only a few hours of training spread over a number of sessions, eight second-grade children were able to communicate using these symbols in a flexible, nonmemorized manner. The article reporting these findings was entitled "American children with reading problems can easily learn to read English presented by Chinese characters."

Rozin's interpretation of his results is highly consistent with the views of acquired alexia propounded here. He believes that the dyslexic child's principal problem, perhaps due to a neurological deficiency, lies in merging a sequence of letters into a known English word. Therefore he recommends that initially a system be used in which arbitrary but easy-to-recognize characters are mapped into speech in terms of words rather than of individual sounds. Since this method will eventually run into the same problem as the Chinese writing system—too many characters to learn—he feels that perhaps a syllabary system, where one visual configuration represents a composite sound unit (e.g., *can, o, pen,* and *er*) might be an ideal point of departure, eventually allowing a smooth transition to English reading, spelling, and writing. Rozin himself is currently experimenting with this method.

Although his success has been unusually dramatic, Rozin is by no means the only investigator who has attempted to unravel the mystery of reading disability and come up with a successful remedial program. Recently, for example, Jay Isgur has claimed great success in training severely dyslexic children to learn the alphabet. Isgur's subjects begin by dealing with specially made objects which have the same shape as English letters and which begin with the correct opening sound (e.g., *M* in M-shaped mittens; *P* in P-shaped pen, etc.). Once they have memorized these forms, the subjects are asked to imagine them with their eyes closed, and eventually to master the actual letter form without any object-linked aids. A few short sessions working with this "Object-Imagery-Projection" technique have enabled an unbroken series of patients at a Learning Disabilities Clinic to master the alphabet, and subsequently to read at the word and sentence level. It is intriguing to speculate whether patients with pure alexia might be able to relearn the alphabet by an analogous method, which would presumably supplement disrupted visual-language associations with spared tactile-language associations. In fact, some evidence (to be reviewed in the next chapter) suggests that alexic patients may well retrain themselves to read by replacing the normal perception of individual letters with exaggerated tracing movements of the head and the hand.

Methods to train in reading abound. Some researchers are convinced that dyslexic children should be taught exclusively by "look-say" methods; others favor drill in phonics, tactile involvement with the letters, use of teaching machines, or even the design of artificial scripts which eliminate the confusing cues of slant and orientation, or feature pictograms or rebuses. A similar if somewhat smaller range of alternatives has been recommended for patients with acquired disorders of reading. Especially promising in this context is the recent success of Michael Gazzaniga and his associates, and also a group of researchers at our own hospital, in teaching an arbitrary symbolic method of communication to severely aphasic subjects. Inspired by David Premack's impressive demonstration that a chimpanzee can communicate using visual tokens, these researchers have first inventoried the patients' cognitive capacities and established his desire to communicate in the hospital environment; then they have designed the new visual language in such a manner that it conforms to the patient's abilities and wishes. While experiments are still in the preliminary stage, it seems probable that a system which bypasses the impaired auditory and oral channels, while utilizing visual configurations less easily confusable among themselves than the Roman alphabet, offers considerable promise as a communication prosthesis for aphasic patients.

Perhaps, in due course, perfected methods for training dyslexic children to read, and aphasic patients to communicate, can be combined into a more comprehensive system which will be helpful to the whole gamut of individuals with reading disability. Yet it is my impression that, just as a variety of methods of teaching creative writing, athletics, or mathematical competence have been evolved to suit widely divergent skills and personalities, so the therapist of reading disorders will similarly require an armamentarium of techniques respectively suited to different kinds of disorders. In any event, whatever signficant strides may otherwise be made, it seems increasingly evident that a complete identification of the components of reading and of reading disorders can only emerge from a fuller understanding of the neural mechanisms involved in identifying visual forms and in relating these forms to objects and phenomena in the environment. When one considers that three major contemporary approaches to reading disorders—Orton's study of lateralization in the brain of the child, Geschwind's focus on the impairment and sparing of various symbolic capacities among the brain-injured, and scattered experiments on the use of pictographic language—were all hinted at nearly a century ago, the prescience of the ophthalmologist Landolt and the neurologist Déjerine seems impressive indeed.

In focusing on the reading process in children and adults, we have examined a capacity which draws heavily on skills of language and on the mechanisms of the perceptual system. Either an impairment in language or a disruption of perception will cause reading difficulties, although, as we have stressed repeatedly, the kinds of problems and the proposed remedies will differ, depending upon the sources of the disability. In the following chapters, we will shift away from capacities which are heavily dependent upon human language towards those which, though sometimes linked to language, are also pivotal in organisms bereft of language. So unthinkingly assumed are the abilities to recognize and to remember that we seldom acknowledge the intricacy and sophistication of these mechanisms; nor do we usually note how dependent upon them we are for our knowledge of the world and our ability to negotiate our way about it. Cases of visual agnosia and Korsakoff's syndrome underscore the centrality of these processes, even as they detail, in a subtle and unexpected way, the relationship between linguistic capacities and other phases of cognition.

# 4 Disorders of Recognition: How Shall a Thing Be Known?

*A polyp would be a conceptual thinker if a feeling of "Hollo! Thingumbob again!" ever flitted through his mind.*

—WILLIAM JAMES

There have been but few genuinely epiphanous moments in the history of psychology. One such, however, occurred in 1890, when the German psychologist Christian von Ehrenfels was inspired to devise the concept of *Gestalt*. Von Ehrenfels's insight became the essential foundation of one of the principal schools of psychology in this century; it also exerted a pervasive influence on other fields of knowledge, and ultimately, by influencing the ways in which medical practitioners viewed certain brain-injured patients, this concept came to alter our understanding of fundamental cognitive processes.

From the vantage point of the present, von Ehrenfels's discovery seems deceptively simple and noncontroversial. Yet he was the first psychologist to insist that the identity or essence of a pattern inhered not in the particular elements of which it was composed, but rather in the relationship among these elements. The melody for "Silent Night," for example, is not adequately described as a pitch of frequency A, followed by a pitch of frequency B, and so on.

Rather it consists of an initial pitch of arbitrary frequency (A or B or X), followed by pitches whose frequency is determined by their relationship to the originally selected frequency—$A + 1$, $B + 1$, or $X + 1$. The actual melody is the entire set of relations ($A$, $A + 1$, etc.). By a similar argument, a chicken which has learned to peck at the darker ($D_1$) of two gray circles, $L_1$ and $D_1$, will no longer peck at circle $D_1$ when it now appears in the company of a yet darker gray circle, $D_2$. Instead, it will shift to the circle that is relatively darker, ($D_2$), embracing a relative, not an absolutist strategy. Again, the crucial psychological unit is a relation; in this case "darker than." This approach undermined the well-nigh universal tendency among *fin-de-siècle* psychologists to regard stimuli as elemental patches of pure sense data: a color, a point, a line, pure tone. Von Ehrenfels introduced a concern with the overall form, pattern, or structure—the Gestalt (German for *form* or *configuration*)—into which these elements were organized, and in terms of which they were related; the isolated elements, then, attained meaning only through being embedded in such a perceptible configuration or Gestalt.

Within two decades of his epiphany, a group of young psychologists in Germany had completely adopted von Ehrenfels's point of view, thereby launching the "Gestalt revolution." At the very instant that an approach in many ways diametrically opposed—the behaviorism identified most notably with the name of John Watson—was coming to hold sway in America, the Continent was falling increasingly under the Gestaltist spell. Patterns, forms, configurations, melodies, pictures, coherent stories, the totalities which had mesmerized Goethe, became the subject of analysis: the notion of isolated quanta of vision, audition, and olfaction was discarded as misleading and artificial.

It is against this background that a young soldier, who came to be known only as Schn. (or, in some publications, as Sch.), became a *cause célèbre* in the world of neurology and psychology.

Until the First World War, Schn. had been a healthy laborer of normal intelligence. On June 4, 1916, while on active duty, he was wounded by shrapnel from a mine and remained unconscious for four days. Medical examination disclosed two wounds at the back of his head, which were operated upon in December of that year. Because of persistent headaches, Schn. entered the Hospital for Brain Injury in Frankfurt in February 1917. There he was seen by Kurt Goldstein, a brilliant neurologist just turned 40, and his colleague, Adhemar Gelb, a skillful and imaginative psychologist.

In most respects, Schn. appeared to be quite normal. His intelligence seemed intact, he had no language disturbances, and his visual acuity was adequate. On gross inspection, his reading and writing also appeared normal. While recuperating, he was trained in the craft of leather goods and later went back to work as a purse-maker.

To their astonishment, Gelb and Goldstein discovered that Schn. was completely unable to identify words and objects when these were exposed briefly on a special viewing apparatus called a tachistoscope. If letters or pictures were shown him with their contours obscured or their interiors marked by cross-hatching, he was also unable to recognize them. Yet, as noted above, his reading otherwise appeared normal. Further observation indicated that the patient's reading was accomplished through a series of slight head and hand movements: he traced with his body whatever contours and angles his eyes discerned. He vehemently denied that this was an unusual procedure—didn't other people all read in the same way? That these movements were indispensable to his reading was proved by preventing Schn. from moving his head and hand, whereupon he failed to read a single word. It was for the same reason that he could not read words which were crosshatched: the gross movements on which symbol recognition depended were thwarted by adventitious lines. (Schn.'s reading strategy may well be the one utilized by other patients who, after an initial period of alexia, slowly recover the ability to decode written messages.)

Schn. found it easiest to identify objects and pictures that contained some clear defining feature; having spotted this telltale cue, he would leap immediately to an answer, not bothering to confirm his hypothesis by tracing the remainder of the contour. A die was recognized by a dot, a clock by its hands. When, however, the drawings had several lines leading away from a single point, chance determined whether he followed the most revealing line. Drawings in perspective posed special difficulty, and a circle tilted away from him was invariably called an ellipse. While four dots arranged in a square configuration ( :: ) are normally seen as a square, this construction eluded Schn., who failed to join the dots into a figure. He had special difficulty in apprehending groups of objects, or making sense of configurations in which the relationship between objects was critical—even the difference between straightness and curvature escaped him. And, most dramatically, he was unable to perceive motion when two elements were presented in rapid succession, as occurs in a film or moving neon light. Indeed, he claimed not to understand what was meant by the "perception of motion."

Given such a severe deficit in interpreting visual input, Gelb and Goldstein wondered how Schn. could find his way around the world. He replied that he always sought cues which provided a more or less unique definition of a given object. Men and vehicles were distinguished because "Men are all alike—narrow and long, while vehicles are wide; one notices that at once." A tree was extricated from its shadow because the shadow was darker. Asked to copy pictures, Schn. did not preserve the details of the model. The head movements he used to spot a "defining" feature of a given object—in one instance, a policeman—did not suffice to enable him to reproduce that particular object; the best he could do was to represent its class or type—i.e., everyman.

The experimenters proposed that Schn. had a selective impairment in his capacity to perceive form, or Gestalt. When confronting a display, normal individuals discern entire objects, as well as the relations between such objects, at a glance; Schn. was incapable even of picking out a single form, except by the lengthy inferential process outlined. He failed to grasp and identify the whole, instead passing back and forth in an aimless way between disparate parts of the presentation. Sensation or elements were noted, visual acuity was adequate, but the capacity to synthesize input into forms suffused with meaning had been destroyed by the lesion in the brain. Goldstein and Gelb's lengthy case report on Schn. stimulated enormous interest. For it described a rare disorder, one alluded to in earlier literature, but seldom if ever observed in such pure form. At the same time it supplied hard-nosed neuropsychological evidence for a cardinal tenet of Gestalt psychology: that the perception of form is a basic, identifiable capacity of the brain. The leaders of the Gestalt movement —Wolfgang Köhler, Kurt Koffka, and Max Wertheimer— quoted copiously from this case study, citing it as decisive evidence for the view they were promulgating. Here was fresh proof that vision (as we know it) is involved not with elements and associations of elements, but with forms and figures, of the type one hapless brain-damaged patient could no longer perceive.

Schn. was an able, willing, and continually available patient. In the years following Goldstein's report, he was studied repeatedly; his case was interpreted both by his diverse interrogators and by those who had merely pored over his protocol. The noted philosopher Ernst Cassirer (a cousin of Goldstein) met Schn. and spoke of "the clarity and sharpness of his thinking, the aptness and formal soundness of his inferences. . . . It was precisely this highly developed activity of discursive 'reasoning' that enabled him in many ways to compensate almost entirely for his gravely impaired power of optical representation and memory, so that for practical purposes, it scarcely made itself known." Later investigators, while not confirming Goldstein and Gelb's findings in every detail, generally endorsed the clinical picture they had presented. These follow-ups revealed that Schn. had certain difficulties in memory, particularly in the visual sphere, in calculation, and in the ability to bring together elements in a variety of domains. There was some disagreement about the extent and locus of his lesion (only an autopsy could resolve this dispute) and some argument about how best to label the difficulty (figure blindness? object blindness? a deficit in simultaneous synthesis?). Over and above these quibbles, however, Goldstein and Gelb's pioneering work was widely acclaimed.

This account of a "Gestalt deficit" had already achieved the status of a classic on the Continent when descriptions of similar clinical symptoms began to surface in England. In 1941 the eminent British neurologist Russell Brain published a report entitled "Visual Object Agnosia with Special Reference to Gestalt Theory," in which he described a fifteen-year-old boy who was able to perceive objects without recognizing their meaning. Like Schn., this boy had adequate visual acuity and could detect elements of sensation. Unlike Schn., however, he did not experience particular difficulty in following the outside line of a figure; that is, his form perception was relatively intact, and he could copy and match figures with adequate skill. His particular difficulty lay in *interpreting* the form —in recognizing its use or function, in relating a rectangular shape, for example, to a book, box, or tray. Here, apparently, was yet another bizarre visual difficulty, one

attributable neither to deficits in elementary visual functions nor to difficulties in form perception; instead, the
deficit inhered in associating a perceived visual Gestalt to
its meaning. Brain attributed the disorder to a woefully
impoverished visual memory which precluded a matching
of the perceived form with "images" or "schemes" of forms
previously seen. Comparison of this case to Schn.'s suggested to Brain the existence of at least three stages of
mental processing: simple sensitivity to lights, forms, and
colors; discerning the form; attaching meaning to the
form. Schn., in this view, was impaired principally in the
second, Brain's own patient in the final stage; but both
cases buttressed the central claims of Gestalt psychology.

Still further support came as one consequence of the
disastrous Coconut Grove fire in 1942. One individual
who suffered from carbon monoxide poisoning, and yet
survived, was a twenty-year-old woman who, upon admission to the Boston City Hospital, was found to be completely blind and speechless. In the following weeks she
slowly recovered to the point where she could talk, wink,
and detect elements in her visual field. There was no permanent impairment of consciousness or intellect; recognition remained intact in the senses of touch and hearing;
yet the patient was unable to identify objects, pictures, or
written materials by sight. Within seven months, she was
able to see parts of objects and straight lines and read
simple materials, but her capacity for visual recognition
and her ability to copy geometric forms were still grossly
impaired. Faces were not recognized, figure and ground
were confused, movies were impossible to follow. Shown
a geometric form, she complained, "When it is curved I
should trace around. But I see other parts and I lose myself. Then I do not see the beginning any more."

A Boston physician, Alexandra Adler, followed the patient for five years, thereby securing invaluable information
about the gradual resolution of such "Gestalt" blindness.

In this particular instance, the basic disturbance—inability to perceive visual form—persisted, yet there was increased facility in identifying forms in daily life. Like Schn., the patient had learned to search for defining parts of objects and to make informed guesses about what she was shown. By using head-and-hand movements *à la* Schn. and through appropriate deductions, she succeeded in reading competently. Still, a strange word like *alluvial* would elude her, for the customary strategies then proved inadequate. In tasks where instruction or self-correction was possible (like reading), steady improvement occurred. However, in areas where there was no ready reinforcement, the patient forgot what she had learned (or relearned). Eventually she married, was able to undertake simple house chores, and had a child. As of 1950, however, she still could not hold a job, decipher handwriting, or calculate accurately; she also needed help in caring for her baby.

The cases reported by Brain and Adler served, as noted, to substantiate the existence of the phenomena described, and the interpretations offered, by Goldstein and Gelb. In the 1940's, however, years after Gelb had died and Goldstein had emigrated to America, two German neurologists tracked down the original patient, Schn. Now middle-aged, he was living in a small town in Germany. Richard Jung, who visited him first, confirmed that the gentleman he was interviewing was really the same Schn., originally seen thirty years before by Goldstein and Gelb. Indeed, the narrowed visual fields and difficulty with brief tachistoscopic viewings remained just as they had been initially described. However, to Jung's surprise, the patient was able to find his way around without difficulty, and to lead a normal social life; he had satisfactory knowledge of his surroundings and could even drive an automobile. Informal testing and observation of the subject suggested that he could see quite adequately and could recognize objects and individuals (including the doctor).

What astounded Jung was Schn.'s behavior when the tests originally administered by Goldstein and Gelb were repeated. Abruptly the patient's manner and demeanor were radically altered. He became stiff and formal, he spoke in a very mechanical, highly stereotyped manner; he moved his head just as described in the earlier reports; he talked as if he were reciting. Occasionally when a stimulus interested or amused him, he would revert to a more natural mien and would dispense with auxiliary movements. Then he would catch himself, assuming once more the bizarre formal behavioral pattern.

In Jung's considered judgment, Schn. was now a normal perceiver who had mastered a special way of behaving during the administration of certain tests. Whatever his original clinical picture, there was no indication that he was any longer unable to perceive Gestalten. He appeared, however, to have invested a significant part of his identity in the assumed role of ideal subject. He had received a large pension for being disabled in the war, and he had gained considerable public attention and fame from the Gelb-Goldstein project. Perhaps because his prior behaviors had been so handsomely reinforced, he reverted to them when the old tests were posed, even though there was now no evidence of them under normal circumstances.

Jung stopped short of any allegation that Goldstein and Gelb had perpetrated a fraud. Instead, he offered the less-damaging interpretation, in line with a well-known pitfall of experimental science, that every examiner found in this curious patient evidence for his pet hypothesis. Reviewing the vast literature on Schn., Jung showed how each practitioner's interpretation supported his own previously formulated theory of higher cortical function. It was natural, then, that two observers wedded to the Gestalt approach should find in a willing subject, Schn., convincing evidence for the truth of that approach.

A harsher conclusion was reached by the other visitor

to Schn., the neurologist Eberhard Bay. Like Jung, Bay noted a disparity between Schn.'s informal behaviors and his mode of proceeding during the readministration of the standard Gelb-Goldstein tests. In addition, however, Bay found the subject to be inconsistent and untrustworthy, sometimes claiming that he could not perceive something, later identifying the same element immediately and without difficulty. Bay could not demonstrate the perceptual difficulties described by Goldstein and Gelb; but he found an abundance of abnormal and somewhat theatrical behaviors. The subject would at intervals issue test phrases that had been learned, employ only sporadically the auxiliary device of head-moving, shift unpredictably from the "schooled" to the "natural" style of responding, and back again. Bay concluded that, originally, Schn.'s difficulties had been greater than conceded by Goldstein and Gelb, probably including intellectual and optical deficits. These had cleared up wholly, or in large part, within a few years. In the meantime, however, the patient had learned to behave in a certain way in order to maintain his comfortable relationship with the neurological establishment of Germany. When seen by two disinterested observers, he was completely unreliable. Falling back on a venerable Teutonic saw to the effect that "He who lies once is not to be believed," Bay concluded that findings based on his testimony had never been legitimate. Goldstein and Gelb had constructed their entire Gestaltist edifice on the foundation of one *false* case. The phenomenon they had described was probably a figment of their imaginations, one amply aided by the witting, semiprofessional collusion of the wounded soldier from Schleisen.

The revisionist views of Bay and Jung notwithstanding, most neurologists would describe patients like Schn. as having selective disturbances in regard to recognition of the visual world—that is, they are agnosic. They can detect elements in the visual realm, in that they react to light, colors, movement, and so forth; but, to one degree or another, they cannot recognize or make sense of meaningful objects and events around them. Theoretically such difficulties in recognition can be due to various factors such as severe intellectual deterioration, language difficulty, or partial blindness. To fall under the classic definition of agnosia, however, the patient must be shown to be sufficiently intact for normal purposes intellectually and linguistically; he must know the identity and use of a given object (e.g., he can use it appropriately when it is handed to him or when he hears its characteristic sound); he must be able to produce its name (e.g., when he hears the sound made by the object or he is allowed to feel it); he must have his elementary perceptual capacities intact (his optic reflexes and ability to spot and track light, colors, and contours must be demonstrated). If all of these capacities are preserved, while the patient remains unable to recognize or identify a particular visually presented stimulus, he merits the diagnosis of "agnosia."

The first hint that such a condition might exist came in the 1870's, when the occipital lobes of dogs were ablated by the physiologist Hermann Munk. As noted in our introductory discussion, these lobectomized dogs could still "see" objects to the extent that they would neither walk into them nor trip over them. Yet they no longer reacted appropriately in these objects' presence: they would attempt to eat stones, defecate in their beds, ignore other dogs, and so forth. Munk spoke of these animals as suffering from *mind-blindness;* and this term, and its Jacksonian equivalent, *imperception,* became the generally accepted labels for this condition.

Two major categories of mind-blindness were initially distinguished by H. Lissauer in 1885. This neurologist characterized responsiveness to sensory elements as "apperception," the linkage of percepts to stored images as "association." Mind-blindness could therefore be either of an apperceptive form (as in Schn., who could not combine elements into forms) or of an associative variety (as in Brain's young patient, who could discern forms, but not appreciate their significance).

Credit for coining the term *agnosia* goes to Sigmund Freud. While still a practicing neurologist, Freud employed this term in a general sense to refer to any failure in the recognition of objects, whether at the earlier stage of form perception (apperception) or the subsequent association of percepts to meanings. In the years following this early discovery and discussions, a plethora of agnosias were reported. There were agnosias for color, sounds, animate objects, inanimate objects, large objects, small objects, persons, faces, music, and so on. Differentiations were even made within each of these realms. J. Delay, for example, spoke of three types of agnosia in the tactile realm, one being the inability to distinguish size and shape of objects; a second the failure to recognize differences in density, weight, and roughness; the third an inability to recognize objects by touch despite adequate feeling capacity and ability to distinguish size, shape, and density. By 1930, neurologists had discerned agnosias for virtually everything that could be known; there were at least as many terms and models as there were well-described cases in the English, French, German, Italian, and Russian literature.

About some of these agnosias, there is little to say. They have been described briefly but once or twice, and their theoretical interest is at best dubious. Others, however, have been described repeatedly and are quite suggestive for the light they cast on the respective natures of pathological and normal functioning. Especially fascinating to many investigators is a recognition difficulty which seems restricted to faces—a condition known as *prosopagnosia* (from the Greek *prósopon = face,* + agnosia). A prosopagnosic can generally identify objects with little difficulty.

His language functions are good and he is most likely intellectually intact. He retains a clear memory of individuals
he has known, and he can recognize them from hearing
their voices, contemplating a verbal description of them,
or noting some telltale mark, such as a mustache, pair of
glasses, or favorite hat.

Where the prosopagnosic fails is in identification of an
unadorned face. Clinical details differ across patients, of
course, but in general there is no feeling of familiarity,
even if the face belongs to a close acquaintance, a relative,
or the patient himself! Told the identity of the face, the
patient will sometimes alight upon a revealing feature.
More often, however, he will express his disbelief, perhaps
adding that the individual (even himself!) has changed
markedly since he last saw him. The prosopagnosic also
fails in recognizing the pictured faces of famous persons;
yet the examiner can sometimes be misled about the patient's impairment if he uses pictures familiar in themselves. The Karsh portraits of Churchill and Einstein, the
seated array of the "Big Three" at Yalta, the Gilbert Stuart
portrait of Washington, the various noted photographs of
Lincoln, pose little difficulty for clever patients, on the
look-out for Churchill's cigar, Washington's locks, Lincoln's beard, or other telltale features captured by the
portraitist. The successful construction of tests of ability
to remember faces or to match them with one another has
proved elusive for similar reasons: patients can often get
correct answers without recognizing the faces, simply
through scrupulous attention to other revealing details of
the representation. Indeed, in some tests, patients diagnosed clinically as prosopagnosic have been known to out-
perform patients with right-hemisphere disease whose face
recognition was clinically intact! In such cases prosopagnosics are reminiscent of color-blind individuals in wartime: they may fail to achieve recognition under ordinary
conditions, but may well spot "camouflage" missed by

those of normal capacities in the given area of perception.

A central issue here is whether such a gross impediment could really be specific to faces. On both logical and psychological grounds, it would seem that it could: the great importance attached to facial expression in social relations, the early emergence of the face as a special cue in the mother-child interaction, the capacity of the eyes or other facial features to capture and hold attention, all tend to buttress the notion of face recognition as a specific, distinctive capacity. And support for this hypothesis has come from some interesting research by Robert Yin. This youthful investigator at MIT studied patients who were known to have the lesion which usually impairs face recognition; this subject group performed more poorly in face-recognition tests than did individuals with lesions of equal size in other areas of the brain. On the other hand, when the faces were inverted, and a similar test was administered, the apparently prosopagnosic patients actually did better than those with other forms of brain damage. Yin has also found that for normal subjects faces are, conversely, more difficult to recognize upside down than are other familiar objects (e.g., inverted houses), but that when presented in their usual orientation, faces prove easier for the normal person to recognize than other objects so presented. These results—this selective ease or difficulty regarding face perception—provide substantial underpinning for the claim that special mechanisms do mediate the cognition of faces.

The precise nature of these mechanisms, however, remains unclear, for the very same reasons that lead us to assume their existence in the first place: the fact that faces are by far the best-known type of visual target and that they are, moreover, so emotionally evocative. The problem is, therefore, whether the brain area in question does uniquely govern face recognition, so that a lesion to this area impairs this capacity alone; or whether any object with strong affective value, or any object seen frequently, would fail to be recognized by a person with that lesion.

Pure prosopagnosics are uncommon, and so opportunities for testing on this issue are hard to come by; but in the few cases which have been carefully studied, recognition of faces does not in fact seem to be the only skill undermined by the lesion. True, these studies have confirmed that most other objects are identified quite easily. When, however, the subject confronts a perceptual realm where very fine discriminations are necessary, such as in differentiating between bird species, kinds of leaves, or painting styles, he seems to exhibit the same kind of difficulty as with faces. Should this finding be replicated in subsequent studies of "pure" prosopagnosia, the view will grow that this condition is simply the most visible manifestation of a general difficulty in making fine discriminations. The fact that prosopagnosia invariably entails lesions in the right hemisphere of the brain, and that this hemisphere appears critical in making such discriminations, may be regarded as further evidence in favor of this hypothesis. It could also be argued, on the other hand, that the ability to make fine discriminations is itself developed originally in relationship to faces; and it might follow, then, that subsequent fine differentiations in other areas would be made on the basis of principles originally evolved with faces. This theory is not as farfetched as it may seem at first airing: birds are often categorized on the basis of their exemplification of different human expressions; and young children beginning to distinguish among painting styles often attend especially to the way that faces are represented, speaking of the various styles in terms of their "family" characteristics.

Even as the facts of a particular agnosia can point up a similarity between two apparently different realms of cognition—here, painting styles and faces—so can they also reveal differences between two apparently similar realms.

Offhand one might predict, for example, that an agnosia for the sounds of spoken language would extend to all other inputs into the channel of the ear. In fact, however, there are at least two independent forms of agnosia in the auditory modality. In "pure word deafness" where lesions characteristically involve the left temporal lobe, the patient's hearing of pure tones is adequate and his ability to recognize and to sing musical patterns is normal. In striking contrast, in auditory agnosia (also called sensory amusia), the patient's linguistic functions are unimpaired while his ability to recognize musical pitches, instruments, the noise of familiar machines, etc., is effectively destroyed. Such lesions generally occur in the right hemisphere, or in areas of the left hemisphere which are not implicated in linguistic processing. The relative "musicality" or "linguisticality" of a sensory element can accordingly be gauged by whether the capacity to perceive that element is spared or destroyed in each form of agnosia. By comparing the profiles of disturbances in these two ideal forms, it should be possible to determine whether consonants, vowels, tone of voice, timbre of instruments, or rhythmic configurations are closer in their "essence" to pure musical tones, or to the sound and stresses of language. Lamentably, such a comparison has not, to my knowledge, been satisfactorily drawn.

Although the agnosias are rare, and the average clinician may see but a handful of "pure" agnosics in his lifetime (while he will see hundreds of aphasics), the existence of these syndromes has been rather generally accepted, and they are invariably described in textbooks. However, in 1950, at a conference in Badenweiler, Germany, Eberhard Bay attacked the whole concept of agnosia, most especially in its visual form. Fresh from his examination of Schn., in the wake of studying fine-grained perceptual activities of other brain-injured patients, Bay had concluded that there were no pure disorders of recognition in the visual mode, and that, indeed, the general notion of agnosia was invalid. According to his new view, only perception was necessary for recognition; the positing of additional "gnosis centers" in the cortex was unjustified and deceptive.

Initially such strong assertions did not fall on sympathetic ears. Bay's neurological colleagues at the conference recalled clear-cut cases they had seen, criticized the tests he had used and the model he had constructed, rebutted his iconoclastic interpretation of the case of Schn.; even if perceptual difficulties *were* present in agnosic cases, they insisted, these were insufficient to explain the degree of recognition difficulty in a classic agnosic. Bay was not dissuaded, however; he has since made it his mission to build the strongest possible case for the rejection of agnosia as a concept.

In broad outline, Bay's argument at Badenweiler ran as follows: One should not speak of or invent a disorder called agnosia, nor of a center of the brain involved in gnosis, if difficulties in recognition can be accounted for on other, simpler bases. Careful reading of earlier cases indicates either that there were language difficulties (which could account for the inability to name correctly, or to recognize the name of, a given object), intellectual difficulties (which would explain the inability to demonstrate the use of an object), or failure by the investigator to report performance on standard tests of linguistic and cognitive functions (which would make it impossible to interpret the case properly). More critically, none of the cases included an adequate screening of perceptual functions—it was this aspect that aroused Bay's greatest pique.

For Bay, perception is far from a simple process which takes place instantaneously and perfectly. Rather, it includes a number of separable components, each of which unfolds in time, and is liable to error. To perceive with complete efficacy, one must have adequate acuity not only in the central visual fields but also in the periphery; one must be able to perceive colors at different positions and of different sizes; and one must be able to adapt to changes in lighting or shading that occur over a certain period of time. In the course of normal perceiving, the stimulus undergoes a transformation by virtue of an active interpretative process. Continuities perceived in object size and shape are maintained by a type of transformation called, in German, *Funktionswandel* ("function change"), a highly subtle and sensitive process that unfolds with precise timing thanks to the integration of its various component elements. Even in cases of severe brain damage, the grossest aspects of perception—detecting an object, a large spot of color, or a salient shape—may be preserved; however, there will be marked difficulty when presentations are under suboptimal circumstances, for example on a tachistoscope, at a distance, or in an unusual setting. There is also a tendency in cases of brain damage for the visual system to fatigue rapidly, in which cases the stimuli will more rapidly drop out of awareness, or will be but partially sampled or incompletely processed. Bay devised a battery of tests for exploring the whole range of perceptual capacities, including the intricacies of *Funktionswandel*. In many patients who appeared on gross "bedside" inspection to have adequate visual perception, Bay was able to demonstrate significant deviations from the norm. This demonstration undermined the assumption that patients labeled agnosic were exhibiting unique difficulties with gnosis. What was called agnosia could be seen, instead, as a perturbation of processes of vigilance that occur throughout the visual nervous system.

At first, Bay's was a lonely voice, but gradually other scientists began to entertain similar views. One of the earliest to concur was the American neurologist Morris Bender, who by the 1960's was regularly and vocally challenging the concept of agnosia. Bender reviewed a large series of cases that were classified as agnosic. In general, he found individuals who could not recognize objects visually yet could identify them manually or by sound; perceived motion and color in the field of vision on standard visual field testing; and displayed no gross evidence of mental dysfunction or aphasia. Scrupulous examination revealed that in no case was there a patient with "true visual agnosia." Every suspected agnosic had alterations either in vision, in other sensory functions, or in mental capacity. A spectrum emerged, with patients having severe mental and mild visual defects at one end, others having mild mental and severe visual defects on the other. Bender conceded the theoretical possibility that one might find a pure agnosic at some point in the evolution of this disease process. However, with repeated testing, prior or future symptoms of the types found in the remaining patients in the series were invariably uncovered. A "so-called agnosia" was more likely to be an accidental symptom occurring at the moment of testing than a veridical reflection of the patient's neurological condition.

While Bay and Bender were the first modern commentators to challenge the concept of agnosia, other investigators who had at one time accepted and fostered it have recently begun to reevaluate their earlier conclusions. The noted psychologist Hans-Lukas Teuber, while conceding that there were certain "higher-level" perceptual disorders, has noted that "the number of such cases [of agnosia] in the neurological and neuropsychological literature has declined rapidly as more defined methods for assessing basic sensory function have become available." Teuber proposes that all perception involves a series of hierarchically ordered stages, from original feature extraction to the recognition and naming of patterns; much of what has been called agnosia is merely a premature termination of this hierarchical process. He goes on to suggest a test of the legitimacy of "figure-agnosia" as classically described, as follows: If a patient has performed well in a test where he had to detect horizontal or vertical regularities in a welter of dots, yet has failed in recognizing familiar objects from their pictorial representation, one may infer a selective loss of the mnemonic traces of an object's meaning. In the absence of such evidence, however, the disorder is more parsimoniously and properly explained as a perceptual disorder, rather than a disturbance of recognition.

The eminent British neurologist Macdonald Critchley has also attacked "The Problem of Visual Agnosia." Once a believer, Critchley is impressed with the evidence collated by Bay, and increasingly uneasy with the early claims of "recognition centers" and "visual memories" for particular objects. He indicates that the particular circumstances under which an object is viewed are critical in determining whether that object will be recognized; a person may appear more or less agnosic, depending on the familiarity of the object, the viewing conditions, the set of alternatives presented, and so on. Critchley reviews the subjective experiences of allegedly agnosic patients, considering their testimony an important source of information about the alleged disorders. Never does such a patient claim that he is seeing the form clearly, even though this should be the case theoretically, at least with associative (as distinct from apperceptive) agnosias; rather, his responses are like those of a normal person viewing an object which is particularly occluded or flashed for but a few milliseconds. He seems involved in a guessing game, in making deductions about the object, based on a partial and imperfect sampling of the field. One such patient is quoted as saying: "At first I saw the front part . . . it looked like a fountain pen . . . then it looked like a knife because it was so sharp, but I thought it could not be a knife because it was green. Then I saw the spokes and that it was shaped like a boat. It had too many spokes to be a knife or a fountain pen." Another characterizes the difference from earlier perceptual experiences in this way: "Previously I'd have said, 'Well, of course, that's a carnation . . . no doubt about it . . . it's quite evident.' Now I recognize it in a more scientific fashion. To get it right, I've got to assemble it." Such testimony, to Critchley's mind, challenges the supposition that the perceptions of these patients are in any sense normal. There are instead faulty constructions of an object out of its component elements, incomplete exploration of the object, subjective anomalies in the experience of seeing. The recognition difficulty is preferably viewed, then, as the result of a more fundamental disturbance in the overall functioning of the perceptual apparatus than as a particular impairment of recognition in the face of fundamentally intact perception.

With the published doubts of such eminent commentators as Critchley and Teuber, the concept of agnosia was placed in serious jeopardy. However, instead of crumbling under this potent onslaught, and succumbing to a dignified burial, it has found robust defenders in a number of quarters. Even as Bay recommended subtle tests in order to demonstrate that perception was not intact, M. I. Botez has stressed precisely the opposite point. He argues that instead of seeking to demonstrate impaired perception in apparently agnostic patients, one should employ special tests to show that their perception *is* adequate. For example, one might display moving objects on the assumption that agnosic patients experience difficulty perceiving a static display yet can correctly construe an array in motion. Indeed, the procedure recommended by Botez has effectively demonstrated unsuspected perceptual capacities in at least one agnosic patient.

Norman Geschwind has rebutted the critics on two counts. First, he suggests that, far from being a product of general brain damage, agnosia of the associative type is better explained (like pure alexia) as a disconnection between two intact brain areas, the language center and the visual center. The patient can see what the object is and can, on other occasions or through other sensory modalities, indicate the object's name. What is disrupted is the transferral of information from the visual to the language area. Accordingly, there exists a two-way naming disorder, sufficient to explain the apparent inability to recognize objects in the face of adequate perceptual, linguistic, and intellectual functioning.

Geschwind also challenges the value of the patient's own testimony about his subjective experiences during perception. If, indeed, there is a partial or complete disconnection between visual and language areas, it would be logically impossible for the patient to provide an accurate description of what he sees, or fails to see. Aware that he is supposed to be seeing, but deprived of information about what is being seen, it is understandable that the individual (as represented by his language area) should *confabulate* a difficulty in seeing. This testimony is no more reliable than that of the patient with a memory disorder who, unaware of where he is, invents a hospital resembling one in which he had previously been institutionalized. In sum, the impaired capacity for recognition does have a distinctive character, based on a particular form of brain injury.

Another endorsement for the agnosias has come from a series of important studies by George Ettlinger. This investigator saw thirty patients who were candidates for a diagnosis of agnosia. They received a battery of tests, including many of those used by Bay to bolster his case against agnosia. Ettlinger found that, indeed, when tested by such subtle methods most of these persons exhibited significant perceptual defects. Totally unexpected, however, was a further finding: that the degree of perceptual difficulty as measured by Bay's tests was unrelated to the clinical difficulties in recognition displayed by the patients! Individuals manifesting severe deficits on Bay's tests

perceived objects without difficulty; persons who performed quite well on Bay's tests displayed clinical signs
of agnosia. These findings led Ettlinger to the conclusion
that impairment of visual discrimination is neither necessary nor sufficient to produce a difficulty in recognition.
The essential defect in agnosia was not (as Bay supposed) a
failure in sensory processing but apparently, instead, one
in making effective use of this input at a central (higher
cortical) level. Bay's tests were really *too* finely discriminating to account for agnosia, which seemed to be a deficit of
another, and not primarily perceptual, order.

Even the most telling logical and theoretical arguments
against Bay's and Bender's position are to little avail,
however, in the absence of convincingly demonstrated
cases of agnosia. While no one would challenge the existence of agnosia-like or "pseudo-agnosic" conditions, the
issue of the concept's validity remains unresolved. It is of
some interest, then, that classical types of agnosia have
been seen and studied in recent years on the Neurological
Service of our hospital. Although neither of the cases that
follow would necessarily fulfill a purist's ideal of agnosia,
they are sufficiently unambiguous to pose a real challenge
to those who would banish agnosia from the neurologist's
classificatory scheme.

One patient whom I had an opportunity to examine
personally in the last year of his life was a physician, A.,
who had suffered a stroke. There were few neurological
findings of interest, except for an impairment of certain
higher cortical functions that suggested a diagnosis of
visual associative agnosia. The patient was able to write
but had difficulty in reading, perceiving colors, and recognizing faces and objects. Colors looked "less vibrant" to
him than they had before, and he frequently misnamed
them. Yet his color vision was entirely normal when tested
by the ability to match "hues"; in addition, he could
always provide the correct color name for an object that

had a habitual hue (e.g., bananas, grass, the sky). A more serious problem was the patient's inability to recognize visually members of the staff, his family, or even his own face in the mirror. He could, however, tell when faces were misoriented or when someone was smiling or frowning. On this difficulty he commented, "They seem somehow out of focus, almost as though a haze were in front of them." In contrast, recognition of individuals by their voices was prompt and flawless.

During the early part of his hospitalization, Dr. A. was also unable to identify common objects. Shown a stethoscope, he described it as a "long cord with a round thing at the end" and asked if it could be a watch. A large match book was called "a container for keys," while a key was termed a "file or tool of some sort." He could never demonstrate or describe the use of an object that he could not name; as soon as the name was provided, however, he would point out the object's defining features and say, "Yes, I see it now." Yet when the examiner suggested to Dr. A. that he, the examiner, might have been misleading him, the patient immediately countered, "I would take your word for it." Reading was done with hesitation, and similar-appearing letters were often confused. Small print and handwriting presented great, sometimes insuperable obstacles.

To rule out perceptual difficulties in form recognition as an explanation for the disorder, a number of special tests were performed. The patient was presented with a variety of objects to draw, including a comb, a bird, a pig, and a train. In each case he produced an accurate, even excellent copy of the object; yet he remained unable to identify it, even after the drawing was complete! He performed creditably on a test where visually presented abstract figures had to be recalled, and was able to pick out predesignated geometrical shapes when these were embedded in more complex illustrations. He could follow rapidly, from origin to end, weaving lines intertwined in a tangled maze. He was even able to scan a page fully, in the process choosing only exemplars of a designated symbol. These performances conclusively demonstrate that, in conventional terms, the patient was able to perceive form accurately.

In a case report on Dr. A., Drs. Frank Benson and Alan Rubens concede that they cannot rule out all perceptual disorders of the subtle type studied by Bay. Yet they insist, with Ettlinger, that such fine differences could not in themselves account for the striking disorders shown by the patient. Certainly, given this individual's above normal intelligence quotient, as measured after his stroke, and his adequate language functioninig, neither intellectual nor linguistic factors can be invoked as an explanation of Dr. A's difficulty. The riddle therefore becomes: how can a patient copy a figure with accuracy, yet fail to recognize or otherwise identify it? The authors adopt the position articulated by Geschwind: a disconnection between language and the visual-perceptual zones. Yet the facts they report, and my own experience with this patient, indicate another, equally likely interpretation. If we assume that the ability to recognize configurations, such as faces and objects, requires the integration over a brief interval of a number of visual elements, then an impairment in simultaneous synthesis—in the capacity to pull the relevant elements together into a coherent unity— would be sufficient to explain the disorder. Because he could see individual parts, yet not synthesize them, Dr. A. could, on the one hand, copy the figures part-by-part accurately, yet, on the other, fail to detect what the figures were. This explanation seems less applicable to the color-naming difficulty; that impairment, however, does not appear to be truly one of recognition, and might be related to a different brain lesion, or perhaps signify some subtle aphasic or mnemonic difficulty.

A major objection to the Benson-Rubens explanation is that, on a fair number of trials, and particularly in the cases of colors and words, the patient was in fact able to recognize elements simply from their visual configuration; whereas if there were a true disconnection between language and visual zones, there should be no correct performance whatsoever. Of course, a partial disconnection can be posited, but this makes matters so nebulous as to preclude any sort of firm conclusions.

A case recently reported by Rubens and his colleagues in Minneapolis suggests another possible explanation of visual associative agnosia. This patient gave characteristically incorrect responses when asked to name objects presented to him visually. If, however, the examiner forestalled an immediate verbal response and instead encouraged the patient first to examine the object visually and to pantomime its use, his performance improved dramatically. The authors suggest that, in responding quickly, and in relying on the injured visual pathways, the patient was likely to arouse an incorrect name; the misidentification, in turn, prevented a subsequent correct recognition of the presented object, perhaps by "jamming the circuits." Procedures, however, which activated alternate sensory paths were far more likely to elicit accurate recognition, which could then be confirmed both by verbal response and by pantomime. This interpretation underlines the advantage of using subsidiary sensory channels when there is a major disruption in one input modality, and points up the different levels and modes of recognition (and nonrecognition) in the patient's functioning.

The second case of agnosia seen on our Service—one, apparently, of the apperceptive variety—was embodied in a 25-year-old soldier who, like Adler's young Coconut Grove victim, entered the hospital after accidental carbon monoxide poisoning. As the patient, Mr. S., slowly improved, he was able to attend to his surroundings and to navigate the corridors in a wheel-chair. He could also identify colors and monitor moving visual stimuli. However, he was unable to name objects placed before him. Some familiar numbers could be identified if they were slowly drawn on a screen. Visual fields were normal under most conditions, although there was a striking abnormality of eye movements during inspection of an object.

As in the other patients we have considered, Mr. S.'s memory, language, and intellectual functions were adequate. He could name objects when cued by sound, smell, or touch. He would often confabulate responses when attempting visual identification, calling a safety pin "silver and shiny like a watch or nail clipper," or a rubber eraser "a small ball." Unlike Dr. A., however, the patient was totally unable to copy letters or simple figures; he could neither describe nor trace the outline of common objects satisfactorily—his drawings of such objects were bizarre, disjointed, and unrecognizable. Matching objects with their pictures and recognition of geometrical figures proved impossible. Exemplars of the same kind of object could be chosen from a group only in the presence of strong color and size cues. With training, a few familiar objects could be named but, as soon as their characteristic guise was in any way changed, recognition ceased.

Explanation of Mr. S.'s agnosia must begin with the observation that his most elementary sensory capacities did remain intact: he was able to analyze and identify colors, differences of aperture size, light intensities, and direction of movement. That he had specific difficulty with the perception of form was strikingly confirmed in a careful study by Robert Efron. Efron looked individually at a whole range of perceptual attributes; he documented that the patient could point to objects, trace their contours, and isolate them from the rest of his perceptual field. With help, he was also able to attend selectively to particular attributes of an object. Efron noted a common factor in all of Mr. S.'s failures to recognize objects, figures, letters, or persons: recognition in all these instances was dependent on ability to distinguish their defining shapes. Efron therefore proposed to make a definitive test of whether Mr. S. was in fact capable of sufficiently fine shape judgments to allow identification of such objects.

To eliminate adventitious cues, Efron resorted to the simplest possible stimuli: squares and rectangles. On some trials, the patient was shown a square and a rectangle; the two figures had identical areas and light reflectance, so that the shape was the only distinguishing aspect; on other trials, the patient was shown identical squares or identical rectangles. In each case he was required to judge whether the two figures were identical. Even when the square was presented along with a relatively long and thin rectangle, Mr. S. frequently erred. And when the differences between the square and the rectangle were not pronounced, the patient consistently failed to detect differences. This task, it should be noted, did not require identification of the shapes, indications of how the shapes differed, or memory of shapes—only a judgment as to whether they were identical. Efron therefore felt justified in concluding that Mr. S.'s "capacity for making this discrimination [by shape] is severely restricted." An incapacity of this sort seemed sufficient to explain the whole raft of identifications and discriminations inaccessible to the patient.

One feature of Mr. S.'s performances still required explanation; although he could not distinguish shapes, he was able to follow a contour or outline. For example, if an individual stood in front of Mr. S., the patient was able to trace with his fingers the person's contour. Efron hypothesized that there is a difference between perception of contours and perception of shapes. A contour is merely the line of demarcation between two adjacent areas which differ in some physical attribute; in contrast, the shape of an object is constituted in the *integration* of its contours:

shape can only be perceived if all the contours and transitions as seen from a particular angle can be combined to form a unity. It is in the execution of this vital task of integration that—if Efron's analysis is correct—Mr. S., and presumably other apperceptive agnosics, are found wanting. At least in the case of Mr. S.'s agnosia, there is no need to invoke deficits of memory, naming, or association. Efron notes, in conclusion, that the normal person can gain a subjective impression of Mr. S.'s perceptual world by attempting to recognize objects seen only in one's peripheral visual field.

While Efron's conclusion here can be translated into the language of Gestalt psychology (Mr. S.'s case is probably similar to those of Goldstein and Adler), Efron has gone beyond their qualitative analyses. On the basis of earlier reports, it was unclear whether Gestalt perception actually referred to identification of objects, of contours, of geometric shape, of joined segments, or of some combination of these features. By controlling other elements (such as overall area and luminence) and parceling out competing factors (such as knowledge of the environment or sensitivity to contours), Efron has systematically eliminated extraneous or redundant explanations and successfully pinpointed the particular function—the perception of object shape—in which the patient's difficulty apparently lay. Such analyses do not, it should be stressed, displace the more classical views of agnosia; Mr. S. remains unique and interesting, even after his disorder is better understood. However, such a careful study as Efron's does reduce grandiosity of claims by specifying exactly which features of perception, recognition, identification, or naming have broken down.

The critical reviews undertaken by Bay and Bender, the conceptual revisions adopted by Teuber and Critchley, and the finer-grained studies done by Benson, Efron, and their colleagues, all call into question the assumption of the early Gestaltists that form and figure were self-evident categories, requiring no further investigation or elucidation. While selected patients do have isolated defects in "recognizing" elements, the expedient of terming their disorder *agnosia* (or *imperception* or *mind-blindness*) does not explain their defect; at best, it pigeonholes it somewhere within a vast, often confusing literature. On the other hand, the attempts of some neurologists simply to dismiss the entire phenomenon of agnosia seem ill founded. True, many so-called agnosias can be explained readily on other grounds. But there is convincing documentation of patients whose recognition disorders are strikingly severe in the face of generally preserved perceptual and intellectual functions; this group of cases merits special study and may well require separate explanatory mechanisms. In particular, the reasons for difficulties in recognizing one or another class of elements—faces, musical sounds, color, shapes, or fingers—are worthy of specific examination for the insights they may provide concerning normal functioning.

As case studies and explanatory models accumulate, however, it becomes increasingly clear that the phenomenon of *recognition,* or *gnosis,* is not unitary in character. The very word itself, *re-cognition,* should give us pause, suggesting as it does a recapitulation of previous cognitive processes. Just as primary cognitive processes are now considered to be complex, multifaceted, requiring intensive study and skilled elucidation, so, too, the whole process of *r*ecognition demands a similarly fine-grained analysis. After all, what shall we accept as proof of recognition? The dog who follows his master, the bird who responds to its mate's song, the child who smiles at the mother's face or voice—are these all safely taken as recognitory acts? Or what type of response by a patient should we accept as recognition? Naming is one candidate, but some aphasic patients who can otherwise demonstrate their correct perception of an object would fail here; selection of the name from among multiple choices is another, yet here we are providing so much information that the correct answer may be forthcoming even in the face of impaired cognition. Ability to demonstrate the use of the object is another possibility, but apractic or motor difficulties may invalidate this index; furthermore, the process of recognition normally does not require an overt action upon an object before the object can be identified. Grouping together various representations or drawings of the object are other possible tests of recognition. Yet, as we have seen, certain patients are able to execute such tasks despite qualifying as agnosic from the classical point of view—i.e., able to appreciate the overall form, while nonetheless being unable to associate the object with its meaning. And so on.

The answer, I submit, is that we search in vain for a simple, single, foolproof definition or test for recognition. From his earliest contact with objects, the infant begins to exercise certain schemes (or generalized forms of actions) in relation to specific objects, and in relation to objects in general. The child first sucks on its mother's breast, then peers at its mother's eyes, then comes to smile in eye-to-eye contact, then cries in the presence of a stranger, then becomes attached to the mother's clothing, learns to associate a photograph of its mother with the real individual, comes eventually to attend to the mother's name, to think of the mother when reading or writing about her, to recognize the mother's handwriting, voice-traces, or presence in a dream (or nightmare). All of these schemes—and their concomitant experiences—contribute to the child's overall concept or cognition of the mother. And the person's exercise of any of these schemes serves to indicate some degree of recognition. Clearly, however, one would credit more complete cognition, or recognition, of the mother, if a variety of these schemes can be activated, and if they can be elicited readily. If only the mother's physical presence elicits identification, the patient is far more impaired than one who can respond with his mother's name or can orient to her when he merely sees her handwriting. Clearly, there are different avenues of recognition and different means of signaling it. Thus, any assessment of recognition should consider the familiarity of the object; the number of channels which can be tested; the kind of schemes in which the object may potentially be involved; the situation of testing, the number of clues given, and the range of alternatives presented to the patient.

Should a patient's full compass of recognitory means and channels be examined, should a cluster of disparate elements and objects be presented under a variety of testing, cueing, and choice circumstances, a more differentiated view of recognition is likely to emerge. Rather than thinking of recognition as a unitary process, either wholly intact or wholly destroyed, it will be seen as a vast gradient, implicated in innumerable ways in normal and pathological processes. Even the most intact individual will show recognition disturbances under some circumstances: encountering a casual acquaintance in a strange setting; turning on the radio and failing to recognize a well-known melody; looking vacantly at a friend's face presented upside down; misidentifying the ingredients of a recipe. And even the most impaired patient will evince some form or degree of recognition: he will suck when a straw is placed in his mouth; turn in the right direction when his name is called; be stirred if he hears his national anthem played by an orchestra. As I was preparing this chapter, I encountered a severely demented patient whose intellectual capacities in general were drastically impaired; he could barely read a word or say his name. It so happened that on the radio at that moment a jazzed-up version of Beethoven's Ninth Symphony was being played. Suddenly the

patient began to sing the melodic line, punctuating it with
foot-tapping and movements of his arm. He did not know
the name of the piece, but he continued to hum it after it
went off the air; certainly, in at least one sense, he had
"recognized" the piece. Yet if he had not manifested that
recognition overtly, we would have had to conclude (erroneously) that there was as little recognition for this form
of sensory input as for the other presentations on which he
totally failed.

Indeed, this moral—the multiple levels and degrees of
recognition—can be drawn equally persuasively for other
higher cortical functions. As we have seen in the earlier
chapters, nearly every aphasic patient is capable of some
reading, writing, speech, and understanding; and even the
well-recovered patient is likely to exhibit latent deficiencies in these areas. By the same token, the patients with
memory disorders to be examined in the next chapter also
retain some mnemonic facility, even as the fabled mnemon-
ists sometimes do forget. In brain damage, as in normal
functioning, absolute abilities and absolute disabilities are
highly exceptional; the special genius of neuropsychological case studies is to help us tease out the component
factors of such broad categories as language, action, memory, or recognition.

Eighty years after von Ehrenfels' epiphany, Gestalt psychology is no longer in vogue. The more durable parts of
its catechism have long since been absorbed into workaday
applied psychology; the less tenable, more exotic claims
are no longer seriously entertained. Similarly, the strongest
claims made by Kurt Goldstein about his patient Schn.
are no longer credible. This is only in part because of
doubts about the particular facts of the case; for it also
reflects the increasing consensus that many so-called agnosic patients do have intellectual and/or perceptual disorders; that somewhat mystical difficulties (like Gestalt

blindness) can be explained by a single, less dramatic property, such as inability to perceive *shape;* and that the patient's overall "score" will vary dramatically, depending on the nature of the test employed, the measure used, the kind of responses or schemes accepted as evidence of recognition. There is fresh evidence that the "sense elements" and "associations" dismissed by Gestaltists may possess physiological and psychological significance; there are receptors in the visual system responsive to the particular atoms of sense (lines, edges) and there are disorders of brain function (such as Dr. A.'s inability to name colors) which seem most parsimoniously explained as disorders of association. Yet these considerations do not, in the last analysis, undermine the importance of the Gestalt tradition, nor that of the study of recognition disorders. From the tangled web of claim and counterclaim, disparate views of the same patient and identical conclusions about different patients, neurological studies of single cases and psychological examinations of matched patient groups, psychometric studies of the perceptual process and clinical observations of patient behavior, should ultimately come a more sophisticated understanding of the processes which mediate knowing; the ways of original cognizing and the ways in which we, like Williams James's epigrammatic polyp, cognize again what we have previously acted upon and known.

# 5 The Loss of Memory

*I consider that a man's brain originally is like a little empty attic and you have to stock it with such functions as you choose. A fool takes in all the lumber of every sort that he comes across. . . . now the skilled workman is very careful indeed as to what he takes in to his brain-attic. He will have nothing but the tools which may help him in doing his work, but of these he has a large assortment, and all in the most perfect order. It is a mistake to think that that little room has elastic walls and can distend to any extent. Depend upon it that there comes a time when for every addition of knowledge you forget something that you knew before.*

—MR. SHERLOCK HOLMES TO
DR. JOHN WATSON

In diseases where appreciable brain tissue has been destroyed, the patient's condition is usually evident, even to the casual observer. Even where there is no paralysis, jerking movement, or drooling, a short conversation is likely to reveal difficulties in expression, in understanding, or in solving problems. Paradoxically, however, one of the most debilitating of brain diseases—Korsakoff's syndrome— may well be overlooked by an interlocutor unaware of its existence and unable to pose the revealing questions. Korsakoff's syndrome may remain undetected for a period because a patient suffering from it may retain a superior IQ, intact language capacities, and the ability to execute well-learned skills at an impressive level. This same patient, however, will be unable to remember any event which has happened in the previous several years and, even worse, has become completely unable to learn new materials. Patients who do not recover from this disease (at least half of those stricken) must therefore be cared for until they die. One such patient was John O'Donnell. I shall now describe a meeting with him several months after his admission to the hospital.

"How are you?" I asked the pleasant-looking, forty-five-year-old man who was seated quietly in the corridor, thumbing through a magazine.

"Can't complain, Doctor," he retorted immediately.

"What have you been doing, Mr. O'Donnell?"

"Oh, just sitting around . . . passing the time of day . . . looking through this magazine."

"What's in it?"

He glanced furtively at the cover, which featured a picture of a recent figure in the news adorned by the headline "Watergate Coverup."

"Oh, politics and all that. I don't follow it much."

"I see there's something about Watergate there," I continued, alluding to the gigantic political scandal which had been dominating the news for many weeks. "What do you think about that?"

"Oh, I don't pay it much mind. I've been busy lately and haven't been keeping up."

"But surely you must have heard about Watergate."

"Oh, yeah, if you say so, Doctor, but I don't have any opinions about that sort of thing," he parried rather vaguely.

"Well, can you tell me anything about Watergate?"

Mr. O'Donnell evinced just the mildest touch of irritation. "Oh, they got some stool pigeon, or something like that. It's all the same to me."

"Good, Mr. O'Donnell. Tell me, have you seen me

before?" (I had been talking with him nearly every day for two months.)

"Sure, I've seen you around. Not sure where, though. You were looking after my leg, weren't you?"

"What's the matter with your leg?"

"Oh, you know, Doctor, I've got these pains in my leg and you're deciding whether to operate."

Mr. O'Donnell did indeed have pains in his legs, but these were chronic, and the decision not to operate had been made over a decade before. Apparently, my question stimulated him to speculate as to why he was in the hospital, and "leg trouble" was the conclusion at which he generally arrived. Occasionally, however, he would simply say that he had been very sick—but today, "For the first time, I'm feeling fine."

"Are you having any other problems, Mr. O'Donnell?"

"Well, sometimes I have a little trouble sleeping, but otherwise I'm just raring to go." He jabbed in the air, playfully, then resumed his vacant expression, as if awaiting my next thrust.

"How's your memory been?"

"*Comme ci, comme ça,*" he said. "O.K. for a man my age, I guess."

"How old are you?"

"I was born in 1927."

"Which makes you . . ."

"Let's see, Doctor, how I always forget, the year is . . ."

"The year is what?"

"Oh, I must be thirty-four, thirty-five, what's the difference . . ." He grinned sheepishly.

"You'll soon be forty-six, Mr. O'Donnell, the year is 1973."

Mr. O'Donnell looked momentarily surprised, started to protest, and said, "Sure, you must be right, Doctor. How silly of me. I'm forty-five, that's right, I guess."

"And who's the President?"

"What, that's a simple question. It's, it's what's his name, you know from Texas, uh, uh, Johnson, Lyndon Johnson."

"And who's his Vice-President?"

"Oh, you've got me, Doctor. I should know that, but it's slipped my mind. Let's see, is it Kennedy?"

"Which Kennedy?"

"Robert Kennedy, I think. Is that right?"

"What about John Kennedy?"

"Oh, he's President, how stupid, how could I forget."

In order to check Mr. O'Donnell's memory for recent events, I hid three objects around the room as he watched: a pen under a pillow, a match near the television set, and a quarter on the window sill. I also asked him to remember the three words *purple, Cadillac,* and *Albuquerque.* He repeated the words several times, and then, on request, told me where the objects were hidden. In this way I could verify that he had perceived, registered, and held on for a few seconds to the information on which his memory would later be tested.

"Now, Mr. O'Donnell, were you in the Service?"

"Why yes, I was. Too young for World War Two, but when the Korean conflict began, I was called up."

"What unit were you in?"

"Third Division, Twenty-third Regiment, Second Battalion."

"Who was your commanding officer?"

"Captain Butters."

"And who was in charge of the operation?"

"Well, we were in Inchon; General Almond was in charge of the operation. MacArthur was in charge of the whole thing. Then Truman recalled him—you remember that big deal."

"When was that?"

"Let's see, summer of 1951, I believe. I was in the Service for three years. After the Panmunjum armistice I came back to the States immediately and entered college."

"What did you study?"

"Well, I first took math, and then accounting. But after I got married we decided to start our own business, so I left school. Everything went fine until we had an accident and the building burned down. The wife and I never really recovered from that."

"I'm sorry. What happened?"

"Well, I went to work at the post office and my wife, she stayed home with the kids."

"Oh, you have children. How old are they?"

"Well, there's two. Johnny—we call him Junior—is seven, and the baby is about two." I knew this was definitely untrue, because Mr. O'Donnell's wife had left him several years before, and his children were both in their teens. However, there seemed to be little point in directing his attention to these errors.

"I'd like to ask you a few other questions."

"Sure."

"When I say, 'Too many cooks spoil the broth,' what do I mean by that?"

"Let's see, 'Too many cooks spoil the broth.' . . . I'd say it has to do with too many Indians, too many people trying to run a show. If you want a job done, it's better to trust it to one competent person. You don't want to have everyone getting into the act. Like in my business. It's small, but we do better that way, just me and my wife."

"Oh, you're in business?"

"Yes, me and the wife, we have a little grocery store."

"How's it doing?"

"Can't complain. In fact, can't wait to get back, you know, there's the Christmas season soon and there are lots of turkeys and chickens and hams we're going to be selling."

"Right. What month is it?"

"It's December, isn't it? December seventh, nineteen hundred and fifty-eight."

"And who's the President?"

"Eisenhower. Good man."

"By the way, Mr. O'Donnell, do you remember a few minutes ago I asked you to remember some words?"

"No, I'm afraid I forgot, I guess I wasn't paying enough attention . . . Sometimes I get preoccupied."

"Well, just to check, let me give you a few hints. One of them was a city."

"Was it Boston?"

"O.K. One of them was a color."

"It was black, wasn't it?"

"And the third was a kind of a car."

"Oh yes, it was a Cadillac."

"Fine. Now Mr. O'Donnell, I also hid three objects around the room. Do you remember that?"

"I'm afraid I don't. I guess I wasn't paying enough attention. Sometimes I just get preoccupied and don't watch."

"Well, let me help you. Look over at that pillow."

Mr. O'Donnell turned toward the pillow and said, "Oh sure, it was a pen." He went up and lifted it, looked over at the window sill, went over there and fetched the quarter. "Now what was the other?" he asked, half aloud.

"The television," I prompted.

"The television," repeated Mr. O'Donnell. "Of course, "you hid some matches there."

"Very good. Let me check a few other things. Can you do some addition for me?"

I gave Mr. O'Donnell a series of mathematical problems to do in his head. He answered very rapidly and always correctly. I also asked him to repeat some numbers after me.

"Can you say seven . . . one . . . five . . . six . . . nine?"

"Seven-one-five-six-nine."

"Let's try six. Two . . . one . . . eight . . . seven . . . four . . . nine."

"Two-one-eight-seven-nine-four, no, I mean two-one-eight-seven-four-nine."

"Let's try seven. Nine . . . six . . . seven . . . three . . . six . . . one . . . eight."

Mr. O'Donnell performed perfectly in recalling seven digits. He even repeated eight digits on another occasion. "What were those three words, again?" I asked him.

"Sorry, I don't remember. I must not have been paying attention. Sometimes I get preoccupied."

"What's the matter with your memory? I just told you those words," I said, raising my voice to suggest annoyance.

"Nothing that I know of. My memory's fine, I think."

"By the way, Mr. O'Donnell, could you name some cities for me?"

"Cities?"

"Yes, cities in the United States."

"Sure—San Francisco, Albuquerque, Los Angeles, Boston, New York, Washington, Chicago, Philadelphia. That enough?"

"Fine. And could you name some colors?"

"Sure—purple, red, blue, green, yellow, brown, orange, red, pink, purple, red, yellow, brown, green, gray and orange and red . . ."

"Very good. I'd like to ask you a few more questions."

"Sure, Doc, any time. I'm just sitting here, I've got all day."

"Did you ever drink in the past?"

"Liquor?"

"Yes."

"Well, I've taken a few nips, a few beers in the evening and when watching the TV. Like everyone else."

"How many beers?"

"Oh, a few. Some, you know, maybe two or three."

"That's all?"

"Well, sometimes more, maybe four or five, all depends on how I feel."

"Do you feel like having a drink now?"

"No, I don't. You guys are feeding me so well here in the hospital. By the way, is it dinner-time yet?"

"Pretty soon."(It was four o'clock, and the patients do eat shortly after that hour.) "Have you any questions for me?"

"No, I don't think so."

"O.K., thank you, Mr. O'Donnell."

"Could I just ask you one thing, though, Doctor?"

"Certainly, Mr. O'Donnell, what is it?"

"How soon will I get out of here? I've got to get back to work because my wife's just had a baby and I've got to tend to the store."

"We all hope it will be soon, Mr. O'Donnell. It all depends on how you're doing."

"Oh, my leg is getting much better—see." He got up and, with his slightly stilted gait, briskly headed toward the dining room.

The conversation just quoted is typical of dozens that I had with Mr. O'Donnell during his months at our hospital. The patient was invariably cheerful, helpful, and considerate. He would patiently execute tasks and respond to questions for hours on end, one major reason being that he had no recollection of ever tackling the task before. The only times in which he displayed even mild annoyance came when I pressed him on a question for which he had no ready answer. Even then, however, any trace of the anger evaporated upon the next question. As long as the conversation was restricted to small talk and pleasantries, Mr. O'Donnell seemed entirely normal. And his knowledge of events of his childhood and the early years of his adulthood, of those spent in the Service, in college, and as a young entrepreneur, seemed generally intact.

From Mr. O'Donnell's estranged wife, and from his previous medical records, we were able to piece together portions of his story. In the early fifties, O'Donnell, a good family man, had launched a successful grocery business with his wife. He had been a "booster" and one of the best-liked individuals in his home town. But then his store, inadequately insured, had burned down, and he had entered a deep depression. Thereafter he had moved aimlessly from one job to another and had begun to drink heavily. At first, his wife tried to be supportive and his friends sought to aid him. But O'Donnell's drinking grew worse, and he withdrew further from social contact. Eventually his wife gave up and left him. After a particularly vigorous binge that culminated in an attack of delirium tremens, he joined Alcoholics Anonymous in a nearby community and, for a few weeks, stopped drinking. However, the unexpected death of his mother, to whom he had been particularly close, aborted this effort; soon he returned with even greater vengeance to the bottle. In February 1973 he arrived in an ambulance at the hospital, having been found in the woods outside town, in a confused and malnourished condition.

When I had first seen Mr. O'Donnell, shortly after his admission, his appearance had been somewhat different than at the time of our conversation above. That is, he had been then unshaven, disheveled, with a noticeable stagger and jerky eye movements. He was unable to keep his mind on any one topic for any length of time, would sometimes mumble incoherently, and once even fell asleep in the midst of a conversation. He was completely disoriented as to the time, place, and reason for his hospitalization. In the ensuing weeks, this gross confusional state cleared up somewhat, but two new elements entered Mr. O'Donnell's clinical picture. First of all, he began to complain that the nurses were taking his possessions and that one of the other patients had struck him in the leg. Neither of these accusations had any basis in fact, yet they were frequently voiced and could not be more than momentarily turned aside by the repeated assurances we gave him. Such a strain of paranoia is not uncommon in patients who are recovering from acute confusional states, who sense that others know something that they do not, and who cannot piece together the disparate fragments of reality they have access to. Since rebuttals of such paranoid ideas are immediately forgotten, the patient may hurl the same accusations several hundred times a day.

The second new facet of Mr. O'Donnell's behavior was not unrelated to this paranoia: When asked questions he could not answer, he would give responses that were patently absurd. Questioned as to where he had seen me before, he immediately replied that we had gone fishing together for many years in Canada. Queried about the name of the hospital, he replied, "Why, this is the Quincy branch of the Massachusetts General Hospital." A question about where he had been before entering the hospital elicited the answer, "Why, I'm just back from Korea, where I've been on active duty."

On the surface, such responses seem to be total fabrications—confabulations in the pejorative sense. It is difficult to avoid the suspicion that the patient is putting you on. Actually, however, there was no reason to think that Mr. O'Donnell's answers were insincere. He was not lying, nor was he spinning a tall tale to amuse or confuse the examiner; rather, he was desperately trying to make momentary sense out of a bewildering situation. Accordingly, he latched on to any fragment of past reality that was accessible and that seemed to fit plausibly into the present context. O'Donnell *had,* in fact, at scattered points in his life, gone on fishing trips to Canada, visited the Massachusetts General Hospital, rested (on his return from Korea) in an Army hospital. What most immediately prompted these anachronistic responses was the association of something in his present environment—my resemblance to a fishing companion, occasional pains in his leg, his Army serial number on his wrist band—to the thrust of a given question. The confabulation, then, represented a legitimate effort to achieve some sense of coherence, some stable orientation that was otherwise, given his gross memory disturbances, unattainable.

By April, two months after admission, Mr. O'Donnell no longer entertained paranoid ideas, and confabulated to only a minimal extent. His health was improving, he was better oriented and less confused, and even his memory seemed slightly better. These developments probably rendered paranoia and confabulation less necessary, yet the reasons for their replacement by a placid, somewhat vague personality are not well understood. In medical terms, Mr. O'Donnell, as a result of an excessive intake of alcohol over many years, and a concomitant deprivation of thiamine (vitamin $B_1$), had first suffered an attack of Wernicke's encephalopathy. This acute confusional state had gradually resolved into the stable, chronic condition of severe memory dysfunction called Korsakoff's syndrome— the bane of alcoholics, and a disorder from which Mr. O'Donnell, like millions of his fellow drinkers, is likely to suffer for the remainder of his life.

As the eponyms suggest, this cluster of diseases was first described in 1881 by Carl Wernicke, the German neurologist whose contribution to aphasia was already well known, and by S. S. Korsakoff, a Russian psychiatrist, in the final years of the same decade. Wernicke's attention was directed chiefly to the severe confusion, and the gross eye-movement disturbances, which accompany the initial stages of the disorder. Korsakoff's interest focused more on the longer-range psychological effects of this "polyneuritic psychosis." During the acute phase, patients were usually depressed, fearful, anxious, and disoriented; sometimes, on the other hand, they were unnaturally cheerful or carefree. They could not concentrate and, as a result, their verbal associations were deficient, if not totally off the mark. With clearing of the confusion, the patient might be able to perceive accurately what was going on in his environment, yet he would continue to suffer severe memory problems. He would have a long *retrograde amnesia*—that is, he would have completely forgotten the period of several years immediately prior to the onset of the disease; in addition, he would suffer from a severe *anterograde amnesia*—he would be unable to retain in memory events that occurred thereafter, or to learn any new materials. Korsakoff believed that some new experiences did deposit "conscious traces" in the mind of the Korsakoff patient, and that, with effort, the patient's memory capacity might be somewhat enhanced. However, he provided little documentation for these views. Finally, Korsakoff stressed that such patients were intellectually intact in other respects: they could speak and reason normally, they could play cards or chess with skill, and their memory of events of the more remote past was entirely adequate. Only if the patient was asked to indicate, say, the date, the name of the current chief of state, or the items on his breakfast menu, would his gross difficulties become apparent.

Whereas many disorders described in this book have engendered considerable dispute, there is a welcome agreement about the fundamental characteristics of the Wernicke-Korsakoff syndrome. Subsequent studies have refined and altered Korsakoff's original observations in some ways; but the general picture, not far different from the original descriptions, is instantly recognizable to any observer of brain-damaged patients. To summarize briefly: Individuals who have habitually drunk to excess over a long period of time, who have sustained for whatever reason an extended deprivation of thiamine in their diet, or who have suffered trauma or nervous disease in certain areas of the diencephalon (a part of the forebrain) are likely to pass through a two-stage pathological process. During the initial stage, that of Wernicke's encephalopathy, they will be

severely confused and beset by both motor and visual deficits. If they survive this acute stage, they will probably
enter the chronic, or Korsakoff, phase. Here the mental
alterations are most prominent and include relatively flat-
tened or blunted affect, virtually total amnesia regarding
the several years immediately past, inability to learn new
materials and form fresh memories, reduction in spontaneity and initiative, lack of desire for alcohol, sex, and
other traditional "reinforcers." Paranoia and confabulation may be found, particularly in the early days of this
chronic stage, but these are not constant features of the
disease. There may also be a tendency to "reduplicate,"
to combine or fuse experiences from disparate periods in
the individual's life. Once constructed, such confabulations and reduplications are difficult to dissolve, since the
patient is likely to promptly forget a refutation of them,
or blithely to ignore it, even when directly confronted
with countervailing evidence. Memory for events far back
in time seems clearer than for more recent occurrences;
and memory for linguistic material seems more impaired
than that for visual experiences.

In a careful study of a group of 245 Wernicke-Korsakoff
patients, including 82 who came to post-mortem, Maurice
Victor, Raymond Adams, and G. H. Collins sought to discover the ultimate fate of persons thus afflicted. Of the
total, 182, or about three-quarters, survived the initial
acute phase, and among the survivors, Korsakoff psychoses
developed in 157 instances. Of these latter, twenty-six percent displayed no further recovery and remained severely
impaired in all the implicated functions; twenty-eight percent showed only slight changes; while twenty-five percent
demonstrated a significant degree of recovery. Only twenty-
one percent—or about 13½ percent of the original group
of 245—achieved a more or less complete recovery, with
the period over which improvement took place varying
greatly in duration. These last were able to go back home

or to resume their jobs, although some pockets of amnesia and some lingering difficulty in acquiring new information could still be detected on intensive examination.

The subjective world of the Korsakoff patient is most difficult to grasp, and it is only rarely that the individual himself will provide revealing clues. At most, he will complain that "I hear things fine, but I just can't remember them," or "When my mind shifts to a new subject, I forget what I was doing before." While such descriptions ring true as far as they go, they do not help us to understand questions of greater substance or subtlety: What does the patient think about during the whole day? Indeed, is his mind occupied at all, or is it as vacant as his expression suggests? What has happened to his sense of self? Why does he display so little motivation to improve his memory, to resume his job, to go back into the world, to strike up friendships with others on the ward? Why, particularly in the case of ethanol-induced Korsakoff's disease, does he no longer crave alcohol?

Even though the difficulty in retrieving past experiences and in achieving a meaningful grasp of new ones is its most striking feature, the Korsakoff syndrome is much more than a simple memory disorder. Profound changes in motivation, incentive, personality, and self-concept, as well as finer alterations in facets of intellectual functioning, are likely. The patient has altered, often in a matter of months, from an individual who may well have been an active, productive member of society to one who shrinks from social contact with others and lives completely in the present in an obscure and sheltered niche of his own. In many ways, he is like someone who is forever arriving in the middle of a ball game and compelled to check the scoreboard to see what is going on; or who is always entering a movie house in the midst of a showing, and forced to attempt to reconstruct the plot. Every time his attention wanders for an instant, there is a new ball game, or a new film; he does not know how he got there, what has happened, and what is likely to occur next. His previous skills and knowledge are retained in principle, in the sense that the right questions or circumstances may elicit them. Yet for most practical intents and purposes they are absent, since he is unable to draw on them to extricate himself from his current predicament. Of course, this is because, with rare exceptions, he is not in any meaningful sense aware of the deficit. After all, how can someone with a shattered memory remember that he has become unable to remember?

Many neurologists, psychologists, and psychoanalysts have wrestled with the question, "What has gone wrong with the Korsakoff patient?"—meaning here not "What can't he do?" but rather "Why can't he do it?" or "What mechanism has failed?" As the syndrome is relatively circumscribed, both in the degree of brain tissue involved and in the area of functioning disrupted, there is a marked temptation (as with other "pure" syndromes) to attribute it to, and to seek out, a single underlying cause. At first, the explanations, as for certain similar "amnesic syndromes" due to strokes or injury, were chiefly derived from observations of patients, formulated in the light of the observer's pet psychological theory, or allegedly based on "common sense." While some of these formulations were quite pertinent, they seldom accounted for all the features of Korsakoff's disease, and none stood out as more persuasive than competing explanations. In recent years, however, experimental psychologists have instituted more intensive investigations of the amnesic syndromes, which have yielded a somewhat finer-grained picture of what is (and is not) wrong with the Korsakoff patient. Even so, what is "fundamentally" wrong with him seems to have eluded these harder-nosed investigators as well—an inconclusiveness that perhaps reveals as much about the inadequacy of our present understanding of memory as about the complexities of the disease.

Korsakoff made his original observations at a time when associationist theories of the mind dominated the field of psychology. Not surprisingly, he viewed his patients as deficient in making associations among new ideas and in connecting present to past experiences. This explanation, however, drew increasing fire from the rival, more "cognitive" school of psychology centered in Würzburg, Germany. The Würzburgers viewed the Korsakoff patient's difficulty not as one of *combining* ideas, but as an inability to solve problems, to plan ahead, to adopt an effective strategy for resolving ambiguities and intricacies. The afflicted person's powers of association were adequate in themselves; it was his capacity to apply his associations in the service of some overarching program of action, or of a coherent and purposeful series of behaviors, that was undermined. This basic disagreement, between an explanation of Korsakoff's syndrome that assumes cognitive capacities to be relatively intact, and one that emphasizes a fundamental deficiency in all ratiocination, has persisted until the present day.

A number of other lines of analysis have emerged as leitmotifs in the Korsakoffian literature of the past fifty years. Those with psychiatric inclinations have stressed the listless behavior of Korsakoff patients and have seen that behavior as reflecting, in the first instance, deficits in motivation. From their viewpoint, the patient's intellect and perhaps even his memory are intact, but he is simply not motivated to learn or to reflect—he has lost the *will* to think. The most extreme statement of this approach has come from certain psychoanalysts who argue that, just like the hysteric who refuses to acknowledge difficult periods in his past, the Korsakoff patient can still arouse past memories but has simply repressed them. This line of argument gains surface plausibility from the fact that many Korsakoff patients have indeed led sad lives, and a few have apparently "recovered" their memories after a successful psychoanalysis dissolved their repressions.

Despite its appeal to those of a psychoanalytic persuasion, however, this theory is clearly inadequate and in all probability wrong. Many patients are quite definitely motivated to participate in activities introduced by the experimenter and indeed will persist for hours in the most aimless tasks. True, perhaps because they are uncertain of the instructions, they seldom take the initiative in such tasks, but this reluctance cannot be equated with a global motivation deficit. Nor does the motivation hypothesis explain why memories of remote events should remain vivid, even in patients whose earlier lives were quite unhappy. But perhaps the most obvious ground for rejecting the claims of psychoanalysis here lies in the typical Korsakoff patient's manifest unsuitability for this mode of treatment, given his inability to remember across sessions and his general lack of interest in talking with others. The few instances where analysis would seem to have been successful probably involved patients who were recovering spontaneously (as some of Victor's and Adams's patients did), or else individuals who were not suffering from brain damage at all but simply feigning a memory deficit. In sum, the motivational theory is consistent with certain facets of Korsakoff's disease, but whatever such deficiencies exist are as likely to reflect cognitive changes in the individual as to be the cause of the memory disorder.

Another recurrent explanation of Korsakoff's syndrome is that the patient has deficient attentional mechanisms. And it is true that in the acute Wernicke's phase many patients seem unable to keep their mind on a single topic, are easily distracted by new information, and cannot in many instances monitor an assigned task. But this explanation is inconsistent with observations of chronic Korsakoff patients. As we have seen, such individuals can attend to a task for an exceedingly long time, provided that no active interference by the examiner is imposed. Once there is such disruption, the capacity to pursue the task will indeed be lost, but this seems to be a defect of memory rather than of attentional processes *per se*. Indeed, in working with such patients I have myself found their momentary attentional processes to be excellent; in answering questions or executing tasks, they draw on whatever evidence is available in their environment (printed signs, facial expressions, subtle gestures). It is only because their attentional mechanisms cannot be directed to past events that they may ultimately fail.

Other alternative explanations have included loss of initiative, loss of will, distractibility, impairment of sense of time, impairment of emotion, loss of libido, repression. For the most part, however, these rationales are either basically synonymous with the ones described above and thus suffer from the same limitations, or are so difficult to define—e.g., sense of time—as to preclude serious critical consideration.

As we have already noted, one major stream of analysis, de-emphasizing motivational and attitudinal features, has highlighted instead the cognitive and perceptual facets of the amnesic syndrome. The partisans of this school have assumed that what is fundamentally wrong is centered in the patient's mental, learning, or reasoning processes— changes in motivation or personality are regarded as a *consequence* of impaired thought processes. Such hypotheses, while not intrinsically more plausible than others, have lent themselves more readily to being tested experimentally. For example, if one claims that the patient has perceptual deficits, it is relatively easy to administer a battery of tests and to compare a Korsakoff population with a normal one, whereas satisfactory tests of a "sense of time" or of "loss of initiative" are more difficult to envisage. The major problem with the cognitive approach, however, is that the competing theories within its framework tend to overlap widely. It is difficult to judge whether a deficit in remembering an elaborate picture should be considered a perceptual or a cognitive or a mnemonic deficit, or some hybrid or amalgam of these. Furthermore, even in the context of any one of these specific hypotheses, distinctions are elusive. Thus, those who describe the problem as primarily one of memory can scarcely claim to have solved it, for critical questions arise immediately: What kind of memory and what phase of memory—memory for things learned recently, for things learned a long time ago, or for all events? Memory for verbal, visual, or musical materials, or for all of these? Is one concerned with immediate, short-term, intermediate, or long-term memory? With the process of storing input just after presentation, of consolidating the information so that it will last permanently, of filing it so as to be readily accessible, or of retrieving it at a later time?

These questions have been debated for many years and at many levels. One can consider memory at the cellular and even the molecular level, e.g., raising issues that could be resolved only in the biochemical laboratory—is the Korsakoff patient impaired in the manufacture of the chemicals which maintain traces in his nervous system? One can consider memory from an anatomical standpoint; e.g., does the Korsakoff patient suffer from a destruction of those brain structures that govern the process of learning, or that relate earlier and later experiences? Experiments involving the creation of lesions in animals would be pertinent here. One may wish to adopt a social or cultural approach: Why is it that Irish-Americans experience so high an incidence of Korsakoff's disease? Is their genetic constitution, their psychological environment, their strongly patriarchal family structure, or their historical background of poverty, the reason they become heavy drinkers and frequent victims? Why is Korsakoff's disease so infrequent, on the other hand, among persons of Jewish and Chinese extraction? This perspective suggests demographic studies and epidemiological surveys.

One can take a psychiatric tack and look at personality structures and motivation; an approach that dictates case studies and psychotherapeutic analysis. And finally, one can raise psychological issues: Are difficulties in Korsakoff's syndrome restricted to verbal materials? to long-term memory? Here we devise experiments that may enable us to decide which cognitive, perceptive, or mnemonic capacities are affected, and in each case to what degree, in the course of the disease. Such experimental research in the past few years has been as valuable for the illuminating controversies it has stirred up as for any conclusions it has suggested regarding the nature of Korsakoff's disease.

Sustained and heavy drinking is the most familiar, but by no means the only, cause of brain injury resulting in mnemonic difficulties of one or another sort. During the early 1950's a number of neurosurgeons were performing radical operations on epileptics whose condition was so severe as to prevent their leading any kind of a normal life. Some of the operations achieved their purpose of controlling the seizures, but others, either because of mistaken judgments about the locus of the disease, or insufficient understanding of its mechanisms, failed to do so. For one brief period, William Scoville experimented with the removal, from both brain hemispheres, of a midbrain structure called the hippocampus. Such an operation had been performed in animals with no noticeable effect. Scoville and his co-workers soon suspended the procedure, however, for it had an unexpectedly dramatic and tragic result: destruction of the patient's capacity to remember.

The most famous patient to undergo bilateral removal of the hippocampus and its related structures was a young man identified as H.M. This patient has become so widely known and studied that his biography is familiar to most workers in neuropsychology; he has even had a whole issue of a medical journal devoted to him, not to mention scores of articles by the Montreal group which originally studied him and by researchers from other laboratories as well.

When H.M., a motor-winder by trade, was operated on initially, he was 27 years old and already so severely impaired by epileptic seizures that he was no longer able to work. After the operation he was drowsy for a few days, but gradually became more alert. His personality was unchanged after surgery, and his IQ actually rose from 104 to 119, presumably because of reduction in the frequency of seizures. He displayed normal memory for the events of his early life, except for a vague period of retrograde amnesia covering one or two years just prior to the operation. Long-standing skills such as reading, writing, and certain facets of his trade were retained without difficulty. But the operation's unanticipated and awful consequence was that H.M., like a severely afflicted Korsakoff patient, was completely amnesic for events which occurred subsequent to it and was totally unable to learn new materials.

Except for Dr. Scoville, whom he had known for many years prior to surgery, he was completely unable to recognize members of the hospital staff; he did not recall and could not learn the way to the bathroom; he did not remember the death of a favorite uncle, although he was reminded of it constantly, and became genuinely upset at each telling.

H.M. was equally ignorant of events around his home. He could not remember his new address, even after six years of residence; he could not master the names of his neighbors, or even recognize them on the street. Although he mowed the lawn regularly, he did not know where to find the lawn mower, even when he had used it the previous day. He would solve the same jigsaw puzzles day in and day out without exhibiting any improvement in performance, and would read the same newspapers over again. He could not even be left alone in the house, for he tended to invite in strangers, thinking they must be friends of the family whom he had failed to recognize.

This last activity indicates that H.M. was aware at least superficially of his memory deficit. He was even known to say explicitly, "I have trouble with my memory." He also did manage to acquire at least a few items of information subsequent to his operation, such as the layout of the rooms in the house, the name of John Kennedy, a picture of The Beatles. Essentially, however, H.M. has remained a man who lives completely in the present, from moment to moment; much of his conversation is vague, qualified, almost embarrassed; only the early years of his life retain any coherence in his mind.

The initial tests of H.M.'s memory regarding nonverbal data and events suggested that his difficulties were equally stringent regardless of the materials utilized. For example, despite 215 trials in three days, he failed to learn a maze, or indeed to display any progress in mastering its route. (By contrast, normal subjects solve the maze in about 20 trials.) Yet when, sometime later, a simpler maze was given to H.M., he eventually learned it in 155 trials. More surprising, he showed partial memory for the path of the maze two years after the initial learning. The ability to learn and retain the solution of this second maze seemed attributable to its shorter length—the latter parts of the maze did not interfere with his memory for the first part. Another apparently contributing factor was that the maze tapped, at least in part, a "motor" rather than a "language" skill. The possibility arose, accordingly, that motor skills might involve different mechanisms of memory than those of language.

This latter hypothesis was dramatically confirmed when H.M. was required to draw a pencil line around the border of a five-pointed star; he was not allowed to observe either his hand or the star by direct vision, but only as reflected in a mirror. Although remaining entirely unaware from one day to the next that he had ever done the task before, he learned and retained in a normal manner this skill of "mirror drawing." Since then, he has been given an extensive series of nonverbal "motor" tasks. Findings indicate conclusively that the acquisition of motor skills does not require an intact hippocampal system.

Another patient with a lesion similar to H.M.'s was more recently studied by Arnold Starr and Laura Phillips. This individual was also of above-average intelligence (an IQ of 135), in this case displaying special talents in mathematics and music. He could repeat nine numbers recited but once by an examiner, eight numbers when they were said to him in one order and he had to repeat them in reverse order. Yet since his illness he had seemed incapable of committing to memory any new information. Indeed, in the course of six years at the hospital, he had managed to learn the names of but six staff members.

Intensive study revealed that certain capacities were surprisingly well preserved in the face of his massive difficulty with memory. Like H.M., the patient was able to learn simple motor skills like mirror writing, stylus tracking, and short mazes. Even more surprising, the patient was able speedily and efficiently to learn to play new pieces on the piano. He would be taught a piece on one day and then be asked to play it again on the following day. At first, he would deny all knowledge of the piece, as well as any familiarity with the examiner or the task. However, once given the opening bars, he could carry through the new composition to completion without difficulty. It must be stressed that these were pieces which the patient could not have known before; the music seemed to be learned as a kind of motor skill, in striking contrast to his impaired memory for verbal information.

Most unanticipated was the discovery that Starr and Phillips's patient could also remember a limited amount of verbal material. As with music, he rarely if ever recollected the occasion of teaching or the nature of the material previously taught to him. Nonetheless, when the conditions of the original learning were repeated, it could be shown that some information had been retained. The patient often would introduce words learned on previous lists into newly administered lists; this "proactive interference"—the frequent intrusion of "old" learning in the midst of "new" learning—was clear proof that some traces of the original task had endured. The patient could also remember certain series well enough to anticipate which word was next; he was particularly helped when the words had been originally categorized according to whether their connotation was pleasant or unpleasant. Finally, after being told a story many times, the patient was able to recall fragments of it, and to convey its general theme, sweep, and flavor, though many specific details were forgotten. Thus some emotional and structural facets of particular literary passages could be retained.

On our Service, we have recently had the opportunity to examine a patient whose memory deficits seem even more severe than Scoville's and Starr and Phillips's subject (if such a *tabula rasa* is conceivable). We also found him able to learn motor tasks at a relatively rapid rate. As this patient was an accomplished pianist, we taught him a piece we had composed; he learned it in a few ten-minute sessions, then retained it perfectly. We next arrived at the idea of introducing lyrics, these containing the same information he was unable to produce in bedside conversation. So we taught him to sing: "Henry's my name;/ Memory's the game;/ I'm in the V.A. in Jamaica Plain;/ My bed's on 7D;/ The year is '73;/ Every day I make a little gain." Except for the final line, which required more intensive tutoring, the words were similarly learned fairly easily, over six sessions of ten minutes each on successive days.

Once learned, the lyrics were retained quite well, though not with the same easy fluency as the music—we sometimes had to prompt Henry with the first word of a line. To our surprise, however, he was able to sing the words without

piano accompaniment and, eventually, to recite them without their being embedded in the melody. He continued
to err when asked to supply isolated points of information
("Can you tell me the date?" or "Where in the hospital
are we now?"), but if the question was phrased in a way
reminiscent of the song lyrics ("The year is . . .?" or "Your
bed's on . . .?"), he was more likely to produce the correct
answer. On a return to the hospital three months after
discharge, Henry produced the song and lyrics with little
difficulty, indeed more accurately than several hospital
personnel who had witnessed earlier training sessions.

These studies prove that nonlinguistic materials are unquestionably easier for Korsakoff or Korsakoff-like patients
to learn and retain than are materials formulated in language. Indeed, in at least one recent study at our hospital,
it was shown that short-term memory (ability, without
practice, to remember an element for eighteen seconds) in
Korsakoff patients is impaired primarily in the realm of
language. These patients are able to remember musical
sequences, visual configurations, and tactile patterns as
adequately as normal individuals, provided only that the
learned materials are not verbal in nature and not easily
described (or "coded") in words. Yet amnesic patients do
appear to have at least a limited capacity for remembering
verbal materials as well, provided that these are rehearsed
frequently, embedded in a familiar pattern, or originally
learned as lyrics for a song.

It seems paradoxical to question whether this manner
of assimilating linguistic materials is genuinely "language
learning." Normally, when an individual learns a new
fact or name, he is able to produce it freely, independent
of any context. For example, the name *Spiro Agnew* is
accessible to me whether I think about the vice-presidency,
the press, Frank Sinatra, plea-bargaining, household words,
or examples for a chapter. This state of affairs, however,
apparently does not obtain for the Korsakoff patient who

has learned a new verbal element: he is able to produce it only when he is transported to essentially the same situation that prevailed at the time of the original learning: in the jargon, his learning is "state-dependent" or "place-dependent." Thus, if made over a period of weeks to memorize a poem including the words *Spiro Agnew,* the patient might emit the name at the appropriate verse, but would remain quite unable to produce it on other occasions or in spontaneous speech. It could even be maintained that the learning of a song, of lyrics, of a list of random words, or of a euphonious Greek name is more akin to the motor learning of a new language than to the assimilation and comprehension of a historical account. The vocal apparatus has been trained to behave in a certain way, but there is little "cognitive" processing. Some support for this view comes from the observation that when Korsakoff patients are reciting learned verbal patterns, they do so in an automatic way, without apparent awareness of meaning. They resemble the young child chanting Hebrew or reciting the Pledge of Allegiance, whose understanding and "recoding" of the verbal materials are extremely limited, if they exist at all.

It is risky, of course, to generalize in an uncritical fashion across a range of memory disorders, since the lesions secondary to alcoholism, trauma, or surgery are by no means equivalent. Our remarks here pertain chiefly to alcohol-induced Korsakoff's disease. In all the cases we have described, however, patients have displayed particular difficulty in recalling verbal materials, and this striking finding requires explanation. Clearly, the same patients can comprehend and understand ordinary spoken language in a relatively normal way, even though they exhibit less spontaneity in initiating conversations and tend to favor brief, often vague responses. Why, then, does so little of what is comprehended linger in the patient's mind, available for retrieval at a later time?

One approach to this question has been to examine what happens to the patient's verbal memory over short periods of time. There is controversy here, as some investigators have found retention of verbal materials to last for at least a minute, while others believe that words fade from the Korsakoff patient's memory within ten or twenty seconds. This dispute might appear easy to resolve conclusively but it is not, because of the irrepressible human tendency to "rehearse." If I ask you to remember a list of four words, you will probably say them to yourself silently as often as necessary, so that you will be able to issue them effortlessly on request. Short-term memory is more purely probed, accordingly, if I can thwart your rehearsing by forcing you to speak of something else. If you are reasonably clever or persistent, however, you may be able to rehearse the words silently (covertly) even while you are ostensibly carrying out arithmetic problems, humming a tune, or executing some other assigned interfering activity. At least some part of the dispute about the efficacy of short-term memory in Korsakoff patients thus depends on the way on which this capacity is tested. Those patients who are better able to rehearse silently, and those tasks which are less demanding on the patients, are more likely to reveal an adequate short-term memory; those tasks where rehearsal is difficult are likely to induce a quick fading of the given verbal materials.

Whatever their degree of efficiency in the short term, however, there is no question that Korsakoff patients are markedly deficient at retaining verbal materials over longer periods of time. Often their memory impairment is attributed to interference: succeeding verbal messages are said to somehow erase, or render inaccessible, information learned previously. This must be true; yet, since the same kind of interference presumably also occurs with normal individuals, we must inquire whether the Korsakoff is simply more susceptible to interference or whether he has some additional problems as well.

Important insight into the Korsakoff's specific difficulty with words has come from experimental work conducted by Nelson Butters, Laird Cermak, and their colleagues at our hospital. In this, patients have been required to memorize lists of words, and the investigators have then studied the confusions and efforts they make, and have sought to determine what sort of cues or devices help the patients retain materials over longer periods of time. Their principal finding is that Korsakoff patients do very little active mental processing on such a task. They encode words merely at the acoustic level (attending only to the sound), rather than, like normal adults, at the semantic level (taking into account meanings and diverse sensory-motor associations). They can echo the word list faithfully, but they make no effort to classify the words by category or to discern any common theme among them. The average person, for example, will have a much easier time learning such a series as *turkey, hungry, family, Thanksgiving* than the more-or-less random sequence *Christmas, tunnel, spoiled, government,* because he will perceive and use as a memory aid the relationship among the items in the first list. The Korsakoff, however, makes no attempt on his own to link the words, to adopt a strategy that will enable him to retrieve them with greater efficiency at a subsequent time, and so for him the two lists pose equal, and great, difficulty. If he is directed to attend to word meanings, he will do so, and this strategy will aid his memory function; but he will not do this spontaneously.

On this analysis, the deficit of Korsakoff patients is preferably thought of as cognitive in nature: it reflects an impoverishment in ability to adopt an intelligent strategy and to focus on the meanings of materials, rather than merely a disturbance in passive responding *per se.* Much the same conclusion has been reached by George Talland, a psychologist who has made the most intensive study of the Korsakoff syndrome. In his widely acclaimed monograph *Deranged Memory,* Talland reports a large number of investigations conducted with twenty-nine alcoholic Korsakoff patients. Talland's subjects performed as well as normal controls when the task required only the immediate apprehension and manipulation of a given set of materials. But if the instruction for the task was changed, if a new set of materials was introduced, if unfamiliar materials were employed, or if recently learned information was instrumental for success—in short, if some flexibility or openness to change was needed—the patients lapsed badly.

Talland concluded that the difficulty in Korsakoff's disease clearly extended to the realm of perceptual and cognitive deficits. Indeed, the best unitary explanation for Korsakoff's psychosis was that it produced in the patient a tendency to close or complete a task in a premature way, without adequately considering its explicit and implicit requirements. Normal individuals tend to consider all dimensions of a problem, to continue a search until a satisfactory solution is attained, to approach a problem by drawing equally on past experience and present considerations—it is this overall synthesizing capacity that is no longer operative in the Korsakoff patient. Like the over-eager young child, the excessively fatigued old man, the bored or annoyed teenager, the amnesic individual goes immediately from the stimulus to the most available, accessible termination point. This means that he is likely to misconceive questions of any degree of subtlety or complexity; in addition, he will have difficulty in the future drawing on recently learned experiences because these have not been adequately categorized in his mind, have not been integrated into his arsenal of knowledge and skill.

This solution to the enigma of Korsakoff's syndrome has elegance and appeal. A description of the patient as a premature "forecloser" in all his activities touches upon the cognitive *and* perceptual features (the patient fails to take into account all relevant factors); motivational and personality features (the lack of will to pursue a problem in all its applications, and an absence of initiative in diverse situations); memory components (failure to incorporate recent experiences which may be relevant to the problem); and attentional defects (missing some facets which should have been considered). In addition, since the neural structures injured in Korsakoff's disease are thought to control the activation or arousal of the individual, it is germane to point out how relatively "deactivated" or underaroused the Korsakoff patient appears.

Talland's position also is consistent with demonstrations that Korsakoff patients remember more than had previously been thought; *if* the appropriate cues are given, they will evince memory of nonverbal materials and even of certain verbal materials. This evidence undercuts the old contention that Korsakoff patients were completely unable to store, encode, or consolidate new information; when an appropriate cueing technique elicits the original input, clearly the information has in some way been stored. The evidence also confirms that retrieval of information is not a unitary process, initiated in but a single way; instead, what is retrieved reflects in large part the kind of question asked and the type of answer accepted. Korsakoff patients are particularly likely to remember if they are shown incomplete representations of words presented previously and asked to complete them; or if they are simply required to indicate which of a large body of materials they had perceived before, and which are wholly new to them. In our own research, we have shown that when a Korsakoff patient is asked "out of the blue" to name instances of a category, he is likely to produce words he was previously told; as with our patient Mr. O'Donnell, this result occurs even though he is unaware that he had ever been asked to remember instances of that category (for example a city or a color). Such findings highlight the fact that memory is inextricably tied in with a whole raft of functions involved in learning and classifying information.

For all its appeal, however, Talland's explanation still seems to me incomplete as it stands. For instance, it does not specifically indicate why verbal materials should pose special difficulties for the amnesic patient, why he should have relatively little difficulty, by contrast, in memorizing music or mastering mazes. Nor does it account for the patient's having such a relatively well-preserved memory for things of the distant past, while so impoverished a memory of more recent phenomena. Presumably premature closure should not be so discriminating against more recent memories, nor in favor of musical sounds.

I should now like to put forward my own tentative hypothesis concerning these puzzles. It seems to me that if the Korsakoff patient were tested in the ways that we test animals—nonverbally, exclusively by tapping motor behavior—he would seem entirely normal. (Indeed, as mentioned earlier, the damage found in his brain is of a sort which produces little if any memory deficit in the monkey.) The reason that the Korsakoff seems so woefully disturbed is because we are comparing him with other human beings, who are primarily "linguistic" (rather than "motor") creatures, and who have preserved and developed a sense of history, that is, of a coherent past.

Let me elaborate: Except in certain ritualistic conversations, where the lines of each interlocutor are preordained, talk between individuals requires a capacity for access to a wide range of information through numerous routes, and for thinking of oneself and of the other person within an organized spatial and temporal context. I, for example, think of myself as someone born at a certain time, possessed of certain preferences, skills, and failings, having undergone certain experiences in a definite order; in the background are explicit goals, means of achieving them, problems, pleasures, defenses, aspirations, etc. In short, I have constructed a *metaphor* of myself, one to which I am continuously making additions and revisions, shaping it in response to my immediate environment, talking (perhaps excessively) about it and thinking of it. I also construct metaphors or representations of other individuals and perform similar operations upon them. When, without prior warning, I am asked about diverse events or persons in my past, I can (assuming I am reasonably awake) run in short order through a mental newsreel, arousing appropriate sensory images or recorded "transcripts"; alighting upon the situation being alluded to, I can relive the appropriate moments. This is only possible, however, because frequently during the past, I have taken the trouble, consciously or unconsciously, to absorb this information and then to fit it in some way into a mental catalogue. Had I not done so, I might still in some sense be said to have "stored" this material, but I would be unable to retrieve it unless externally aided in resurrecting the circumstances or the states during which the material was originally learned. And unless my interlocutor knew something of this original state, or I could somehow bootstrap myself into resurrecting it, this memory would remain inaccessible to me, at least until I happened to find myself in a situation where, like Proust partaking of a childhood aroma, the original "images" or "tapes" would be spontaneously "played."

The Korsakoff patient is able to perform such operations on materials from the distant past which were at one time well learned, consolidated, incorporated into his personal metaphor. At a certain point, however, the shaping of this metaphor has been interrupted or thwarted, presumably because beyond that point he can no longer retain information long enough to alter his total picture of himself. Thereafter, at best, certain vague fragments dangle from various end-points on the metaphor's structure; for the most part, it remains moored at an earlier epoch. He is able to master new things, particularly of a nonverbal nature, so long as he is not expected to trot these learnings out on request or to "access" them spontaneously. Such requests are only rarely made, however. Rather, like an animal being tested, the subject of a nonverbal learning study is simply introduced into situations where he has the opportunity to reveal his earlier learning. The more accurately the original learning situation is re-created, the more likely that memory of the event will appear to be present. And, within the verbal sphere, when the original learning conditions are faithfully re-created (i.e., the framework within which the given words were learned is repeated), there is much higher probability that the patient will be able to reactivate what has been learned. The more "motor-like" and less "language-like" the manner in which the verbal materials are treated, the greater the likelihood that memory will appear to be intact. This is, of course, in stark opposition to the case with the normal human adult, who has difficulty in remembering materials in their precise original form, precisely because he has actively encoded them for meaning, even as he has assimilated them into his personal mental metaphor.

This brief exposition scarcely suffices to resolve the fundamental problem of the Korsakoff syndrome. However, it does underscore the fact that the deficit the syndrome embodies is primarily and distinctively human, one only perceptible because, by its existence, it throws into sharp relief the mechanisms which account for the amazingly comprehensive memories most humans can demonstrate. Whereas an experimental animal learns a task only through repeated rehearsals over many trials, the human being is the example *par excellence* of one-trial and even no-trial learning. Told only once that Raquel Welch (or a comparable male superstar) favors black undergarments and that they should be sure to remember this fact, it is unlikely that most individuals will have to be reminded again. Or, simply instructed to look at the number of traffic lights at the next intersection and promised ten dollars if they will phone the correct answers to their local newspaper, most individuals will do so even without any practice or any prior reinforcement. These behaviors are only possible because of human beings' remarkable capacities for encoding and decoding verbal instructions in a plethora of ways and for building up and adding constantly to mental metaphors of themselves and their past and future behavior. Each retelling and each utilization of this metaphor strengthens and stabilizes it; hence the memories become sharpened and entrenched with the passage of time.

Why, however, does the brain injury in the Korsakoff patient have a particularly devastating effect upon the *verbal* memory for isolated facts? One hypothesis is that the information given to the patient is no longer capable of arousing strong affective reactions or sensory-motor associations and is therefore never fully assimilated. Data about Raquel Welch or ten dollars is likely to be learned by the normal person because there are strong pleasurable reinforcements associated with its mastery. Should the Korsakoff patient, perhaps because of injury to the brain region involved in "primary" reinforcement, be diminished in the possibility for such reinforcements (as his generally lowered affect and lack of interest in sensual experience suggest), then this information would be no more likely to be remembered than a phone number, which most of us forget about as rapidly as a Korsakoff forgets a list of words or the promise of a reward. As regards motor sequences, on the other hand, a different kind of learning-reinforcement circuit—one akin to the pathways aroused in animals—may be involved. So long as this circuit has not been disrupted (as it may be by damage to the frontal lobes), the patient should be able to remember nonverbal information at a reasonably adequate level. It seems, then, that the Korsakoff differs from the normal person primarily in his inability to transfer to the "verbal-symbolic" level the kinds of mnemonic mechanisms adequate for recalling music or maze patterns but unsuited for daily news or the names of new acquaintances. This lack, in turn, freezes his mental metaphor at an earlier moment in time. Crippled by the lowered potential for reinforcement, the patient becomes unable to incorporate the new information essential for ongoing revision of the mental metaphor.

While Korsakoff's disease is the most spectacular memory disorder encountered in brain-damaged patients, other mnemonic anomalies are worth citing as we attempt to arrive at a satisfactory conception of the progress of memory. In diametrical contrast to those patients who are unable to remember anything are those scattered few nonpatients who, for one reason or another, are unable to forget anything. I refer here not so much to those "memory experts" who have invented systematic training methods for improving an average or subpar mnestic skill, as to those occasional geniuses or *idiots savants* who seem effortlessly to retain everything. The most astounding example is the mnemonist S. described by A. R. Luria— a man literally unable to forget the most trivial detail, the longest arbitrary list, the most complex and most remote of his experiences.

S.'s feats almost defy the imagination. He could remember lists of numbers or words of any length, reciting them either frontwards or backwards on request; years later he could produce the entire copies of previous lists, without ever confusing any two of them. Even if information was presented to him in a language with which he was unfamiliar—such as the time he was shown long passages of *The Divine Comedy* in Italian—S. had no trouble committing these to memory and recollecting them some fifteen years later. His faithful memory extended back to earliest childhood: he recalled being placed in his crib, lying there and staring at the wallpaper, feeling sensations of comfort and warmth, when less than a year old. This accuracy of memory persisted day by day until middle age, so that S. was an unbelievably rich repository of experiences and recollections.

Over the course of some thirty years, Luria developed considerable insight into the mnemonist's methods. The key to S.'s astonishing ability apparently lay in the powerful sensory imagery that inevitably accompanied all his activities and that was spontaneously triggered by any allusion—by himself or others—to an earlier event. His essential procedure was to listen to a word or phrase, watch a picture or a scene, and then simply allow an incredible variety of sensory associations and feelings to emerge, thereby enlivening and eventually solidifying the experience in his mind. For all the numbers and letters he had standard images; moreover, every tone of voice elicited a characteristic feeling and sensation. For instance, exposed to a tone pitched at thirty cycles per second, S. saw a narrow strip like old tarnished silver; then it receded and was converted into an object that glistened like steel. Next the tone took on the color associated with twilight, while the sound continued to dazzle because of the silvery gleam it shed. The number *1* was pointed, firm, and complete, while the number *2* appeared flatter, rectangular, whitish in color, and sometimes almost gray; *1* also reminded him of a proud, well-built man, while *2* was a high-spirited woman. Even when he was merely imagining a scene, his electroencephalogram exhibited the typical pattern of an individual attending to a visual display.

This very richness of associations to every sensory input exacted its price, however; S. sometimes failed to recognize a voice on the phone or a face in the crowd because the individual appeared slightly different on this occasion and a wholly new set of associations was engendered. Such paradoxical difficulties offer an important clue to the limitations of S.'s intellect: so overpowered was he by the particular imagery of concrete experiences that he was severely impaired in generalizing across situations, in classifying together members of the same category, such as variations of the same voice, or different glimpses of the same visage. This susceptibility to the accidental, and concomitant insensitivity to the general, proved not infrequently a serious handicap.

Indeed, Luria's investigation dramatically demonstrated how this condition could be overtly dysfunctional. The inability to forget means that the individual, like Sherlock Holmes's fool, is carting about an unbelievable amount of useless information; furthermore, this information actively thwarts the perception of aspects and situations in a new light. The mnemonist was unable to appreciate a line of poetry or an abstract argument because he always responded to any concrete item by dredging up his disparate sensory associations, including countless irrelevant and interfering ones. He was also impaired in deciding what was better overlooked or omitted; every conscious experience immediately occupied his attention and aroused his overly keen sensory apparatus, even when it was better left unobserved. His ultimate fate was tragic: increasingly unsuited for any occupation where cognitive powers—the ability to organize, classify, evaluate, and dismiss—were required, he became a professional curiosity who made his living traveling from city to city, demonstrating to strangers that he could remember yet a longer list of random numbers or table of grocery items. He achieved little in life, for so powerful was his capacity to dream that he was seldom aroused to action in the "real" world. Paradoxically, S.'s vastly superabundant possession of the faculty lacking in Korsakoff patients handicapped him in a very similar manner: whereas the Korsakoff is unable to integrate novel events into his storehouse of knowledge because of lack of sensory and affective arousal, S. was so overwhelmed by such associations that he, too, was unable to winnow out the vital from the trivial.

Luria's report lends support to those who have argued that the human mind is—or at any rate can be—a receptacle of all the experiences the individual has ever lived through. Similar evidence comes from Wilder Penfield's amazing findings about recall during the course of brain surgery. When parts of the brain are electrically stimulated by the surgeon, the patient appears to remember with great vividness and fidelity experiences from early childhood. The reason for this strange occurrence is not yet clear. Perhaps Penfield has shown that all of us have the gift of the mnemonist, but that this skill is only evident under atypical circumstances. It is at least arguable, however, that patients are not remembering a particular experience at all, but rather a general set of experiences, of the sort that populate recurrent dreams. In other words, there need not be TV cameras whirring in our heads preserving on a mental videotape everything we have ever seen, heard, or done; rather, we may learn to extract regularities from sets of experiences and incorporate these regular configurations into our personal metaphors as a kind of "generalized memory" on which we can subsequently call. What is being electrically stimulated is not an instant (or long-postponed) replay but rather an archetype or prototype which was actually realized in multifarious ways at diverse times. Instead of a particular collie, terrier, or spaniel, there is a generalized dog; instead of one particular scene with Lassie, there is an idealized picture of the collie for all seasons; instead of one performance of Beethoven's Ninth, there is an amalgamated rendition which one can turn on in one's mind's ear at the breakfast table or the concert hall.

As yet, there is insufficient evidence to indicate whether it is the "videotape" process or the abstraction and generalization process just described that more accurately represents our storehouse of old information. Perhaps, indeed, we have the potential for both kinds of memories. A bizarre power called eidetic imagery is found in about eight percent of young children: youthful "eidetekers" appear to be able to remember whole scenes with uncanny accuracy; this capacity generally atrophies in adulthood, but is present with reasonable frequency among brain-injured individuals, and occasionally surfaces as a "photographic memory" in highly intelligent persons. The documentation thus far on eidetic imagery would appear to support the Penfield position; yet, again, it is possible that its possessors are merely able to "reconstruct" a faithful replica of an earlier scene, rather than reading it off the screen of their mind's eye. Another plausible view is that a photographic memory is a primitive capacity available to some immature organisms but that, for adaptive reasons, this capacity atrophies in most individuals. Support for this speculation comes from the fact that when eidetekers comment on or otherwise categorize a scene during its initial presentation, the scene tends to fade and they are no longer able to remember its visual facets afterwards. (Luria's mnemonist related similar experiences.) On this view, a superbly faithful memory—founded on incredibly rich sensory associations or on an internal "camera"—may be present in early life; but the disadvantages of such a capacity are sufficient so that a tendency toward abstraction, generalization, and omission of irrelevant details takes over in most of us. The mnemonist (and some artists) emerge as persons who have accentuated the primitive capacity, scientists as individuals who have developed the abstracting memory, while the hapless Korsakoff patient retains neither of these rival mechanisms.

Brain damage can produce other peculiar quirks of memory. In transient global amnesia (sometimes called the "Mini-Korsakoff" syndrome), a patient will suddenly cease to hold on to any information for more than a few seconds. All past memories up to a few hours before the start of the attack will remain intact, and for brief intervals, memory and immediate perception will be unaltered; but the patient will not remember what is happening from one minute to the next. He can drive a car but not cook an egg (unless he is watching a clock and has written down the time the egg was placed on the stove). Such an attack generally lasts about a day and then gradually clears up. In most cases the patient eventually returns to normal, except that he has complete amnesia for the period of the attack and for perhaps half an hour preceding it.

This phenomenon suggests the existence of at least three phases in memory: (1) an immediate memory lasting a few seconds, which, as in an attack of transient global amnesia, is never impaired; (2) a period of consolidation, or short-term memory, in which the electrical activity in the neural circuits becomes converted into patterns in which memory is permanently stored; (3) a long-term, remote memory, which depends upon widespread representation in the brain, at least in the relevant gyri. In transient global amnesia, the consolidation process appears to have been disrupted; the total length of time forgotten before the start of the conscious attack is hypothesized to equal the length of the consolidation process.

Individuals who become aphasic from a stroke or tumor may also experience various kinds of memory disorders. In amnesic aphasia, for instance, the patient has a selective difficulty in remembering the names of objects, faces, and events; usually he can pick out the correct name from among multiple choices, and so he is rather like the normal individual who can read but not speak or write in a foreign language, or who fails to recall the name of a long-lost friend. In conduction aphasia, there is particular difficulty in repeating information. The patient's under-

standing and his ability to express himself spontaneously
are usually good; he can understand what is being said,
but has a selective difficulty in reproducing it immediately
after hearing. The crucial issue in both of these aphasias is
whether the difficulty is primarily mnemonic, in the sense
that the patient has forgotten what the desired words are,
or whether the deficit is better thought of as linguistic in
nature. In the latter case, what is lost is not the particular
concept or meaning of the word, but rather the knowledge
of how to produce it as a linguistic (phonological) entity.
A generally reliable test is to determine if the patient can
paraphrase what is desired and if he can rectify, or at least
evince awareness of, his own mistakes. If he can, then his
strictly mnemonic capacities have not been impaired;
they are only incapacitated as a result of a more fundamental difficulty in producing language. It should be
pointed out, however, that some investigators would will-
ingly "collapse," or identify with each other, certain
aphasic and mnemonic disturbances. Here is one area in
which a more detailed understanding of the anatomical
connections subserving speech, language, comprehension,
and retrieval of past information would be invaluable.

One final quirk of memory encountered among brain-
injured patients has been mentioned before: reduplication.
Particularly in disease implicating the right hemisphere
and in the early stages of Korsakoff's disease, patients
may begin to speak in all earnestness about a person,
building, event, or object which does not actually exist
but which is in all essentials identical to one that does
exist. A frequent occurrence is the patient's insistence that
he is in a particular hospital, one very much like the one
he is actually in, but which is nonetheless a figment of the
patient's imagination—e.g., there is no Quincy Branch of
the Massachusetts General Hospital, no Brooklyn Extension of Mount Sinai Hospital. The mechanisms involved
in this peculiar disorder are exceedingly obscure; the pa-

tient may be trying to make sense of a feeling of familiarity that he has in a given context, together with at least a fragmentary suspicion that he is not exactly in the same situation again. The conflict between his own feeling that he is in Quincy or Brooklyn, and the external indications (such as doctors' coats or relatives' comments) that he is actually in Boston or Mount Sinai, is resolved by reduplication, a kind of mental merger between memory and reality.

As with most disorders of cortical functions, some reflection uncovers analogous situations in normal life. When one is totally preoccupied with an issue, and one's spouse or child says something, the resulting phenomenon is somewhat like Korsakoff's disease. The Korsakoff (like you) hears the sound, and may even come up with a relatively automatic response, but the question is never really pondered or processed completely; and in the absence of active encoding, it will, like an unused phone number, soon be forgotten completely. Similarly, as Proust so compellingly demonstrates, the sudden encounter with a smell or feeling from early childhood can instantly conjure up a wealth of long-forgotten experiences in a particularly vivid way. At such times we momentarily share the experiences of Luria's mnemonist or of the patient whose temporal lobe has been stimulated. When we search for a word, finding it on the tip of our tongue but finally resorting to an available paraphrase, we are like the amnesic aphasic. When we get the gist of what someone has said, but cannot for the life of us repeat it, or when we hear a new name, yet cannot re-create the name's unique phonemic characteristics, we are somewhat like the conduction aphasic.

Finally, there may even be examples of reduplication in our own lives. When we arise at night in a strange hotel room or when we awake in a novel position in our own bed, we feel that the place is strange, yes, but also that we have been in the same situation before; a hybrid mental construct may well be devised to reconcile these contradictions. I recall a particularly instructive instance of this phenomenon in my own experience. I was sitting in a new library at Harvard, one I had never visited before, but whose seminar rooms resembled those of a nearby building, Larsen Hall, with which I was quite familiar. Unconsciously, I came to feel that I *was* in Larsen Hall—so that when I looked through the window and actually saw that building, for an instant I thought to myself, "My God, Larsen Hall has another wing, just like the one I'm sitting in." My confusion was resolved only when, through access to the up-to-date revision of my own metaphor and to a memory of my very recent activities, I came to realize the truth, and how I had been momentarily led to deceive myself.

Occurrences such as that related above offer yet further confirmation that there is no unbridgeable gap between normal mental processes and those encountered on the neurological ward. The difference, of course, as in the case of disturbances of language, reading, and recognition, is that what occurs occasionally and transiently in the normal individual becomes, alas, the way of life for the victim of brain injury. We have reviewed in this chapter a variety of mnemonic processes—short-term, long-term, verbal, motor, photographic, and schematic—and have explored the various kinds of impairment to which they are subject. This may suggest to some that the term *memory* is too diffuse to be useful; and indeed, in psychological writings, one often finds classified as "mnemonic" everything from knowledge of how to digest food to ability to speak correctly. One of the chief virtues of neuropsychological study is that we gain perspective on which features of a widely acknowledged psychological process are most central. And in this context, it seems most useful to consider the two kinds of capacities which are so impaired in Korsakoff patients: (1) the ability to so understand and encode linguistic input that it can be brought out later under conditions quite diverse from those in which it was originally introduced; and (2) the ability to integrate information into metaphors of ourselves which we have developed over the years and into the sense of the passage of time contained in it. The core of human memory, in other words, should be viewed as a highly structured cognitive process, intimately dependent on man's linguistic and intellectual powers. It differs from memory in all other organisms, even as it is distinct from the mnemonic processes in our own body—ranging from "how to breathe" to "how to tie our shoes"—all of which endure and even thrive in blithe ignorance of our personal metaphor and our sense of time.

# 6 The Gerstmann Syndrome: Fact or Fiction?

*Why do all men, both foreign and Greek, count in tens? . . . it is because all men have ten fingers.*

—ARISTOTLE

Despite their undeniable differences, the case studies and conditions reviewed in earlier chapters all share important common features. In most instances a normal middle-aged adult has suffered a stroke or other form of brain injury, one which affects a significant, but discrete, area of his brain. As a consequence of this injury, he has become impaired in one or more important faculties—speech, understanding of language, reading, recognition of objects, memory for verbal materials—yet has retained appreciable competence in many other high-level cortical functions, e.g., spatial perception, musical ability, mathematical competence. The study of such relatively "isolated" disorders is of special interest to the psychologically oriented observer, for it may lead to significant, even pivotal, revisions in our understanding of such issues as the relationship between language and thought or the links between acquired and congenital disorders of reading.

Yet, even with reference to the disturbances revealed heretofore, there has often been significant controversy. We have seen, for instance, that a diagnosis of visual agnosia no longer satisfies certain analysts: they reduce this "higher-order" deficiency to a more elementary (and pervasive) problem in visual perception or intellectual acuity. Similarly, the relatively clear-cut taxonomy of aphasias to which I myself subscribe is anathema to followers of Pierre Marie. These investigators hold, with their master, that there is only one "true" aphasia; all the varied syndromes are merely distorted or imperfect versions of this central difficulty. Although it is tempting to dismiss these squabbles as merely academic arguments, tempests in a terminological teapot, they are in fact of crucial import for the effort undertaken here. Would that we could simply describe the results of brain damage and say "this is how it is." But what we see, and how we talk about it, is never based on pure, naive, veridical perception; rather, it is inextricably bound to what we already know, what we're looking for, what we're trying to prove. Just as a proper appreciation of contemporary art demands familiarity with the fashions and approaches of earlier eras, so the study of brain damage is inseparable from consideration of the hypotheses of earlier clinicians, the categories and syndromes they devised and, lamentably, the facts they distorted or overlooked.

Up to this point, we have stressed the reasonableness of traditional classifications. In so doing, however, we have ignored the tension between the "objective" results of brain damage and the interpretive statements made by clinicians. It is time to give the floor to the other side, by subjecting one of the "purest" of higher cortical disorders to a critical review. In so doing, I have deliberately chosen a syndrome about whose very existence I have some doubts. Yet I have tried to be just to both sides of the issue, to bring out the legitimate points raised by the partisans of the particularistic "syndrome approach," as well as by those skeptical about its validity.

In 1924, Dr. Josef Gerstmann, a young assistant in neurology at a Viennese hospital, examined a 55-year-old
woman patient who had recently suffered a stroke. In addition to the usual signs, Gerstmann detected a most unusual symptom—the patient was totally unable to name,
or by any other means indicate recognition of, the
several fingers on either hand. Excited by this unexpected
finding, Gerstmann wrote up a brief note on the case for a
Viennese weekly medical newsletter. In the next few years,
Gerstmann and other colleagues in the German-speaking
world encountered several patients who presented a similar clinical picture. At the same time Gerstmann had detected a number of other unexpected symptoms which
seemed to accompany the difficulty with fingers. By the
early 1930's, this cluster, already enshrined as an established clinical picture, was becoming known as the Gerstmann syndrome.

During the years following its proclamation as a syndrome, neurological students and residents were routinely
instructed about Dr. Gerstmann's findings. Dozens of articles in various languages verified these findings; nearly
every neurological textbook referred to it as a routine
clinical syndrome following a stroke, tumor, or accident
in the left angular gyrus region of the brain. Yet, by the
early 1950's, doubts had begun to arise. Certain scholars
who went back to the early papers were surprised to find
in these what they regarded as serious defects in procedure
and reasoning. Other scientists applied powerful statistical
tests to large groups of patients and became yet more dubious about the reality of the Gerstmann syndrome. Macdonald Critchley, one of the world's most eminent neurologists, published a penetrating review called "The
Enigma of the Gerstmann Syndrome," in which he retracted much of his earlier enthusiasm for this hypothesis.
And Arthur Benton, a younger and more outspoken critic,
summarized the conclusions of his statistical investigations

in "The Fiction of the Gerstmann Syndrome." When Josef Gerstmann died in 1969, the last manuscript found among his papers embodied a final attempt to shore up the validity of "his" syndrome, amidst the growing signs that it was no longer a viable neurological diagnosis.

As no one has seriously maintained that a certain kind of patient seen in Vienna and in many other places in 1930 had suddenly vanished from neurological clinics throughout the world, something else must account for the sudden rise and gradual fall of the Gerstmann syndrome. A review of this interesting chapter in medical history may not only serve to unravel the significance of this peculiar difficulty in identifying fingers, but may also clarify the relation between clinical medicine and neuropsychological research, as well as illuminating some pros and cons of the "syndrome approach" in general.

Gerstmann's original excitement stemmed from the fact that his patient performed essentially at a normal level on most routine bedside tests. Her ability to move her body as she desired and to see, hear, and feel was undisturbed. She could speak perfectly, and understand and repeat what was said to her. She was also able to read satisfactorily, although, like other brain-damaged patients, she sometimes became fatigued after a while.

As a routine part of the neurological examination, Gerstmann designated in turn the various parts of the patient's body and asked her to name them. She did so promptly and without difficulty—until Gerstmann came to the fingers: she completely failed to name her thumb, forefinger, middle finger, ring finger, and little finger. Gerstmann then gave the patient these names in turn, each time asking her to point to or to raise the appropriate finger. Again she failed. Finally, he simply asked the patient to match fingers: to lift up the same finger on the left that he touched on the right; to lift up the same finger that the examiner himself had raised; to lift up the finger that was portrayed in a picture. On none of these tasks was the patient successful. Yet, surprisingly, when doctor and patient discussed the structure of the hand and the location of the fingers simply in the abstract, the patient seemed to have retained her "concept" of these bodily parts. Failure came when knowledge was tested in a concrete situation.

Gerstmann noted in passing that the patient could not carry out a number of other tasks, including writing out a message (agraphia) and distinguishing the left part of her body from her right. However, he did not realize the significance of these deficiencies until some time later, and he thereupon wrote, in 1927, a second paper. Whereas the first had simply been called "Finger Agnosia" (inability to recognize fingers) and had dwelt on this anomalous difficulty with digit recognition, the second, entitled "Finger Agnosia and Isolated Agraphia: A New Syndrome," was more ambitious. Gerstmann reviewed four cases, including one published by two other neurologists. He pointed out the now persistent coincidence between difficulty with finger recognition and inability to write, and argued that both deficiencies arose from a disturbance of the "body scheme"—the patient's appreciation of the detailed composition of his own body. Gerstmann stressed that these difficulties could not be attributed to the more general sort of impairments which usually affect brain-injured patients: problems with language, recognition, or purposeful action. Instead, there was a specific zone of the brain, probably in the posterior region of the left cerebral hemisphere in most individuals, in which one's knowledge of the body in general, and the structure of the hand in particular, was contained. Destruction of this zone, for whatever reason, would produce the clinical picture now encountered in four separate cases.

With publication of a third "classic" paper in 1930, Gerstmann had formulated his final views on "his" syn-

drome. Now there was a tetrad of symptoms—finger agnosia, right-left confusion, agraphia, and acalculia (inability
to perform mathematical operations)—alleged to invariably accompany a circumscribed lesion in the parietal
and occipital lobes of the left cerebral hemisphere. Supporting evidence had now accrued from several medical
services and, as far as Gerstmann was concerned, the existence of the syndrome was now beyond dispute. His attention turned instead to a more precise localization of its
source and to an attempt to solve its puzzle—i.e., to discover a single underlying function, a basic connecting
link, among the four key symptoms of the syndrome.

The interest that Gerstmann's work was arousing was
typical of the fascination that any new syndrome holds for
neurologists—a fascination that inheres in the *unusual
combination* of symptoms it represents. If a right-handed
patient suffers a stroke in the left hemisphere of his brain,
we know that the patient will in all probability experience
language difficulties—indeed, it would be remarkable and
"publishable" if he did not. And once there are language
disturbances, it is routine to expect difficulty with many
language-related functions, such as repetition, spelling,
verbal memory and naming, understanding of metaphors,
and so on. Just because it is so evident that all these functions will be either destroyed or spared together, there
would be little point in linking together any four of
them and declaring the set a syndrome. The neurologist and the neuropsychologist direct their attention, instead, to those unexpected clusters of symptoms—the apparently improbable collection of dissimilar features—
which on occasion are spared or impaired simultaneously,
and for just that reason seem potentially most fruitful for
the elucidation of the links between mind and behavior.

Gerstmann had detected a symptom that had seldom before attracted any interest: the inability to name, recognize,
or match fingers in the face of adequate recognition of other

body parts; and he then had linked unanticipated features to the finger agnosia: the inability to express oneself in writing (in the face of normal oral expression), the inability to distinguish left from right on one's body (in the face of normal left-right discrimination in "extrapersonal" space), the inability to perform mathematical calculations (in the face of otherwise normal intelligence). It was possible, of course, that these four symptoms appear together only coincidentally, that they might represent damage to four totally discrete functions which just happen to be located near one another in the brain (as are, for example, the centers which respectively mediate movement of the articulatory organs and movement of the limbs). Yet for Gerstmann and others it was a virtually irresistible temptation to speculate about the possibilities of a deep, underlying structure that tied together all four symptoms. As a result, during the years following widespread acceptance of the syndrome, Gerstmann and his colleagues put forth a number of hypotheses about "The Reason" for its existence.

Gerstmann's own hunch was that these factors all reflected an inadequate "body scheme." Knowledge of each portion of the body, he reasoned, was separately represented in the brain; accordingly, that portion related to hand and finger knowledge might be selectively impaired. The hand, moreover, made a particularly significant contribution to mental processes: through the fingers one learns to count and then to calculate; furthermore, nearly all tool use, including manipulation of a pencil in writing, depends upon the ability to utilize the hand; finally, the hands also serve as the means whereby various concepts, such as direction and left-right orientation, are generally introduced. If the hand is indeed the "means" for these various "ends," a severe impairment of one's finger-and-hand concept would suffice to produce a Gerstmann syndrome.

Other neurologists developed other hypotheses. Some

stressed that all the component symptoms involved the ability to orient oneself in space, to relate elements within an integrated spatial framework. Others emphasized the "directional" aspect: while the ability to orient oneself in space was intact for practical purposes, there was impaired knowledge of the meaning of direction, leading to the Gerstmann tetrad. A few investigators, following the same line of reasoning as Eberhard Bay in his critique of visual agnosia, suggested that Gerstmann had merely devised a particularly sensitive and sophisticated test (one of subtle discriminations among fingers) for language impairments, or for general disturbances of recognition and action; this test sifted out patients who had suffered mild strokes, or who were almost recovered from their disability, and so might be overlooked by grosser testing methods. On this view, Gerstmann's "syndrome" was nothing more than a "slight" degree of aphasia, agnosia, or apraxia.

This last group of critics, however, was definitely in the minority—most neurologists were convinced of the new syndrome's validity. And there now followed a familiar phenomenon. For once an entity has been defined and endowed with an eponym, numerous case reports inevitably seem to ensue. Whereas until 1924, no one had ever commented on this cluster of symptoms, nearly every year now brought new cases into the literature. In some instances, Gerstmann's findings and his theoretical views were simply quoted; in others, new explanations or modifications were suggested. Robert Klein reported a case of unilateral finger agnosia—a patient who could recognize fingers on one side of his body, but not on the other. S. L. Rubins described a Gerstmann patient with a new symptom: he was able to perceive pinpricks but was insensitive to pain; when jabbed with sharp tools, he did not protest. Paul Schilder claimed that there were five separate kinds of finger disorders, each of which could be localized at specific points in the brain. As for Gerstmann himself, he sometimes demurred at this or that amplification, but in general he was content to let the evidence accumulate and the explanations proliferate. Writing in 1940, at the height of the syndrome's "vogue," he declared with pride:

Investigations in a large number of cases of this type have so far failed to reveal any evidence of psychic, particularly of intellectual disorder: of aphasia, apraxia or other manifestations of agnosia, or of motor or sensory changes, to which the symptom complex of finger agnosia or its individual features could be related. . . . [Having cited twenty-five papers, he concludes] it may be said that in all publications up to the present my data on finger agnosia and its association with disorientation of right and left and isolated disorders in writing and calculating as a special cerebral complex have been confirmed so extensively and unfailingly that the syndrome may now be considered as established.

With the coming of the war, Gerstmann had moved to the United States, where he entered private clinical practice. In the meantime, the war was providing additional pertinent data. Millions of recruits were receiving intelligence tests as well as other forms of psychological and neurological screening, and neurologists who knew of the Gerstmann syndrome (Pasteur's "prepared men," as it were) began to notice a peculiar symptomatology in certain soldiers. These were generally individuals of normal (in some cases, superior) intelligence who suffered from selective disorders—they might display difficulty in learning to read maps, distinguishing left from right, orienting themselves in space. Often such symptoms appeared in the context of some linguistic difficulty. For example, the person could read and write adequately, but had required many years to learn; even in his twenties, he continued to exhibit extreme difficulty in spelling or in efficiently processing written (or Morse code) messages. After several reports describing such phenomena had appeared, the idea gradually arose that there might be a "developmental" form of the Gerstmann syndrome.

In any fairly sizeable group of individuals, a small portion will deviate from the norm—given persons may be color-blind, or tone-deaf, or mechanically clumsy, possess total recall or total amnesia for phone numbers. Usually, such disabilities serve more as a subject for amusement than a matter of real concern; under certain circumstances, however, they can become seriously disabling. Thus, an individual who has difficulty in reading maps or in discriminating left from right may have coped adequately until his induction into the army; suddenly, however, he stands apart from his peers and may feel remarkably uncomfortable, if not wholly incompetent. Students of the Gerstmann syndrome claimed that neural anomalies analogous to those which produce mechanical clumsiness or tone-deafness may also yield a particular difficulty with spatial and ordering tasks *à la* Gerstmann. The individual may have greater difficulty with initial learning, may perform these tasks at a much slower rate, or only with great difficulty—as may in given cases be true. At any rate, once the idea had gained currency that otherwise normal youngsters might experience specific problems with orientation or mathematical reasoning, reports of the Gerstmann syndrome began to emanate from military installations, institutions for retarded children, and even the more enlightened school systems in Middle America.

If the components of the syndrome were indeed related in brain-injured adults and in certain otherwise normal children, further study might yield insights about the ways in which writing, calculation, left-right, and finger recognition occurred in normal individuals. Psychologists interested in child development, for example, began to wonder whether knowledge of one's fingers was a prerequisite for competence in arithmetic; whether the ability to write (and to spell) presupposed knowledge of left and right; whether these various factors emerged at the same time (perhaps due to a single underlying operation) or in a given order in all children (one element constituting a logical prerequisite for the other). This line of reasoning fitted in well with the growing interest in children's cognitive development; it was particularly consonant with the theoretical perspective of Piaget, who had minimized the importance of language in thinking, postulating instead the centrality of spatial and logical operations in a range of intellectual capacities. Other scholars also entered the fray. Anthropologists pointed out that counting on one's fingers was common in primitive societies, and that numerical systems were nearly always built upon the base of ten. Linguists noted the intimate etymological relations between body parts and numerical systems in many languages. Thus the word for *one* is often that for *finger;* the word for *six* is *hand-one* in Malayo-Polynesia; *ten* is *hand-hand* in Aztec and *both hands* in Melanesian. Such relations can even be discerned in our own language, where *digit* applies to numbers as well as body parts, and the terms *hand* and *writing* are generally united. All these considerations supported—or were at least consonant with—Gerstmann's views on the underlying links between the component elements of his syndrome.

Interest in a syndrome where the individual's sense of number was selectively impaired inevitably raised the question whether this sense might, under different circumstances, be spared in isolation. Could there indeed be a patient whose linguistic and perceptual capacities have been vitiated, while at the same time he retains the skill of working with numbers and numerical operations? Or are mathematical operations inherently so complex that they can only be executed by an individual who is otherwise intact?

There has been to my knowledge no patient who remained capable of high-level mathematical operations in

the face of massive brain damage, though scattered anecdotes do exist concerning mathematicians who still plied
their trade in the aftermath of an aphasia. Occasional reports have surfaced of individuals who have lost the ability
to perform mathematical operations in one sensory modality—for example, on auditory presentation—while retaining the ability to perform the same operations when
the materials are presented in purely visual form. Indeed,
one such patient seen on our Service was essentially unable to attach meaning to orally presented numerical concepts: he would shake his head when he heard the words
*seven* or *eleven*, repeating them with only the bare awareness that they related to numbers; when, however, complex
addition or multiplication problems were presented to him
in written form, he solved them promptly and usually without error.

The most intriguing examples of isolated mathematical
ability are, of course, those of the *idiots savants*—individuals of deficient, often extremely low, intelligence who
emerge as uniquely gifted at certain mathematical tasks.

L. was one such individual. This boy, eleven years of
age at the time when he was most intensively studied, had
an IQ of 50, placing him in the severely retarded range.
Deficiencies of information and reasoning capacity notwithstanding, this freakish youngster could perform all
manner of numerical feats. He was able to remember end-
less series, such as railroad timetables and newspaper financial columns. He could immediately state the day of the
week for any date between 1880 and 1950. Given twelve
two-place numbers to sum, he came up with the total the
instant the presentation was completed. His speed and
accuracy at other arithmetical challenges were equally impressive.

A team of neuropsychologists studied L. for several
years. They described a youngster whose forte was recognized at a very early age and pursued with a single-minded

zeal. When only three, the child delighted in counting objects and showed remarkable interest in all aspects of number and music. At age four he played with the sounds of words, both real and nonsense, learned the alphabet, and listened indefatigably to music. "Only while spelling, counting or listening to musical recordings does he become quiet and somewhat restful," reported the observers. At the age of five he could count by 2's, 4's, 8's, and 16's; and by the age of seven he could make all kinds of monetary change.

The examiners concluded that L. was mentally deficient in visual and motor tasks but possessed superior auditory perceptual and mnemonic capacities. This made it possible for him to learn to speak and to echo faithfully in English and other languages, to spell words both backwards and forwards, to recognize all pitches played for him, and to memorize and perform pieces of music on the piano. His musical proficiency was entirely by ear; he would not (or could not) learn to play from a score.

Awareness of his superior auditory capacities, more especially in the face of such grave deficiencies in other areas, apparently motivated L. to "show off" in the spheres of number and, to a lesser extent, spelling and music. On meeting people, he would immediately ask for their birthdays, then stun them by announcing the correct day of the week on which they were born. Yet when asked how these feats were accomplished, he became tongue-tied: he was a slave, not a master, of his bizarre genius.

As the investigators indicate, L.'s skills must not be confused with those of a truly intelligent person. All of his impressive performances were robotlike; at no point did he reveal any real understanding of the realms in which at first glance he excelled so spectacularly. His musical performances were devoid of emotion; his conversation was stilted and limited; his application of arithmetic to meaningful situations in daily life was slight. The same child who could perform complex calculations was unable to indicate which of two individuals was older.

L.'s skills were based on a prodigious memory in the auditory sphere, a strong motivation to impress others, and a few tricks of computation that he was capable of using while remaining at best only dimly aware of doing so. He was at the opposite pole from a great mathematician; some of the very greatest mathematicians, indeed, have been indifferent calculators. The precocity of such geniuses as Galois, Abel, and Gauss, each of whom made mathematical discoveries of the first order while still in his teens, was based rather on a profound intuition about the realm of numbers, the nature of arithmetical and mathematical operations, an awareness of the central issues in mathematics, and the means for solving them. Such an understanding and intuition were completely lacking in L., who depended exclusively on an awareness of number series arranged in concrete patterns. The noted historian of mathematics Tobias Dantzig has expressed well the differences between these two orders of numerical wizards:

No two branches of mathematics present a greater contrast than arithmetic and the theory of numbers. The great generality and simplicity of its rules makes arithmetic accessible to the dullest mind. In fact, facility in reckoning is merely a matter of memory and the lightning calculators are but human machines, whose one advantage over the mechanical variety is greater portability. On the other hand, the theory of numbers is by far the most difficult of all mathematical disciplines.

What does characterize the individual with a special gift of mathematical intuition? My guess is that, like L., the gifted mathematician initially exhibits precocity in the performance of certain mathematical tasks but that, in contrast to L., the future topologist or algebraist becomes intrigued with the reasons for his feats, the explanation for the fascinating properties of numerical systems. He does not simply operate upon objects and numbers; he reflects upon the meanings of his operations and, eventually, attempts to formalize these impressions. Jean Piaget relates the story of a talented mathematician, who attributed his choice of career to such an experience as a youngster:

> When he was a small boy [the mathematician] was counting some stones and he counted them from left to right and found there were ten. Then he counted them from right to left and lo and behold, there were ten again. Then he put them in a circle and, finding ten once again, he was very excited. He found, essentially, that the sum is independent of the order. This is a discovery. It is a reflective abstraction stemming from his own actions. The order was not in the stones themselves.

The "compleat mathematician," then, emerges as one who, over and above his gifts in the auditory and visual spheres, has a keen interest in his actions upon numerical phenomena, and a curiosity about the reasons for their particular effects. Such capacities would seem to depend upon the capacity for critical detachment, and for comparisons among patterns and actions, which emerge only in the later years of childhood, when the sensory cortexes have long since matured, and the frontal lobes already play a prominent role in the individual's intellectual functioning. In all probability, the skills required for ultimate mastery in the mathematical sciences, then, presuppose the development (and intactness) of a number of cortical zones, including the primary sensory areas, the frontal lobes, and those parietal regions implicated in the Gerstmann syndrome. Put differently, a sense of one's own fingers and one's own body, a developed orientation in space, skill at manipulating graphic symbols, and a mastery of number systems are necessary prerequisites for both the normal individual and the *idiot savant;* but the future accomplished mathematician requires as well a persisting curiosity about the early fruits of his mathematical explorations which drives him to constantly experiment, devise, prove, test, reject, revise, and strive for elegance in his formulations.

The above discussion may well appear as a digression from our consideration of the Gerstmann syndrome; and yet it is precisely these kinds of issues which confronted those investigators seeking a basis for mathematical acumen in the brain of the normal child, and an understanding of the differences between the youthful Gauss and the young *idiot savant*. Whether, in the end, it turned out to be the use of one's fingers, the relations between ordinary language and the number system, the child's reflections upon his manipulations of objects, or some combination of these which gives rise to mastery of arithmetic remained to be determined; but the promulgation of the Gerstmann syndrome had spurred the search for behavioral antecedents or anatomical prerequisites for the important skills of number manipulation and numerical mastery. Such speculation, though by no means dependent on Gerstmann's discovery, reinforced the impression that he had hit upon a fundamental unity in human cognition; an intriguing link had been propounded between the organization of the nervous system and the evolution of language and culture. To those of a structuralist bent, the initial prospect of an underlying connection between Gerstmann's tetrad of symptoms and the eventual hope of relating cultural achievements to man's biological heritage, was heady wine indeed. Paradoxically, however, it may have been the very attention focused upon the Gerstmann syndrome by those not primarily concerned with its immediate medical implications which began to undermine the case built up for it over the years. For, by the early 1960's, reservations about the Gerstmann syndrome were being widely voiced and its proponents were clearly on the defensive.

The primary challenge came from Arthur Benton, an Iowa-based psychologist who for many years had worked with children and brain-damaged patients. Benton's attack took three forms. First of all, he severely criticized the early reports which had been the original basis for the establishment of the new syndrome. These reports, starting with those of Gerstmann himself, had been unacceptably sketchy in their accounts of patient examinations. The investigators would neglect to mention which tests they used and how often they had been administered; they would toss off without elaboration phrases like "slight finger agnosia," or "questionable right-left disorientation" or "no noteworthy constructional apraxia"; they failed to indicate whether they had tested for this or that feature sometimes associated with the syndrome. As a result, it was nearly impossible to relate the findings of diverse investigators to one another and so to assess the overall validity of the syndrome in terms of such questions as: Is there anything special about the four elements? Do they really occur together more often than any other set of four elements? Are they localizable in a particular region of the brain? Is there some underlying structure or psychological dimension linking them with one another?

Second, Benton pointed out that Gerstmann was not the first physician to have observed finger agnosia! The French ophthalmologist Jules Badal, for instance, had described a similar patient in 1888. Badal's patient had displayed difficulty in identifying which fingers had been named or touched, and this deficit was attributed "chiefly to a profound alteration of the sense of space." Though conceding that Badal's case had presented many other symptoms, and that the report was not widely known in European neurological circles, Benton argued for due acknowledgment of the precedence in this area of a forgotten figure of an older generation.

Benton's final line of criticism was the most fundamental. He argued that, given the obscure reporting in
earlier cases, it could not in fact be determined whether
the four key features of the Gerstmann syndrome did have
any special interrelationship. It was necessary, therefore,
to conduct a fresh investigation, which he proceeded to
do. A large group of patients was given a battery of tests
designed to probe all manifestations of finger gnosis, writing, mathematics, and right-left orientation, as well as a
number of other capacities—not considered by Gerstmann
—which might possibly be associated with the so-called
syndrome. These latter included reading, memory for
visual figures, and the ability to copy two- and three-dimensional designs. If Gerstmann was correct, the first four
elements should "co-occur" more frequently than the
other possible sets of four elements.

Careful review of his data indicated to Benton that all
seven of these capacities correlated highly with one another. Indeed, the correlation among the four Gerstmann
components was actually lower than that between each of
these four symptoms and various deficits outside the classical syndrome. Clearly these findings offered no support
for Gerstmann's hypothesis—although, as Benton acknowledged, they did not undermine that hypothesis either,
since Gerstmann, after all, had been describing a disease
in a specific locus. Benton therefore examined the twelve
patients in his test population who had disease in the same
region of the brain as Gerstmann's cases. Even within this
subgroup, however, there was no evidence for a special
association of the four elements of the syndrome. Benton's
conclusion was unequivocal and direct:

Judged from the standpoint of behavioural analysis, the
Gerstmann syndrome is a fiction; it . . . is simply an artifact of
defective and biased observations. Objective unbiased observation discloses a large number of combinations of parietal deficits. Since all these combinations appear to be equally strong

with respect to their internal associative bonds, and frequency of occurrence, either all or none should be designated as syndromes. . . . the syndrome has perhaps served a useful purpose in the past in certain respects but it now carries the hazard of retarding advances in the understanding of the organization of abilities and disabilities in patients with cerebral disease. . . .

Once Benton had raised his challenge, other practitioners began to reconsider their earlier views. Additional large-scale statistical analyses were conducted and, in each case, the Gerstmann syndrome did not survive the computer print-out. A number of investigators, in Germany, Austria, and Indiana, concurred that the four symptoms did not correlate with one another sufficiently to warrant the positing of a syndrome combining them. Only the Glonings in Vienna, friends of Gerstmann, were willing to argue that there might still be some usefulness in referring to an "enlarged" or "diluted" Gerstmann syndrome.

How fair and how decisive was this line of attack on the status of the Gerstmann syndrome? This question can be examined from two viewpoints: the force of particular arguments, and the reaction of the neuropsychological community at large.

I have read most of the original cases described by Gerstmann and his colleagues during the first third of the century. An unmistakable air of enthusiastic discovery remains detectable on these now-yellowed pages. First one, then a second, then many other investigators uncovered— in otherwise unremarkable patients—a profound disability in recognizing fingers, as well as a circumscribed set of related (or relatable) difficulties. The raft of findings at this time certainly seem to me to have justified extensive discussion in the clinical literature.

At the same time, I could not but note how sketchily those parts of the examination not related to the Gerstmann tetrad were outlined; and it was amazing to discover that *in every single case* other, associated signs were present which yet did not find their way into the syndrome as ultimately constituted. Thus, of Gerstmann's first cases, a number were unable to recognize and name colors, one had visual and another sensory disturbances, two had difficulty in copying designs. Mild naming defects, difficulty in copying figures, problems with spelling orally, general spatial disturbances, and other minor aphasic, agnosic, and apraxic symptoms also abound in these pioneering reports. One is forced to conclude that a distinct element of accident or randomness entered into Gerstmann's choice of four particular deficits as the key features of his syndrome, to the exclusion of other possible elements and combinations.

The effort to transfer credit for the Gerstmann syndrome to some earlier figure seems rather unnecessary. No scientific discovery is completely without antecedents; a major portion of the credit should go to the individual who was first to make explicit claims about the discovery, who drew out its implications, and who was able to impress its significance upon the rest of the scientific community. On these counts, Gerstmann compares favorably with many other medical practitioners whose names adorn a specific disorder. It is interesting that in his published answers to the growing questioning of the syndrome, Gerstmann is most critical of the effort to wrest this discovery from him: personal recognition seems to be as important as scientific vindication.

The nub of the controversy, however, clearly inheres in the meaning of the extensive statistical analyses conducted by Benton, Gloning, Heimburger, and Poeck. These studies have established that, when large-scale studies of sizable groups of patients are conducted, the Gerstmann syndrome dissolves or fades away. Yet even then the question remains, whether this may be a case of the one diamond in the coal mine being overwhelmed by hundreds of chunks of coal, or whether, instead, the alleged diamond itself is just another piece of coal on which special status has unjustifiably been conferred.

Those who continue to argue for the validity of the Gerstmann syndrome have generally taken the diamond-in-the-rough tack. In science, they say, it is irrelevant whether there are many imperfect examples of a condition, or whether the condition gets lost when surrounded by numerous nonrelated diseases. The crucial issue is: can we find one, or a small number of cases, which present a particular clinical picture in pure form? If so, the syndrome is genuine, its clinical and neuropathological significance justified, its diagnostic value established. It is not surprising that a random set of patients will present a random cluster of symptoms, for the brain can be injured in innumerable ways. To disprove the Gerstmann syndrome, one would have to prove that the hypothetical lesion in the angular gyrus does not really cause it; and even if one case of the syndrome were produced, the entire counterattack would collapse.

A variation of this argument stresses that, of course, if one looks hard enough, one can always find "something else" wrong with the patient. What is crucial about the Gerstmann syndrome is that its four components do stand out. The patient may have naming problems, to be sure, but why the particular difficulty naming fingers? Certainly he may have some visual problems, but why can he read words yet not manipulate numbers? The syndrome has no claim to legitimacy in the first place if one must perform elaborate statistical tests either to confirm or to refute it. Rather, the four difficulties should be so manifest, so strikingly more apparent than "rival" symptoms, that any qualified neutral observer, given a half-hour for examination, should be able to determine whether the patient has Dr. Gerstmann's syndrome.

To my own mind, this latter argument strikes at the

heart of the controversy. It is indeed desirable that within a half-hour a harried and overburdened physician should be able to determine a patient's principal complaints and difficulties. And in such circumstances the Gerstmann syndrome, *if valid,* would most certainly come in handy. For, given a patient whose general perceptual, intellectual, and practic functions are relatively spared, it would indeed be useful to be able to point up four or so related severe difficulties in a brief compass of time. Only if the examination stretched to one, two, or three hours, or even over a few days, would other deficits be likely to emerge, causing what had been a syndrome to dissolve gradually into a diverse set of individual symptoms.

The fact is, however, that the more one ponders the symptoms originally isolated by Gerstmann, the more they seem themselves to constitute a nebulous and undefined lot. First of all, difficulty in any of these areas can be found even in normal individuals if the task is hard enough. Simply try to solve a number of long multiplication tasks; to recognize fingers when the examiner sits opposite you, crosses his arms, and then interleaves his fingers; to keep directions straight on a long and complex finger maze or in a reversed mirror. It becomes necessary, in short, to define just when the particular difficulty begins to emerge in order to make a proper assessment of the presence, or absence, of brain damage.

Even more to the point, each of the symptoms is simply a name: the actual tasks failed by patients could be described in wholly different ways. For example, a patient unable to write a dictated passage might be said to have *spelling difficulties;* a patient who cannot multiply because he no longer knows his times-table may be said to have *memory problems;* a patient who fails at sums because he cannot keep the column of figures straight can be said to have *difficulty in spatial alignment;* a patient who confuses fingers might be said to have *impairment of fine discrimi-*

*nations* among highly similar objects. Only if one establishes independently that the patient can spell perfectly in the auditory sphere; that he knows his times-table and other relevant "old" information; that he can maintain graphical elements other than numbers in a straight line; that he can match two sets of sticks aligned in a fingerlike way, can one legitimately draw the particular conclusions propounded by Gerstmann.

Not only is there no evidence that Gerstmann ever instituted these necessary controls, but in my own experience with the Gerstmann syndrome, I have found that patients given this diagnosis generally encounter difficulty with most of these related tasks: spelling, drawing and copying three-dimensional figures, placing elements like matches in a prescribed order or sequence, and responding appropriately to time-and-space-related antonyms like *up/down, in front of/behind, early/later,* and so forth. Again, this finding does not preclude the existence of a patient who fails all Gerstmann tasks and passes all "check" tasks; it only raises the question whether any such patient has ever been reported.

At this point it may well seem that we have all but demolished the Gerstmann syndrome. Yet not so—for, given enormous individual differences, imperfect examining procedures, symptoms changing over time, and so forth, it seems reasonable, in the final analysis, to accept as a genuine syndrome any set of separable symptoms which occur in relative isolation and which can be related via a common neuropsychological factor. Adopting this standard, I conclude that it is justifiable to speak of a Gerstmann, or at least "Gerstmannesque" syndrome, but not defensible to enshrine the four symptoms originally posited by Gerstmann; rather, there seems to be a somewhat wider (or more diluted) set of symptoms, including (but not necessarily restricted to) spelling difficulties, ordering difficulties, and difficulties in copying and drawing, as well as minor difficulties in naming and in understanding complex linguistic messages. This clinical condition can result from a relatively discrete lesion in the left parietal (angular gyrus) region or as a later stage in the resolution of a more widespread lesion. When these symptoms co-occur, the chances are extremely high that there will be pathology in this region, and not in another one. On the other hand, occurrence of a single disorder (e.g., writing) or even of two Gerstmann components is insufficient to localize the patient's lesion. Support for the viability of the Gerstmann syndrome comes from the paradoxical fact that a lesion in the neighboring area (the distribution of the posterior cerebral artery) can produce a complementary set of disturbances. In these cases, writing (and analogous linguistic functions), spatial orientation, left-right orientation, and finger-gnosis may all remain relatively intact, but the abilities of reading, naming colors, and remembering visual presentations are impaired. It is just such juxtapositions of lesions and syndromes that are so valuable in diagnosis and treatment. Faced with Gerstmann's set of symptoms, the neurologist will locate a tumor or stroke in a different area than when he is confronted with the posterior cerebral signs.

What may, at the outset, have seemed a dispute over the facts of the syndrome may now be viewed in another light. The usefulness of Dr. Gerstmann's syndrome comes from the fact that, given a certain cluster of symptoms, one may be able to determine with some precision the locale of the sufferer's brain disease. (Much the same justification can be advanced—in my view with much greater warrant—in support of other so-called pure disorders, like alexia with agraphia or visual agnosia.) The flaw in this is that, in giving a name to the various symptoms, one is necessarily making enormous and highly risky assumptions about the factors operative in mathematical calculations, left-right localization, or the writing of paragraphs. As we come to understand better the factors that contribute to such activities in both normal and brain-injured individuals, the components may well be replaced by less flashy, more purely descriptive terms (e.g., difficulty in distinguishing spatially aligned elements which differ in only one discriminable feature; or, inability to coordinate a large amount of graphic information). If this should happen, one should then be able to devise wholly new tasks (e.g., to distinguish between similarly colored egg-cups arranged in a given order) and to predict the performance of a "Gerstmann" patient on them. Such a predictive method would seem to be the ultimate test of the viability of a syndrome. In the meantime, we confront a situation where the Gerstmann syndrome is likely to remain useful to certain practitioners, while becoming increasingly distasteful to scientific "strict constructionists." While, for the physician "to be able to call a demon by its name is halfway to getting rid of him," to the scientist bent on explanation,

Once these special categories have been established, there is a tendency not only to use these in the observation and description of subsequent case material but also to allow them to determine to some extent which behavioral events are selected for study and report and which not.

The chief scientific justification for positing a syndrome, then, may be the impetus this very positing provides for eventually dissolving the syndrome through an unraveling of its operative mechanisms.

In 1970 the *Viennese Journal of Neurological Treatment* published "Some Posthumous Notes on the Gerstmann Syndrome," by Josef Gerstmann. This short piece was based on notes that had been made by Gerstmann just before his death the previous year, collated by his widow, and edited by a sympathetic critic. In the article, Gerstmann once again cites the numerous reports that support his position, chides Benton for persisting in an error that Gerstmann had earlier "pointed out" to him, and seeks to correct Critchley's impression that some of Gerstmann's colleagues had dissociated themselves from his position by the early 1930's. Gerstmann remained convinced until the close of his life that he had made a major scientific discovery; he insisted that "impure" forms of the syndrome constituted no evidence against its existence in pure form. For an epigraph to the article, Gerstmann quoted Churchill: "The truth is incontrovertible. Panic may resent it; ignorance may deride it; malice may destroy it; but it is there." Few would today echo Gerstmann's belief that his discovery was impregnable to attack or revision. Yet, to the extent that his undeniably brilliant intuition has helped lay the groundwork for a better understanding of higher cortical functions, he indeed made an important contribution to the advancement of scientific knowledge.

We have taken a searching look at a particular neuropsychological syndrome, one that has engendered more than its share of controversy, only to conclude that both the announcement of its birth and the reports of its demise have been somewhat overstated. Dr. Gerstmann's syndrome is far from all (and only all) that he claimed; but neither is it simply a horrid mistake, to be excised instantly from all medical textbooks and scientific chronicles. The realization that even imperfect entities have diagnostic value for clinical practitioners is important: this practical use alone would justify the continued resort to such diagnoses as *auditory agnosia* or *transcortical motor aphasia,* even if belief in pure instances of these disorders could no longer be sustained. At the same time, we stand warned that clinicians' impressions are often insufficient for scientific purposes. If disease entities are to be considered scientifically valid, their existence must be placed in "experimental jeopardy"—that is, a clear definition of the entity must be propounded and empirical investigations launched, these either substantiating the proposed syndrome and uncovering its neurological basis, or calling it severely into question.

The precariousness of the Gerstmann syndrome should, moreover, not be construed as a critique of all "pure" neuropsychological syndromes. Disorders like Korsakoff's disease, conditions like pure alexia, aphasic classifications like Broca's or Wernicke's, have proved far more robust in the face of critical examination. Indeed, in each of these cases, increasingly "hard" experimental evidence has now been uncovered in support of both the clinical symptoms and the neurological substrate of the alleged disorder. Here, then, is the merit of the searching critique à la Benton: it may, on the one hand, undermine the classical syndrome, but, on the other, it may also place decades of clinical intuition on a much firmer scientific basis. And when clinical impressions and experimental findings reinforce one another, then the claim for a specific neuropsychological disease entity is compelling indeed.

With our review of the Gerstmann syndrome, we conclude that portion of this book devoted primarily to isolated disorders of higher cortical function. Our concern now shifts to more general disease processes, which affect the gamut of cortical functions; and we consider certain pivotal questions about brain disease, such as its effect on artistry, its implications for the sense of self, and the revelations it yields concerning the anatomical division of labor between the two hemispheres. To begin with, we shall focus our attention on a collection of breakdowns markedly different in character from those so far encountered in our inquiry.

# 7 The Breakdown of Mental Processes

*I fear I am not in my perfect mind.*

—KING LEAR,
ACT IV, SCENE 7

A common thread runs through the tangled web of disturbances we have reviewed heretofore. In nearly all cases, the patient has suffered an insult—usually a stroke—to a specific part of his brain, leading to the loss of particular functions, against a background of many more-or-less spared functions. Such lesions yield invaluable information about how capacities are organized, and which are fundamentally akin, in the normal brain. Yet, in some ways, the brain may be said to resemble a brick building, which can be destroyed in numerous ways. A missile may strike a single window or office, leaving the rest of the structure intact. Or it may devastate an area of comparable size at the foundation of the building, thereby toppling the whole structure. There may be simultaneous attacks on a variety of sites in the building, making repair very difficult; or an equally extensive series of attacks, taking place over a long period of time, each of which is individually thwarted so that the overall structure remains in reasonably good shape. There may be a slow disintegration of the mortar, sufficiently gradual that it may not be noticed, until at last the building has become so fundamentally rotten that one day the entire structure abruptly disintegrates. And so on. While no exact parallel is intended between edifices of brick and of nerve cells, the processes by which the mind can break down are equally varied, the results equally disparate, and ofttimes informative about the manner of original construction.

In this chapter we shall look at some typical patterns of breakdown, due to disease processes, old age, and other onslaughts on the nervous system. By relating them to one another, and by contrasting them to the construction of the building blocks of the mind in the young child, we shall attempt to make some sense of these breakdowns. First, we shall encounter four individuals whose mental breakdowns each reflect a highly characteristic pattern.

E.J., aged 58, is a former bookkeeper and amateur musician. Up to three years ago he was an active member of the community, a good family man, a performing violinist at the local symphony orchestra, and an efficient, hard-working accountant with a successful wholesale business. One day, while on an outing, E.J. amazed his family by getting lost and being unable to read a road map. Gradually thereafter, he began to withdraw from other persons, and to deteriorate intellectually. He stopped playing his violin, complaining that he was making too many mistakes. He found his work increasingly difficult to do and was constantly making computational errors; finally he and his employer agreed upon a voluntary retirement. He had particular difficulty in remembering actions that he was supposed to carry out, and in mastering new names and facts.

At first, E.J.'s family clung to the hope that his condition merely represented a temporary depression or setback. But one day, when it became clear that he no longer knew the name of the President, they took him to a physician. After he had made the rounds of specialists and undergone a plethora of tests, he was tentatively diagnosed as suffering from Alzheimer's disease, an irreversible degenerative disease of the brain that was in effect making him prematurely senile. His condition continued to deteriorate, so that after another year he could no longer remain at home. His memory was now so poor that he would forget when something had been placed on the stove; his ability to control his actions was so impaired that he burned the furniture and himself with cigarettes; his speech was so impaired that he could hardly express or understand anything. One day while in the shower, he panicked completely when unable to open the door—only the timely arrival of his daughter averted a major crisis. It would seem but a matter of time before his deterioration is complete; within one or two more years, his death will likely follow.

I asked E.J. to come into my office to speak with me. He answered to his name but appeared confused about what was wanted until I beckoned him to follow. He stumbled down the hall, sighing heavily and sat down opposite me.

Though dressed only in simple hospital garb, E.J. remained an impressive figure. He was well groomed, with hair cut and nails trimmed; he had a neat mane of white hair, his glasses were clean, he sat relatively straight and maintained a thoughtful, if mildly disturbed, expression. Observed at a distance, he might have appeared indistinguishable from a patient on the surgical or medical wards.

I asked him to spell his first name, Elmer. "El . . hu, M-E-R . . . no, that's not, E-L-R-E, . . . oh, never mind," he replied, over a two-minute period in which we both grew extremely uncomfortable. I didn't ask him to spell his last name but instead requested his age.

"I really don't under . . . ," he replied.

"Where do you live?"

"In El . . . mer," he said, rather relieved to have gotten something out at least.

"No, where is your home?" I corrected. "Is it in Boston?"

"No."

"Dorchester?"

"No."

"Cambridge?"

"No."

"Belmont?"

"Yes," he responded immediately, evincing marked satisfaction at a successful communication. I asked him to name some objects about the room. Of all those to which I pointed, he only named "glasses" correctly on his own. When he was supplied with terms to choose among, his performance improved, but he still gave the incorrect answer, or no answer at all, on half of the items selected.

We tried some simple calculation problems. Again, he was unable to provide a single answer on his own. After I had repeated the sum $5 + 5$ many times, he did succeed in raising both hands, displaying ten fingers. But the question "$2 \times 2$" elicited only a sheepish "Oh, boy, oh, boy," repeated over and over again. When I posed a third problem, he protested: "I just don't . . . you have people who make . . . and so forth . . . and so forth . . . and it becomes . . . I just don't like it"—each phrase accompanied by a helpless wave of the hand. As before, he failed on the name of the President, but when I supplied it, he retorted, "That's it, a real bastard."

"Why?" I asked.

"Because, I don't like him. He's a cookie, what you call it." E.J. also selected the vice-president's name from among multiple choices, adding the comment, "That's one of them." However, he was unable to pick out the names of the mayor of Boston or the governor of Massachusetts from such lists.

Examination of his language skills revealed that E.J. was better at repeating sentences than at any other task; he was completely unable to write, and could only read single-digit numbers and a few familiar words. He echoed a number of sentences correctly but then began to perseverate on earlier items and I had to discontinue the testing. His naming of objects was abysmal but more often than not he did assent when offered the correct name. Rarely could he express an idea verbally, but sometimes one was able to decipher the intended meaning from his tone of voice and accompanying gestures.

Tests of his ability to carry out simple actions produced very pitiful performances: He could neither draw any objects nor copy any figures, not even when I sought to guide his hands. He was unable to light his own cigarette or to comb his hair until I placed his hand in the right position. Given an envelope and a letter and told to place the letter in the envelope, he did not grasp the intent of the command despite numerous explanations and supporting gestures on my part. He did "salute" when I issued the command, but was unable to show me how he waved goodbye, or coughed. Given the appropriate props, he was able to brush his teeth but, when through, he didn't know where to put the brush. And he retained the paste in his mouth, unable to swallow it or to spit it out. He was somewhat better at imitating gestures that I made with my body but, as with the sentence-repetition task, he quickly reverted to a reenactment of prior sequences and was unable to break out of this "set."

I was unprepared for E.J.'s excellent perfomance in one area—that of duplicating various rhythmic patterns. Once he had grasped the basic idea, he succeeded in reproducing rhythms of some complexity, and his performance was qualitatively different than it had been at other tasks: he responded immediately and energetically and displayed remarkably few perseverations. His success in the musical sphere stood in stark contrast to the depressed level of his other functions. Although he could neither name melodies he heard nor produce melodies whose names were given, he was able to continue almost any motif which I began, never with the words, but consistently with appropriate rhythm, pitch, and phrasing. Here was a severely demented patient with relative sparing of at least one higher cortical function, possibly due to the great prominence this function had assumed in his earlier life, or to his unusually potent motivation in that domain.

Mr. A.P. was an eighty-three-year-old man who entered the hospital not because there was anything particularly wrong with him, but just because he was "getting old" and "my sister can't take care of me any more." This description was essentially accurate. Until the death of his wife three years before, he had been a healthy, well-contented retired schoolteacher living in central Florida. Thereafter he had moved back North to live with his sister in a Boston suburb. There he had helped with the household chores, played cards with the neighbors, and gone on little walks around the neighborhood. None of these activities ceased completely, but the pace at which they were carried out and his general liveliness and alertness slowly diminished. Eventually, with his sister becoming increasingly arthritic, and his niece having moved away, he could no longer remain in his sister's home. Aware of his eligibility as a World War I veteran, and in consideration of the gradual decline of his faculties, the family succeeded in having him admitted to our Unit for observation.

Upon learning that Mr. P. was a card player, I pulled out a deck and asked him if he'd like to play a game of gin rummy. Slightly suspicious of a doctor who played cards, but no doubt happy to have something to do, he agreed. I gave him the cards to shuffle.

He shuffled the deck dexterously and dealt out two hands. In the first games neither of us played with particular distinction, but we both avoided major errors.

After about fifteen minutes, however, Mr. P.'s performance steadily deteriorated: he began to discard cards he should have saved and, on two occasions, confused his hearts with his diamonds. "I'm not myself today," he said, and we stopped playing.

"Does that happen often?"

"What was that?" he asked.

I repeated the question and he said, "Well, I don't know. Come to think of it, I do forget the cards sometimes but usually I play better. We'll have to play again later. That is, if it's all right with you, sir."

I explained to Mr. P. that I wanted to ask him some questions and administer a few tests. He readily agreed. "That's what I'm here for, I suppose," he said modestly.

At this point, I began to administer a standard intelligence test, the Wechsler Adult Intelligence Scale. I use this test with patients like Mr. P. not because I have faith in its accuracy in quantifying that somewhat mystical entity, the intellect, but because it contains various measures of linguistic, numerical, mnemonic, and cognitive capacity that together serve as a convenient aid in an initial assessment of the patient's abilities and disabilities. (As regards intelligence in general—assuming any really precise definition is possible—it might be more accurately measured, in my own view, by the use of items not included in the Wechsler Scale; my "ideal" test would certainly tap the capacity for operational thinking so properly emphasized by Piaget, or the ability to learn new materials, an element almost completely missing from standard IQ instruments.) The Wechsler has the indisputable advantage of providing effective norms for gauging performance relative to age, educational background, and type of brain disease, among other factors. Without the test, to be sure, a sort of intuitive, rough-and-ready judgment on the patient's competence could still be made, based on a compound of training and experience. But after administering the Wechsler,

I can conclude with some confidence that the patient is doing either well, adequately, or poorly for a person of his status and condition, and that he exhibits expected or unanticipated strengths and weaknesses.

Having determined that Mr. P. tired quickly, a factor that might have interfered with a fair assessment of his capabilities, I made two modifications in the procedure. First of all, I administered the test in a number of short sittings; second, I did not time his performance, but simply scored him right or wrong on each item. I also gave him a standard memory test (designed by the same man, David Wechsler, who devised the Wechsler Scale proper).

Let me quote a few items in order to convey the flavor of Mr. P.'s performance. Asked to define the Apocrypha, he gave virtually the exact answer found in the Wechsler manual: "A number of books of the Bible whose authorship is disputed." Queried on what praise and punishment have in common, he again came up with an excellent response: "They're both ways of conveying to someone else what you think of what they are doing." On the digit-symbol test, where each number on a written sheet has to be paired with an arbitrary symbol, he proceeded very slowly but, after ten minutes, completed the whole exercise correctly. On the memory test, he was able to provide information about his early life rapidly and with complete accuracy.

On other parts of the test, however, Mr. P. fared much less well. He was able to repeat only four successive numbers after me, consistently failing when required to remember a five-number series. He had difficulty in assembling jigsaw puzzles which, when completed, depicted a hand and an elephant; and he failed dismally in copying a series of designs made up of nine blocks colored red and white. He kept looking back and forth between the model and the blocks, muttering, "I never did anything like this before." One of his worst performances occurred on a part of the memory test where he had to acquire a list of new and quite arbitrary associations to a set of familiar words. Though told five times that the word *cabbage* was supposed to be associated with *pen,* he consistently said "lettuce" for that item. And when asked to remember a rather detailed story about a scrubwoman who lost some money and was helped out of her difficulty by the local policeman, he recalled the gist of the story but failed to retain many of its details, such as the lady's name, the area where she lived, her family circumstances, the way in which she had lost and recovered her money.

All in all, then, Mr. P. performed most successfully on items where he was required to draw on knowledge acquired earlier in life, such as general information, the definition of words, and the relationship among concepts. He also performed creditably, albeit very slowly, on any task where painstaking accuracy was demanded. Where he did not distinguish himself was on the few items where he had to remember new information—and he was particularly poor when he had to combine a series of arbitrary elements into a new configuration, like a block design or an unknown puzzle. This profile was borne out in his scores: his verbal IQ was 115, a sign that he had once been of above-average intelligence; his IQ on the nonverbal or performance part of the test was 85, a huge drop; and his memory score was equally wide of his former intellectual level, at 83.

In the ensuing days, I came to know Mr. P. well and had the opportunity regularly to observe his behavior around the ward. He was unfailingly kind and courteous, greeting me each morning with a friendly hello and a smile. I concluded that he recognized me, for, while courteously nodding to everyone, he only spoke to the regular personnel on the ward. But he was never able to remember my name without prompting, though I told it to him a dozen times; he would always recall it, however, as soon as I gave him the first letter or asked him to pick it out from among multiple choices. We played cards again several times and, as Mr. P. himself had indicated, his performance was extremely variable. On some days, particularly in the morning and when the weather was good, he would play with considerable skill, speed, and accuracy; on other days, he would perfom even worse than on the first day, committing elementary errors and giving up as much in resignation as disgust. I observed a similar pattern when he played the piano. Sometimes he could perform "The Blue Danube Waltz" and "Für Elise" with accuracy and aplomb; on other occasions, a plethora of errors would creep in, his hands would get all fouled up, and he would abruptly close the keyboard. One day his sister came to the hospital and he enthusiastically requested that I meet her. We conversed for half an hour, and Mr. P. was in very good form. He was laughing, telling jokes, and reminiscing with (I learned later) complete accuracy about their childhood together in Ohio. But discussion of current affairs was not so easy for him: he was uninformed about what was going on in the world, and he had forgotten that his sister's daughter had moved away, for he asked, "Why didn't you bring Cathy along?"

"Why, dear, what's happened to you?" his sister exclaimed, with what seemed a knowing glance at me. "Cathy moved away from here three months ago."

Mr. P. stopped for a moment and looked around despondently. "My goodness, I plumb forgot. I must be getting old."

Mr. J.L. has been a patient on our Service, off and on, for two years. When he first came to us, he was slowly recovering from a severe automobile accident in which the front of his head had been badly bashed in. He had been comatose for several days, and two operations on his frontal lobes had been necessary, during the second of which the surgeons had had to remove approximately ten cubic centimeters of tissue. He had been in the insurance business before his accident, and his numerous trophies, photographs, and letters from friends during the initial postoperative days confirmed our impression that he had been a vigorous, active individual, an exemplar of the successful insurance salesman.

During the months after his surgery, J.L. gradually returned to normal—or so it appeared to those who had observed him from the time of his life-and-death struggle. His memory, which at first had been devastated by an amnesia extending back over several years, gradually recovered until he recollected everything he had experienced up to a short time before he had lost consciousness. At the same time, his ability to acquire new information, such as the name of the hospital, the day of the week, the names of the various doctors and therapists, also returned to near-normal. He was able to walk well, could take care of himself more or less normally, regained some weight, and had no difficulty either in speaking or in understanding speech. Indeed, he was able to play cards with skill, he regularly listened to the radio and watched television, and it seemed but a matter of months before he could return home to his family, resume his active career, and look back on the accident as merely an unfortunate episode, however painful.

It was not to be so. Two grave symptoms suggested to us that J.L. might never again be as he once had been.

First of all, he slept all day. While this is a familiar reaction in patients who have had severe trauma, there is usually a gradual resumption of the normal sleep-waking cycle, and a return of motivation to put one's affairs in order, to make and consummate plans. J.L. persisted in his diurnal slumber, however, while all through the night he would remain vigilantly awake, pacing the halls, watching television.

Second, he invented a bizarre account of his injury on

which he adamantly insisted, despite our continual explanations to the contrary.

"Well, I got it in a baseball game, Doctor. I was hit by a baseball."

"Look in the mirror, Mr. L——. You can't get a hole like that from a baseball."

"Well I did, I remember that I did."

"No, that's not true. You were in an automobile accident and you had to be operated on to get rid of the debris and to close the wound."

"Well, that's what you tell me, Doctor, but I know that I was hit by a baseball."

As far as we could determine, J.L. had indeed played baseball a few days before his automobile accident, though no one is sure whether he was actually hit by a ball. In any event, he had seemed all right until the accident. An initial inability to remember the cause of injury is common and not in itself remarkable; it was the sheer unyieldingness of J.L.'s insistence on his baseball game, despite constant assurances to the contrary by his family, friends, and physicians, that signaled that his recovery was not proceeding as it should.

The pattern into which J.L. fell is, alas, that in which he remains mired to this day. Engaged in casual conversation, he appears well; indeed, he displays a ready wit and is reasonably well informed about current events. On all standard intellectual testing he performs above average, presumably at about (though perhaps slightly below) the level he held prior to his accident. Deficits can be shown on a few highly specific tests, particularly ones which probe ability to shift mental "set" or to follow a new direction quickly; but one must be careful not to place undue emphasis on such marginal findings. As noted, he plays cards well, can master new information easily, and behaves more or less appropriately when confronted by physicians, family members, and the decreasing circle of old friends who still come to see him.

His intellectual integrity notwithstanding, J.L. is a completely changed man. Gone are the enthusiasm and drive that molded him into a successful salesman. Instead, we have a quiet, retiring, somnolent individual, who seldom speaks except when spoken to, who exhibits no desire to return home (though, if pressed, will claim that he does), who passes the time watching televsion, solving crossword puzzles, or just sitting, and who, during daylight hours, remains (perhaps to avoid contact with other people) Oblomov-like in his bed, resting if not sleeping. We ask when he expects to return to work and he invariably assures us, "Very soon." But he never does, nor does he even initiate the slightest steps to do so. His family has lost interest in having him at home, and he walks around generally uncombed, disheveled, unshaven, his appearance announcing to the world what is also clear from his conversation, that he no longer cares very much about anything. Yet he is not devoid of feeling. When provoked, as with the story about how his accident occurred, he will get angry. And one day he commented to one of us, "Why, you know me, Doc, I'm just an appendage around here. I'm just a vegetable."

The fourth patient I will briefly sketch is an individual whom I never met personally, but who has gained justifiable notoriety. He represents the first modern example of a "callosal disconnection," an exceedingly uncommon disorder which was occasionally described in the classical Continental literature in the field. P.K. was a forty-one-year-old policeman when he was admitted to the Neurology Service of our hospital in March 1961. During the previous month he had begun to develop dull headaches, frequently in association with nausea and vomiting. The members of his family had also observed personality and behavior changes, including increased forgetfulness, apathy, confusion, and abrasiveness in social relations, particularly at work.

Neurological testing indicated the presence of a tumor, and the patient was immediately operated on. After surgery he showed a severe paralysis on his right side and a marked aphasia. He improved steadily in linguistic and motor functions, but continued to display a variety of cognitive deficits in memory, calculation, and abstract thought. In the course of routine testing, it was discovered by Dr. Edith Kaplan that the patient could not write with his left hand. This wholly unexpected finding prompted a detailed examination of his clinical picture.

At the time of these special tests, the patient was only mildly aphasic. Asked to write with his right hand, he performed quite normally. Letters, words, numbers, and sentences were correctly written to dictation, and he was able to copy printed material, converting it (as do most individuals) to script in the process. His performance with his left hand, however, offered the sharpest possible contrast: His letters were either incorrect or completely unrecognizable; when requested to write particular words or sentences, he would produce an altogether illegible scrawl. He could copy printed materials, but instead of converting to script, he would faithfully imitate each detail of the block letters. When allowed to view these error-laden productions, he was quite astonished. Yet he could not spontaneously correct his errors as long as he was using his left hand.

P.K.'s left-hand performance was tested further by requiring him to recognize objects by touch with that hand when he was blindfolded. His answers, given orally, were hardly ever correct, and indeed, generally went absurdly far afield: a ring was identified as an eraser, a padlock as a book of matches, a watch as a balloon. But when told, instead, that he should simply indicate how to use the object—for example, make pounding movements to signify a hammer—he did so correctly. Even then, however, he would punctuate this correct demonstration with such grossly inappropriate asides as "I would use this to comb my hair with it." When he was presented, still blindfolded, with an object which was then taken away, and he was thereupon asked to retrieve it from among a group of objects in a box, he was able to do this successfully. Most dramatically, he was even able to make a correct drawing with his left hand of an object that had earlier been placed in that hand and subsequently removed.

According to Drs. Norman Geschwind and Edith Kaplan, who investigated this patient intensively, those functions governed by the right side of the brain (the control of the left limbs) and those governed by the left side of the brain (the control of the right limbs and all linguistic behaviors) appeared out of contact with one another. "He appears to behave," these investigators argued "as if there were two nearly isolated half-brains, functioning almost independently." This surmise was strengthened by a demonstration that objects placed in either hand could not be identified by the other hand, and that a task learned by one hand (such as a simple maze) had to be completely relearned by the other—whereas normal individuals routinely "transfer" learning across limbs and across cerebral hemispheres. Carrying out commands with the right hand, such as drawing a square, waving goodbye, or pretending to brush his teeth, posed no problems; these same commands, however, could not be executed with the left hand. Asked to draw a square with that hand, he drew a circle. Instructed to point to the examiner with his left index finger, he pointed to his own eye with his left index and middle finger. Commanded to pretend to brush his teeth with his left hand, he on one occasion pretended to lather his face, and on another, mimed combing his hair.

Just how the patient's left hand (or right hemisphere) knew what act to perform, or even that it was to perform any act at all, is a perplexing question, given the a-linguistic nature of the right hemisphere. Either some information (a degraded signal) was coming from the left hemisphere;

or the right hemisphere *was* comprehending language to some degree, or, more likely, nonverbal cues or other efforts to put the patient into the "right set" were partially effective. This puzzle has not received the attention it deserves.

The phenomena observed by Geschwind and Kaplan were in themselves unambiguous and compelling. Their interpretation in terms of disconnected hemispheres, however, was controversial; to support it, they had to cast doubt upon rival explanations for P.K.'s bizarre left-side performance. The possibility that his inability to name objects was due to tactile difficulties was ruled out by his ability, when tested in this sense modality, to match objects and to act out appropriate sequences with them. Only when verbal identification was required did the patient fail. Nor could the inability to write be attributed to elementary motor difficulties, for P.K. drew quite well with this hand and was able to copy letters without difficulty. There was always the possibility that the patient was hysterical or else malingering, but his general behavior did not fit either of these diagnoses; in addition, the restriction of the disorder to *one* side of the body was incredible as a psychological defense. The possibility of a general spatial or perceptual disorder, resulting from a lesion in the right hemisphere, was also excluded, given the fact that the patient performed satisfactorily on spatial tasks as long as no verbal components were included.

Having thus eliminated the more plausible alternatives, Geschwind and Kaplan concluded that P.K.'s condition was explicable as a display of autonomous behavior on the part of the two hemispheres, each behaving as if physically disconnected from the other. As long as stimulus and response were both confined to the same hemisphere, whether left or right, there was correct performance. As soon as a response required the coordination of the two hemispheres, however, there was failure—for example, when an object placed in the left hand had to be named, or when an object placed in one hand had to be selected from a group by the other hand. This daring hypothesis of a split between the hemispheres was confirmed when the patient died the following year. Inspection of the brain revealed a large lesion in the frontal portion of the left hemisphere (where the tumor had been), and a marked thinning of the corpus callosum, the band of tissue which connects the two hemispheres, resulting in a "cerebral disconnection syndrome." There was no involvement of the right hemisphere. Shortly afterwards, Professors Bogen, Vogel, and Sperry at the California Institute of Technology reported a program of surgery in which they had disconnected the two cerebral hemispheres of selected patients in order to stop the transmission of epileptic seizures from one hemisphere to the other. In their careful studies of patients (further described in chapter 9), these investigators have confirmed many of the findings originally reported in the "naturally occurring" history of P.K.

Four patients, four different patterns of breakdown. There is the former accountant-violinist, E.J., who has sustained severe dementia in every area, with the possible sparing of his musical capacity; the old man A.P., who still retains his faculties in substantial measure, but is beginning to decline sharply in a number of cognitive and memory domains; the salesman J.L. involved in an accident, essentially normal on conventional testing, who has nonetheless undergone a profound personality change; and P.K., the policeman with a brain tumor, whose left side is no longer in contact with the right side of his body. Numerous other cases could be cited, each representing a different pattern of breakdown, an alternative way of dislodging the bricks comprising the structure of the mind. But these four cases do provide a kind of capsule panorama of the manifold ways in which cognitive capacities may be altered by diseases of the brain. Let us now examine the nature of the disease process that was implicated in each case and trace the kinds of deficits that accompany it.

In 1906, at a meeting of the Southwest German Society of Alienists (*alienist* being the old term for *psychiatrist*), Alois Alzheimer recounted his findings in the case of a fifty-one-year-old woman. This patient initially presented the symptoms of defective memory and increasing disorientation in time and space. These were followed by increased depression and hallucination, then by a profound dementia in which the full range of mental abilities—language, recognition, understanding, execution of voluntary movements—was gradually devastated. When the woman died and Alzheimer examined her brain, he found that the entire cerebral cortex—the outer mantle where the highest levels of mentation are thought to be mediated—had atrophied. When further cases of this type had been described, and the neuropathological picture confirmed, Alzheimer's name became attached to the disease pattern he had been first to identify.

Alzheimer's disease is a form of pre-senile dementia. Whereas most older persons undergo a slow, perhaps even dignified, decline in mental abilities, a few individuals have the misfortune of sustaining a more pernicious and rapid form of dementia at an earlier time in life. These pathologies—Alzheimer's disease as well as such other dementing processes as Pick's disease and Jakob-Creutzfeld disease—involve an active degeneration of the nerve cells of the brain, particularly in the cortex, leading to a rapid decline in mental skills. Paradoxically, at least in the case of Alzheimer's disease, elementary reflexes remain normal and the patient's general demeanor is unremarkable—at least in these senses, even Alzheimer's disease is "selective." Neither prevention nor treatment for these diseases is known. For certain ones there do appear to be familial or ethnic predilections; as in most other areas of health, a careful choice of ancestors can forestall great misfortunes.

Although these dementing diseases of middle life have certain similarities, each features a more-or-less characteristic pattern, and can usually be distinguished by observation of the patient's behavior. Alzheimer's disease makes its appearance gradually over a period of one or two years, during which the patient's memory declines, he experiences naming difficulty, and finds increasing difficulty in finding his way around and in handling other spatial tasks; there may also be personality changes, including a pronounced lack of spontaneity and a tendency to flair up in anger, only to calm down with equal speed. The second stage involves more serious manifestations of decline, such as clear-cut linguistic defects in expression and comprehension, increasing difficulty in recognizing and remembering, growing incapacity to carry out sequences of actions. There may be spurts of jealousy and paranoia, but, as cognitive functions decline, disorientation and lack of awareness supplant these more "organized" reactions of the personality. The patient, who may look presentable and whose former station in life will often still be perceptible, will increasingly spend his time resting or sitting quietly, looking perplexed, answering questions in the halting and stumbling manner of E.J.

Finally, in the concluding or terminal phase of the illness, the patient is completely unable to perform any sort of intellectual function. There may be cerebral seizures, as well as a kind of generalized primitivization known as the Klüver-Bucy syndrome. This behavior pattern—first identified in monkeys whose temporal lobes had been removed by researchers Heinrich Klüver and Paul Bucy—includes total inability to recognize anything in the visual modality (visual agnosia), a tendency to touch every object in sight and to introduce it into one's mouth (hyperorality), diminution of emotion to the point of complete dullness and apathy, and, in certain cases, hypersexual activity, with the patient indulging in the full range of sexual behaviors, including self-play and both homosexual and heterosexual relations. By this time, needless to say, the patient is so demented that there is no question of conscious planning or pursuit of pleasure involved in these activities; rather, like Klüver and Bucy's lobotomized monkeys, he is at the mercy of the "brutish" parts of his brain.

It is the temporal and parietal lobes that Alzheimer's disease attacks with particular perniciousness. This is the region of the brain that governs many higher-level intellectual activities, such as language behavior. The frontal lobes of the brain are relatively spared until the concluding phase of this disease. In contrast, another dementing process, called Pick's disease, begins by attacking the frontal lobes. Comparative observation of victims of these conditions, therefore, offers dramatic evidence of the respective behaviors mediated by the parieto-temporal and frontal lobes. The Alzheimer patient, as already noted, is socially appropriate in behavior and may retain an impressive personal appearance, even when his cognitive abilities are already severely debilitated. The Pick patient, on the other hand, is socially inappropriate in behavior and appears disheveled and unconcerned virtually from the onset of the disease, at a time when his parietal and temporal lobes are still spared and his intellectual functioning appears relatively adequate.

In some respects, at least, a sufferer in the early stages of Pick's disease resembles our patient J.L., whose cognitive capacities cannot be faulted, but whose personality has undergone profound changes and whose attitudes and behavior have degenerated. J.L.'s condition, resulting from his accident and the surgery that followed, is also reminiscent of that of various individuals whose frontal lobes were removed, in whole or in part, some years ago, at a time when this radical surgical procedure was a fashionable cure for chronic schizophrenia. Frontal (or the more selective pre-frontal) lobotomies came into vogue precisely because they appeared to spare the intelligence while eliminating the most severe psychotic symptoms. Yet it had in fact been determined over a hundred years before that frontal lobotomies were not without their cost.

The first frontal lobotomy was not performed by a surgeon at all, but was the result of a freak accident. In Cavendish, Vermont, in 1848, an explosion sent a huge rod—13¼ pounds, 3½ feet long, and 1¼ inches in diameter—smashing through the head of a young construction foreman named Phineas Gage. The rod passed through the front of his skull, from his left cheek to the upper right portion of his head. Although survival seemed unlikely, Gage in fact sat up a few moments later, touched his wound, and asked, "Where's my rod?" Defying the fears of the attending physician, one Dr. Harlow, Gage not only survived the night but went on to live for another twelve years. His personality, however, underwent a profound alteration. In place of the softspoken, reliable foreman he had been, there now stood a loud-mouthed, obnoxious soul who cursed continuously, exhibited little sense of purpose, and wandered aimlessly until his death in San Francisco in 1860. IQ tests were not available at the time, of course, but it seems fairly safe to assume that Phineas Gage's intelligence was altered to a much smaller extent than his personality. For, despite their prominent location, the large convolutions of tissue just underneath the front of the skull seem to be less involved with an individual's ability to handle delimited problems and tasks than with his capacity to plan ahead, to monitor and tend to his personal appearance, to care about the impression that he makes upon others, and to make his mark in the world.

This is not to suggest that the frontal lobes play no role at all in cognitive functioning (though that was the prevailing wisdom at the time when lobotomies were regularly performed). It is more precise to say that the kinds of functions tapped by IQ tests are relatively spared by removal of the frontal lobes, while other intellectual functions, of a more subtle but equally significant sort, *are* clearly implicated. The frontal lobes in man are the last to develop in a physiological sense and presumably are also the last to be integrally involved in the mental life of man. They seem to assume crucial importance for just those aspects of thought which emerge only in adolescence or adulthood: the ability to think about oneself as a separate individual, to make elaborate plans and to see that they are carried out, to alter goals when that seems appropriate, to form a model of the world and of one's relationship to it, to behave and respond appropriately across diverse social situations, to mediate between the pressures of the outer world and one's own inner promptings.

It is noteworthy that all other parts of the brain have elaborate connections with the frontal lobes—Nature's hint, as it were, that this is where "it's all put together." Thus the individual without frontal lobes may appear to have his various subparts functioning adequately, and hence will perform well on a variety of tests. Where he fails is in coordinating his life into an organized whole, an ability extremely difficult to capture in a paper-and-pencil test but, by the same token, one more important for successful living than the digit span or paired-associate learning of the psychologist's laboratory. As these subtle and vital functions of the frontal lobes came to be increasingly confirmed, the clamor for lobotomies died down. Whereas at one time these operations were done "with an icepick" (sometimes literally)—some fifty thousand being undertaken over a single ten-year period, 1945 to 1955, in this country alone—they are hardly ever performed anymore. There are now more delicate operations, as well as powerful drugs, which control seizures or emotional disorders

without blunting such higher sensibilities as abstract thinking, or the power to plan and dream.

The essence of frontal-lobe functioning is epitomized
not only in the Alzheimer patient, who in some sense remains himself despite the atrophy of his intellect, but also
in certain severely aphasic patients who nonetheless retain
a rudimentary ability to express themselves. These individuals display keen insight into their condition. They
know what has occurred; they are appropriately hopeful,
or depressed, depending on how their condition alters
daily; their behavior and attitudes and their appearance
are entirely appropriate; and they often can put into
words, though in admittedly fragmentary form, a correct
understanding of just what is wrong with them. I have in
mind a man named Zasetsky, studied by Luria and described in detail in Chapter 10. In a diary kept over twenty-
five years, Zasetsky produced a marvelous account of his
own shattered world; I also think of a conduction aphasic
whom we have carefully studied on our Service: his understanding and expression remain imperfect, but he is nonetheless able to appreciate what is wrong with him and
what is to be done. He tells me: "I was at zero but now
I'm coming back. I could read nothing; I could say, speak
nothing. Numbers, no good either. But now I'm coming
back. Already I can talk, say what I want to say, see. The
reading, that's next. I can read books for little kids and
then it's going to be fourth grade, fifth grade, right on
there. The writing, that's coming good too. Numbers,
that's still a problem. But can't do them all at the same
time. First the words, then the numbers. I keep track of
what I'm doing. See. And here's the paper from last week
—I still forget how to write that letter, what's it called,
but I've learned to spell 'basket' and 'elephant' and some
other words. I know it's not going to be perfect for a long
time, but I've got time. A year, two years, go to school

every day, I'll be able to go back to my job." The patient
is a lab technician, and it does appear likely that he will
eventually be able to resume his work.

The status of the frontal lobes is, in sum, crucial. Indeed, even the specific locus of injury within these lobes
is an important factor in determining the level of behavior
that can be anticipated in a year or in twenty years. Patients in whom injury or removal occurs in the lower or
orbital surface are less likely to have intellectual deficits,
though they will exhibit a characteristic lack of concern.
Those with destruction in the superior portion of the
frontal lobes are more prone to develop difficulty in discerning relations among disparate elements, sustaining
attention, shifting their mental "set" or "orientation"
rapidly when so required. Still, it should be stressed that
these differences, however significant as regards the diagnosis and prognosis for individual sufferers, are really matters of degree—of variations in the relative prominence
of the several elements in a syndrome (using that term
loosely) shared by all "frontal" patients. In general terms,
then, the frontal patient lacks the ability to organize a
number of elements into a smooth sequence; he fails to
recognize that, on the one hand, the sequence can be carried out, while, on the other, it can be modified or even
scrapped if circumstances warrant it. So particular difficulties arise where a shift in "set" is necessary, or where
impulsive changes intrude.

As for the realm of personality and social relations, the
patient's behavior appears purposeless, meaningless, mis-
guided, conferring a quality of disjointedness or discon-
nectedness on his behavioral repertoire. This may be
because, as lesion studies have documented in other primates, the frontal lobes are crucial for behaviors bearing
on the individual's relation to other members of his social
group, such as grooming, family relations, and codes and
rituals of sexuality, play, and self-assertion. Since the fron-

tal lobes have extensive connections, both to the cortical areas which subsume specific intellectual functions, and to the subcortical areas concerned with feeling and motivation, it is not surprising that severe pathology in this region (such as that suffered by J.L.) exacts a devastating toll on the "whole man."

Whereas the patient with injury to his frontal lobes may be transformed into an entirely different person, the ordinary individual, as he ages, is likely to become ever more entrenched in his habits and style of living. If he is short-tempered and selfish, these tendencies will be heightened; if given to paranoid ideas, he is likely to feel yet more persecuted; if kindly and generous, he may conceivably give away all his possessions and spend his last days rocking softly and contentedly on someone else's back porch. As our patient A.P. noted himself, he was not particularly ill; he was just getting old. His personality, basically cheerful and sunny, became confirmed in his old age; though well into his eighties, he continued to pursue his interests of card-playing, walking, and music-making. True, he had slowed down a bit and his hearing and vision "weren't what they used to be," yet his personality and "identity" remained unchanged to all who had known him in years past.

Our particular interest lay in following a pattern of intellectual deterioration which accompanies the general process of aging. Mr. P. presented a typical, indeed a classic, pattern. The accumulation of years was least evident in those tasks in which acquired information and general linguistic functioning were at a premium. So long as tasks stressed accuracy, not speed, he performed at a high level. Remembrance of things past was remarkably keen, tending to confirm the not uncommon observation by older persons that their memories of remote events become actually more vivid, while the events of the present cease to have much importance, and are only irregularly attended to and absorbed.

Other aspects of intelligence are marked by a sharper decline with age. Especially fragile are such functions as the learning of new information (such as a list of numbers or a set of paired associates) or the placing of elements into an unfamiliar configuration (copying block designs, assembling unfamiliar puzzles). There is a tendency to fall back on tried-and-true methods, to cling to old habits, so that tasks that require a new use for an old skill, or the attainment of a new skill, pose special difficulty for the older person. Sensory acuity, of course, also declines with age and there may be a generally lower level of excitability or arousal; as a result, a more powerful stimulus or more extensive opportunity for responding are required before the aging person will react to a particular situation. Exceptions occur when the aging person is expecting a specific event, like the arrival of a dear friend, or is strongly attached to a particular possession (like a Bible or a cat); under such "heightened" circumstances attention or vigilance remains high and is directed exclusively at these targets.

Research on older persons has yielded a number of other findings, not all of which support the "old wives' tales" about the old. True, women tend to perform better on most tests of intelligence during later life, though the healthiest males perform as well as the most vigorous females. There are vast individual differences among older persons, with some functioning at an optimal rate until well into their 60's or 70's. For the most part, an apogee in intellectual and physical powers is achieved in the decade or two after adolescence, but the decline in performance thereafter is marginal, and can often be counteracted by compensating mechanisms (e.g., accuracy supplants speed). It is noteworthy in this connection that highly educated and intellectual individuals generally perform well until late in life.

When more severe declines begin, usually in the seventh or eighth decade of life, the changes are benign at first. Names are difficult to recall, dates are often confused, there is gradual waning in facility at reasoning and in the ability to learn new materials. The patient becomes increasingly concrete and pragmatic in his approach, responding with what emerges most readily and most habitually, rather than viewing the situation from a novel or unaccustomed perspective that might be more appropriate. Even when new responses are particularly called for, as in the memorization of a fresh word association, the patient is as likely as not to continue producing the word he habitually produced before. Among the factors determining the rate of intellectual decline are the patient's health, his overall physical condition, and his motivation; difficulties in any of these areas are likely to hasten the deterioration in performance. In sum, an inability to learn as well (or, conversely, a heightened tendency to forget) is nigh on to universal in old age, but whether this is due more to a difficulty in processing new information, to interference between competing patterns of information, or to an impairment in retrieving adequately stored information remains strenuously debated.

At some point, these benign and essentially universal trends of old age may be replaced by a sharper, more malignant decline. A precipitous decrease in intellectual functions is Nature's declaration that something is seriously amiss. Sometimes the patient's decline may be due to a depression, brought on by external circumstances perhaps, or by practical or emotional difficulties of one kind or another; if the depression should lift, the patient will regain his earlier cognitive level. Usually, however, some sort of disease process, such as multiple strokes, has set in. Signs of more malignant aging include a severe amnesia which may lead to periods of clouding, confusion, and general diminution of consciousness, delusions and delirium, and inability to assimilate new experiences. Eventually, a terminal phase is signaled, in which the mental and physical decline is completed. The patient loses virtually all awareness of his surroundings and death seems a natural and inevitable dénouement.

Our patient A.P. is in a benign phase of aging. It is entirely possible, of course, that he will eventually succumb to a more malignant form, but equally likely that he will live for many more years, or will perish for some reason unrelated to the aging of his brain.

Why some people age rapidly and die early, while others fully retain their cognitive capacities until they reach the century mark, is a perennial puzzle, on which gerontologists are busily working. Appropriate answers will probably include many well-established principles—the necessity of keeping active, the importance of long-lived antecedents—as well as more specific information about advantageous diets, activities consonant with the aging process, the compensatory mechanisms most profitably adopted. The same question in terms of personality—why some people age gracefully, while others become increasingly desperate, unpleasant, or tyrannical—is also, obviously, of more than academic interest. Finally, the diverse effects of aging on assorted careers and life-styles begs further investigation. George Talland has expressed well the central issue in this regard:

> . . . the contrast of the athlete who, at thirty, is too old for the championship, and the maestro who, at eighty, can still treat us to a memorable performance on the concert stage. . . . Are our aged masters freaks of nature, paragons of self-discipline, or do they but demonstrate the inadequacy of our present notions about the effect of age on human capacities?

We have described persons displaying general declines in abilities, either due to pernicious pre-senile diseases, or to a gradual diminution of powers attendant upon the inexorable onset of old age. We have also observed an individual whose intellectual functions are essentially unchanged but whose personality has undergone major alteration. Our final case, the patrolman P.K., has been cited primarily because of the bizarre split between the two sides of his body, with the resultant gross disparity in their respective capacities to function. In these circumstances, as Geschwind has pointed out, it becomes almost meaningless to talk of *the* person, *the* individual, as if one were describing an inviolable whole. One has, in effect, two persons, or two brains, within one skin, and securing an adequate reply depends upon tapping response mechanisms within only one of these two: One talks not to the patient but rather to the left hemisphere; one shows an object not to the patient but rather to the left or to the right hemisphere.

The radical difference between this latter kind of "disconnection syndrome" and the other forms of general breakdown described here must be stressed. With the two dementing patients, E.J. and A.P., there is more or less widespread atrophy throughout the entire cerebral cortex. In the case of the frontal-lobe patient, there has been damage or removal of a significant body of tissue, one which presumably mediates vital integrating processes in the normal individual. The lesion in a case like P.K.'s, on the other hand, need not be a widespread one, nor need there occur vitiation of any part of the brain mediating a particular function (language capacity, visual perception, personality integration, etc.). Instead, a bundle of connecting fibers that in itself appears to mediate no pattern of behavior, but rather to transmit information from one part of the brain to another, is no longer functioning properly. Thus, the functions served by particular individual regions of the brain seem to be intact, and the functions impaired are just those that can only be accomplished by the transfer of information from a locus A to a locus B. And it takes the accidental discovery of a bizarre phenomenon and the administration of special tests to demonstrate that something is amiss. Once it is discovered, however, a whole set of abilities—those which depend upon the orchestration of centers connected by the association tracts—can be shown to be selectively impaired; for the range of tasks involved, the patient is better thought of as two distinct, separately functioning entities, rather than as a single person who has sustained a certain degree of injury.

Having now completed a review of assorted cortical disorders and disconnections, we may well ask whether there is some pattern among the collection, some coherent overall picture; or whether, instead, the brain can break down in an infinite number of ways, each having little relationship with the others. I believe that a certain coherence does exist, and in this connection it should, I think, be helpful to review some facts about cognitive development in children, and specifically to examine the effect of brain injuries in the developing child.

Certain broad trends seem to characterize the process of mental development. At first rigid and rather unadaptive in his approach to externally imposed tasks, the child becomes increasingly flexible; initially indefinite and diffuse, he learns to give answers which are articulated, definite and precise; given to lability and syncretism in his approach, liable to shift strategies without reason, the child gradually embraces a more stable orientation. The eminent developmental psychologist Heinz Werner has summarized this process by saying that children's behavioral systems become increasingly differentiated—capable of ever finer and more appropriate distinctions in responses to their environment—even as they become hierarchically integrated—organized into a systematic totality whose parts complement one another and can operate in synchrony.

Somewhat more elaborated than Werner's formulation is Jean Piaget's view of cognitive evolution, in which the course of development of the ability to perform particular actions and mental operations is delineated. The child's actions unfold initially in an effort to deal with the world of sensory-motor experience (the manipulation of physical objects); during the middle years of childhood, the child becomes capable of directing the same actions toward mental representations or images of these objects, and so is able to carry out such "operations" in his head; finally, at the advent of adolescence, the child becomes able to execute operations not only upon objects and their images, but also upon verbal and mathematic descriptions of objects and actions. He has now reached the point where he can enter into scientific or logical debate, for he can set up an axiomatic system and proceed to make deductions and inferences from it.

Any experience with the objects or elements of the external world involves at least two potential reactions. The individual may either retain the initial sensory experiences in as pristine and unchanged, or "photographic," form as possible; or he may transform the sensory input in a more or less radical way, arriving at fresh configurations which present the initial information in a novel form. Following Piaget, we may call the "photographic" processing and faithful remembrance of sensory information a "figurative approach"; and the "card-catalog" categorizing or reclassifying of information, an "operative approach."

One finds that the child of seven or eight is already as capable as the adult at figurative forms of thought. Given sounds to hear, sentences to learn, pictures to attend to and remember, he will perform as well as, or even better than, his elders. When, however, the task is one of transforming the initial input in some way, converting the shape of something felt into its visual configuration, or setting some words to music, the older child performs at a significantly higher level. For him, in contrast to the younger child, reclassification and recoding represent relatively natural processes, habitually resorted to because of their efficiency and economy. In sum, figurative processes develop early on in the child's development, perhaps peaking in the years immediately preceding adolescence; operative processes, involving translation across sense modalities or systems of symbols, develop relatively slowly and continue to improve at least through the adolescent period.

The build-up and perfection of various sensory and motor skills is another crucial milestone of childhood. The pre-adolescent child can easily attain a modicum of skill in diverse realms, ranging from bicycle riding to skiing, from learning a foreign language to mastering multiplication tables, from playing the piano to operating a television camera. Youngsters during this period are willing to practice these skills continually, and the more they do, the more accomplished, subtle, and supple their performance becomes. Indeed, so strong is the proclivity of the child to mimic the essential aspects of these acts and to acquire facility in a relatively short time, that the pre-adolescent years may represent a critical period for skill-learning, the time when acquiring skills is easiest. Certainly this conclusion seems safe for the learning of new languages, a phenomenon widely observed, but I suspect it pertains equally well to such "nonlinguistic" skills as piano-playing or skiing, which can also become superlatively "differentiated" and "hierarchically integrated" during this period.

But what happens to the behavioral repertoire of the child or the adult when his brain is injured? From the standpoint of scientific inquiry, it would be more elegant were the process of development simply to be undone, or rolled back, like a film which, though shown in reverse, continues to be plausible. Yet such reversals are in fact fairly unlikely—disintegration at times of stress or in cases

of brain damage seldom follows a simple backward un-
winding of the laborious developmental process. Instead,
certain facets are dramatically transformed, while others
prove relatively resistant to injury.

The form of degeneration that most closely approxi-
mates development-in-reverse is perhaps that occurring in
pre-senile dementias. Recall that in these situations the
primary sensory receptors of the patient remain relatively
intact, while abutting cortical zones concerned with higher-
level capacities, such as recognition, naming, calculation,
or abstraction, decline more rapidly. In Alzheimer's disease, for example, the patient can still repeat what he
hears, find his way about in a familiar setting, or groom
himself; yet he fails on nearly any task in which some
kind of more active mental operation is required. Indeed,
he frequently fails to understand what is being called for.
Such patients seem to have better-preserved figurative
senses: they can more readily perceive and retain than they
can transform or recode what has been perceived.

Still, even in such cases the reversal of the developmental
process is by no means exact. For instance, the early loss
of memory in Alzheimer's disease contrasts strongly with
the excellent recall exhibited by most young persons. And
on the other hand, we should keep in mind the case of
E.J., who, though afflicted with drastic deficiencies in other
high-level skills, retained considerable proficiency in the
performance of music. I suspect that we have here an instance of a skill developed to a very high level during early
life, perhaps during the pre-adolescent years. Such skills
may achieve an independent, autonomous status, so that
they can "run off" or function smoothly even when the
brain is otherwise deranged. As Anton Pick pointed out
many years ago:

Occasionally on an accidental basis, the greater automatization of later acquired functions provides an exception to the rule

and shows that it is not age itself but rather its resultant degree of automatization that determines the increased resistance.

To be sure, even the musical function here will eventually atrophy, but its robustness signals that it will be among the last skills to decline and disappear.

Also partially reflecting childhood development are those benign changes which at first accompany the aging process in all individuals. Our patient A.P. had the most difficulty with tasks in which information had to be altered in order to form new, unfamiliar configurations; his performance was far better when he had simply to utilize configurations already known, such as word definitions or facts. In contrast to the situation with the developing child, however, his performances were often subject to imperfections caused by the inappropriate intrusion of old habits and ways of approaching tasks. The deployment of overlearned habits is, of course, a prominent characteristic in the mature organism; such "perseverative" intrusions are less probable in the immature organism, which is as likely to evolve new habits as to exploit old ones. Nonetheless, there remains a certain parallel between the rigidity of the young child who insists that a certain thing must be done in a certain way and that of the old person who clings to established procedures while resisting the intrusion of any new *modus operandi*.

The greatly reduced speed and the painstaking accuracy of the older person also distinguish him from the young child, who, if anything, is likely to attempt tasks at too speedy a rate, to be excessively impulsive, and hence make errors. These differences in tempo may reflect fundamental properties of the nervous system, such as rates at which impulses fire or the degree of resistance met at synaptic boundaries, at different periods of life. They lead to the familiar (and not unjustifiable) observation that the older person exhibits better judgment and more wisdom, while youth is speedier and more flexible. Providing that the older person's frontal lobes are reasonably well preserved, and he can continue to draw on his prior experience, he may indeed display that perspicacity treasured in elder statesmen.

When the aging process becomes less benign, and significant lags in intellectual functioning become evident, the developmental process appears in rather more striking ways to undergo reversal. Many of the problems designed by Piaget have been administered to senile, demented patients, and the progression of stages found in normal children—sensory-motor operations followed by concrete operations, topped by formal operations—is indeed reversed with these patients as the dementia takes its course. It has also been established that, during the final days of life, the neurological condition of the old person reverts in striking ways to that of the young child: infantile behaviors like the grasping reflex and the sucking reflex recur; the individual no longer feels both pinpricks when he is stimulated simultaneously at disparate loci; babbling survives longer than talking.

And yet, even during more malignant phases, the older person cannot be said to become a mirror image of the child, for many of his oldest, most developed skills will remain preserved. Thus, the pianist does not become totally unable to move his fingers across the keyboard; instead, he can sometimes play a whole passage with skill, while at other times he finds himself unable even to place his fingers in the right position. His recollection of his whole life may at times be clouded, while at other times he will exhibit vivid reminiscences, particularly of his earlier years. His well-developed skills and his picture of himself are not completely shattered by the aging process; instead, parts remain preserved and can sometimes appear in intact form, given the right conditions, appropriate arousal, and a little bit of luck. Until the last stages, aging undoes development in a selective way—some highly developed skills, accompanied by more primitive proclivities, are likely to endure until the last.

With somewhat more limited brain lesions, such as those which give rise to frontal syndromes, aphasia, or agnosia, parallels with development are extremely tenuous. In the typical focal syndrome, due to a stroke, missile wound, or the early stages of a rapidly growing tumor, the individual remains fundamentally unchanged except for the more-or-less complete destruction of a particular capacity. The individual with Broca's aphasia can hardly express himself at all in words; yet he may draw pictures with a high level of sophistication and skill, and his intellectual functioning may be otherwise impressive. The visual-agnosic patient will recognize objects and phenomena successfully in other sensory modalities and may exhibit little or no linguistic or intellectual deterioration. And the individual with a frontal syndrome, like J.L., will perform normally on most tests of intellectual functioning, while at the same time emerging as a new person with minimum motivation, disheveled appearance, decreased sense of self. We have in the case of focal injuries an analogy to the building where a single office has been bombed out; the rest of the edifice may remain totally preserved even as the functions directed in that one office have been annihilated (unless they can be assumed by a neighboring agency).

With lesions to a circumscribed area of brain tissue, there is often the destruction of a figurative capacity in the face of preservation of the ability to perform complex operations. An individual who becomes deaf for words or blind for objects is able to accomplish equivalent functions when information is presented in a different modality—e.g., the word is instead presented in written form, or the object is perceived tactilely. The fundamental capacity to perform the operation has not been disturbed, but a figurative channel in which it would ordinarily be perceived and retained has been dammed up. An especially peculiar figurative impairment is that caused by disconnection syndromes, such as the one which befell the patrolman P.K. In this case, both of the requisite "higher level" functions —the operations—were intact: linguistic capacity in the left hemisphere, recognition and perception of objects in either hemisphere. But the potential for transferring a configuration or bit of information to that part of the brain where it could be appropriately utilized was disrupted by the placement of a lesion on the pathway connecting the centers. Providing that the information could be transmitted successfully, there was no problem in achieving the correct answer. But given the unusual injury, special methods often had to be used to transmit the information. Interestingly, such freak injuries do occasionally have parallels with certain congenital anomalies in children, and in this regard, at least, there does exist a relationship between development and dissolution.

Focal lesions, to be sure, sometimes do cause operative as well as figurative losses. In the case, for example, of a small lesion strategically placed at the intersection of the visual, auditory, and tactile "association cortexes," an entire range of fundamental capacities becomes impaired. The patient becomes unable to orient himself in a visual-spatial matrix, loses the ability to carry out mathematical operations, and can no longer comprehend complex utterances involving linguistic-logical elements. He can neither put A on top of B nor indicate the sex of "my mother's brother." The capacity to relate elements to one another in a new configuration has been destroyed, whether these elements be aspects of the spatial world, or substantives manipulated in a sentential frame, or a set of numbers. In contrast with figurative impairments, no substitution through other sensory channels or motor sequences seems possible. Rather, we must acknowledge an operative breakdown in the presence of relatively well-preserved figurative capacities. So too, in certain other lesions, such as the one producing the Gerstmann syndrome, there arises a fundamental difficulty in ordering elements: the arrangement of letters in words, fingers in the hand, left and right in space, numbers in a mathematical problem, are equally impaired. Again, no alternative way to carry out these functions seems possible; here, too, an operative impairment is consequent upon a circumscribed focal lesion.

To sum up the discussion thus far, neither the clinical patterns produced by dementing processes nor those resulting from more focal lesions mirror in any simple way the patterns of human development. Dementing processes more closely resemble a reversal of developmental processes, but particularly in the case of highly specialized or automatized skills, the pattern of dissolution may deviate markedly from that of development. Focal lesions can lead to a vast range of clinical pictures. Perhaps the majority entail preservation of operative capacities in the face of a singular decline in figurative cognition; certain equally circumscribed lesions, however, particularly those implicating cortical areas that connect the primary sensory regions, are prone to produce operative disturbances. The latter conditions, such as the Gerstmann syndrome, present a picture somewhat reminiscent of the young child whose figurative capacities are more or less intact but who has yet to attain higher-level operational skills. All told, in considering the relation between development and breakdown, we seem—as J. de Ajuriaguerra has pointed out—to be confronted with two essentially distinct, though unquestionably related processes:

In the infant, after all, we are studying a subject in the course of self-creation; in the aged individual we have a subject who has also acquired in his adult life a degree of mechanization in his pattern of conduct and whose disintegration tends to move from voluntary action to automatism; taking into account the fact that at least some portion of his voluntary control has less mobility having already been partially mechanized . . . disintegration is not always a mere reflection of integration. Whereas mobility is one of the notable characteristics of infantile evolution, rigidity is a characteristic aspect of the persistence of structure in cases of dementia.

Discussion of breakdown in adults inevitably raises the question of alteration of behavior in the child who has suffered an injury to his head. There have been—fortunately, we may say—fewer children with damaged brains to study than adults; and, since there have also been fewer post-mortems, evidence on localization of function in the child is practically nonexistent. Nonetheless, a few principles do seem to emerge from the studies that have been reported, and these are sufficiently suggestive to merit repeating here.

Nearly any form of brain damage produces *general* regression in a young child. He is likely to become tired, withdrawn, isolated, reluctant to interact with others. Most functions seem dampened at first; a mental and emotional trauma has occurred across the board. The younger the child, the more pronounced the regression; but the younger the child, the more likely (other things being equal) that there will be significant, perhaps even complete, recovery. This is because, as we noted early on, capacities seem to be much more widely and diffusely represented in the brain of the young child than in the brain of the adult. All the child's experiences and behaviors seem to be registered, at least to some extent, in both hemispheres—the right hemisphere, for instance, is integrally involved in language functions, the left hemisphere equally so in visual and spatial functions. In the adult brain, by contrast, there is a specialization of function such that circumscribed areas subserve individual functions, so that injury to a small area may produce profound difficulty in regard to one particular function in the face of the relative sparing of others; whereas in the child, whose full range of functions is widely dispersed, nearly all of them will be affected by any lesions, but the degree to which any given skill is affected is often slighter.

By middle childhood, dominance of one cerebral hemisphere over the other has been firmly established (though, even now, not quite so firmly, apparently, as in the mature adult brain—see below). This means, in most cases, that the child has become clearly right-handed (or left-brained) —his executive functions, from language to piano-playing, are now mediated by the left hemisphere. This emergence of dominance signals the relative recession of the right hemisphere's role in language as this region concentrates increasingly on visual and spatial functions.

The younger child can sustain extensive destruction in, or even total removal of, his left hemisphere without appreciable permanent damage. Recovery sometimes occurs so rapidly that it becomes unreasonable—if not impossible —to maintain that the right hemisphere has been acquiring language for the first time. Rather, the engrams for language appear to have been laid down in the right hemisphere as well as the left during initial language learning; now they must simply be aroused so that the left-hemispherectomized child may talk again. The situation is totally different in the event of extensive left-hemisphere disease in the older person. Here the right hemisphere takes over but slightly, if at all. At some time in the process of development, the right hemisphere has evidently lost its ability to engage in linguistic activities: this is the price we pay for dominance. It is perhaps at this point in development that the "localizing" view becomes more tenable, and the "holist" orientation correspondingly less so.

There are no records of fluent, or Wernicke's, aphasia among children below age ten. Such youngsters never speak fluently at rapid rates, nor is their speech peppered with the perseverations, paraphasias, and stereotypes of adults with lesions in the posterior sections of the left hemisphere. Instead, disabled children almost invariably express themselves in a terse, telegrammatic style, just as they did in early childhood. Reading and writing are invariably severely disturbed, presumably because these activities have not yet attained that independence from spoken language which may occasionally characterize reading and writing in more accomplished adults. Curiously enough, the comprehension of language seems to be better preserved (relatively speaking) in children than the ability to express language. Perhaps speech comprehension is especially widely represented in the brain of the child, while there is already some specialization for the expression of language in the left hemisphere.

Notwithstanding the apparently remarkable recovery we have described in children who have suffered significant brain damage, a certain note of qualification must be sounded; for there appears at least some reason to doubt that such children can ever realize their full potential. Recovering enough to "get by," to talk, read, write, and calculate adequately is not, after all, equivalent to fulfilling all of one's potential talents, becoming a skilled poet, singer, businessman, or athlete. One reason for skepticism in this regard is that, while children who have had strokes or hemispherectomies may pass the easier versions of tasks, they often display residual difficulty with more complex items, such as those requiring mastery of linguistic syntax, or the ability to negotiate tricky mazes. Particularly in the case of children with left-hemisphere lesions, language functions appear to be assumed by the spared hemisphere at the cost of a diminution in visual and spatial mastery. It may well be, of course, that with time these difficulties too will disappear altogether. But it may also be that so much time is spent in recovering, that so much "uncommitted" brain has to be utilized to lift the child "by his bootstraps" to an adequate level, that he will not be able to profit fully from that period in which skills are readily learned by the normal child. The particular difficulties exhibited by these brain-injured children in learning new functions is disturbing evidence that their brains may lack the suppleness, adaptability, and potential for higher organization of the uninjured brain. We may hope that such a pessimistic hypothesis will ultimately prove completely unfounded, but the best that can be said at this time is that the evidence seems inconclusive.

The fate of brain-injured children is of profound concern not only as regards their own rehabilitation, but also as regards what can and should be done for the far more prevalent brain-injured adult. We shall touch on this question at greater length in the last chapter; what needs to be stressed here is the potentially crucial implications, for all those thus afflicted, of the relationship between early learning and brain damage. If, as the evidence suggests, learning in the first years of life involves the whole brain, and language acquisition takes place initially in both hemispheres, then the fate of these early engrams is of vital significance. Should these traces disappear completely, of course, little can be done. Consider, however, the child of nine or ten who superficially appears to have reached the stage of complete hemispheric dominance in the language area (and otherwise), but who nonetheless recovers more or less completely from injuries to that area—an instance where the right hemisphere was already linguistically silent, but its potential for language was still exploitable. My mentor, Norman Geschwind, has summarized well the lesson implicit in this fact:

It would clearly be a remarkable advance if every adult aphasic could recover the level of speech of the nine year old. The number of permanently severe aphasic patients who do not recover even close to that level is enormous. Here is an instance where understanding what is going on in the child is vitally important. If we knew the mechanisms involved in the child, perhaps some way could be found to "attack" the right hemisphere of the adult in order to make the language learning manifest.

Just as the pattern of recovery in the child may present compelling lessons for rehabilitation of the adult, knowledge gained from the brain-injured adult may have critical implications for the child. A most striking fact, one reviewed earlier in some detail, is the range of reading disorders which may occur following focal brain injury in the adult. Some of these mirror quite faithfully the developmental disorders found in certain young children who, in the face of normal intelligence and motivation, are unable to read. Similar parallels can be found between lesions which cause specific difficulty with mathematical, musical, artistic, mnemonic, or visual-spatial capacities in the adult and the patterns of learning disabilities which befall a small, but nonetheless significant proportion of children.

The sudden emergence of such conditions in adults, against a background of otherwise normal functioning, provides an invaluable opportunity: we can study the brain anomalies which lead to these conditions; we can experiment with alternative ways (different symbol systems, modalities, media) for presenting the information which has suddenly in one modality become inaccessible. The adult's condition is stable; his alternative pathways of learning have been well developed. Lessons drawn from such studies can be invaluable for aiding the child, who, owing to congenital or hereditary reasons, seems unable to learn a certain type of material in the customary way. Alternative channels open to adults can be shown or taught to the child; the earlier this is done, the more likely that the child's difficulty can be completely circumvented.

Here, the degree of organization and specialization attained in the adult brain has helped to clarify the child's difficulty, and also to define the ways in which the problem can be obviated. In sum, we see that even if the processes of development and dissolution do not completely mirror one another, the lessons learned may be extremely valuable in the rehabilitation of any individual who has suffered brain injury.

# 8 The Pathology of Art

*I wish to God that some neurologists would sit down and figure out how the improviser's brain works, how he selects, out of hundreds of thousands of possibilities, the notes he does and at the speed he does—how in God's name, his mind works so damned fast! And why, when the notes come out right, they are right. . . . Composing is a slow, arduous, obvious, inch-by-inch process, whereas improvisation is a lightning mystery. In fact, it's the creative mystery of our age.*

—ALEC WILDER

Brain damage, as a consequence of a stroke, tumor, or accident, may befall any individual at any moment. Detailed case studies collected over many years have revealed certain regularities in the effects of these "insults" upon a varied population. We know, for example, that most patients who have a stroke in that portion of the frontal lobe of the left hemisphere called Broca's area will be able to understand language adequately but will speak in a broken, telegrammatic manner; and that patients who sustain injury in the posterior portions of the right hemisphere will speak and understand language adequately, yet may lose their way or fail to dress themselves properly. At present, in fact, we may be said to have a thorough knowledge of how brain injury affects the "average" person, whether in the form of localized lesions or of the more diffuse forms of brain injury.

But what happens to those skills which are not widely represented in the general population? What of the individual who has a special talent or an unusual way of looking at the world? And what of the individual whose skills have developed to an exquisitely high degree in the years prior to his lesion? Do these atypical capacities prove particularly brittle in the wake of brain injury, or do they, to the contrary, serve as a robust shield, protecting the individual against the usually devastating effects of injury? Such questions can only be approached through the study of gifted individuals whose abilities prior to injury were well documented, and, further, through a comparison of their performances with those of appropriate "control groups."

Of all the effects of brain injury, perhaps the most intriguing are those involving artistic performance or expression. In the artist we encounter an individual who has developed a communicative skill to a very high level, who possesses the ability to affect other individuals in a profound way, who derives and elicits strong intellectual and emotional satisfaction from involvement with a symbolic system. How, then, will *he* react to injury to the brain? Will the virtuoso musician remain more nimble following a stroke than the desk-bound executive? Is the painter more likely than the accountant to retain color discrimination or spatial orientation? Is the brain-injured writer able to express himself more effectively than others similarly afflicted who have lacked these specialized gifts? In short, are the artist's characteristic emotional state and his unique and idiosyncratic ways of perceiving the world altered in the same manner as those of other afflicted persons?

The investigation of these questions requires several steps. First of all, one must make a preliminary assessment of the status of these skills in the normal population, and then determine how such individuals are affected by brain injury. Then, it is necessary to test a group of brain-intact artists on these same functions in order that *their* customary level of performance can be established. Only then can one focus in upon the unfortunate artist who has suffered brain damage, interpreting his current situation in the light of whatever knowledge has been obtained about his skills, emotions, perspectives, goals, and tensions during the years of his most accomplished achievement.

Regrettably, we are as yet equipped to make but modest headway in the exploration of these provocative issues. Highly skilled artists, for one thing, constitute a tiny minority; for another, such individuals are less likely to appear under circumstances where they can be intensively studied and (perhaps understandably) less willing to subject themselves to such scrutiny. Most neuropsychologists, moreover, lack special skills beyond their own discipline; comparisons with normal individuals are difficult to sustain and interpret. For these and similar reasons, there is at present little definitive knowledge about just how brain injury affects the accomplished artist. Further, what information does exist illuminates the elements or bases of technical competence—the painter's spatial sense, the composer's rhythmic capacities, etc.—rather than the artist's unique motivations, inner feelings, themes, and aspirations.

Still, the findings of a number of investigators who have probed the level of artistic skills in the normal population do constitute at least a useful point of departure. In addition, a few insightful neurologists have studied accomplished artists who sustained brain injury and have presented their findings in one or another forum. Moreover, reports describing the effects of brain damage on the literary and the pictorial artist seem relatively consistent with one another and so permit some tentative, though sketchy, conclusions. Less of a consensus obtains regarding the effects of brain injury on the skills of musicians; yet even in this heatedly debated area, important issues have at least been delineated and are now susceptible to testing. And so, while definitive descriptions of the fate of improvising skill, or the robustness of sketching capacity, are not yet at hand, there are sufficiently pregnant hints in the literature to provide something of a preliminary view of artistic functions in the normal and the gifted victim of brain injury.

Injury to the central portions of the mantle of the left hemisphere in normal individuals almost invariably causes disturbances in language. As we have seen, those sustaining injury in the anterior portions of the hemisphere are likely to speak in a terse, ungrammatical, substantive-laden mode; in contrast, those with defects in the posterior portions of the hemisphere will be extremely voluble, with syntax relatively intact, yet with few meaningful substantives punctuating their speech.

Disturbances in oral language are accompanied in practically all cases by equivalent or greater difficulties in written language. This is because writing seems to be "parasitic" upon the capacity for oral communication, and also because writing is about as complex a skill as most normal individuals possess. Entailing linguistic, motor, and visual competence, the capacity to organize thoughts logically while simultaneously coordinating the mechanical aspects of the graphic act, writing is more likely to be impaired than other linguistic skills, irrespective of the site of injury. Theoretically, a patient who is clearly aphasic and yet can write normally is at least conceivable; to the best of my knowledge, however, no convincing report of such a case exists. In fact, should one actually encounter such a patient, whether an ordinary individual or a skilled man of letters, the suspicion would immediately arise that he is not truly aphasic, but is instead either deaf—and thus can monitor his writing but not his speech—or else malingering.

Even if the aphasic recovers well, returning to a normal level in casual conversation, he will rarely be able to resume literary communication with any degree of ease or fluency. On the other hand, it is quite possible, at least in principle, that someone with literary talents could in fact sustain considerable injury to the nonlinguistic right hemisphere while remaining capable of distinguished work in the literary arts. Although I know of no actual recorded cases of continued distinction in creative writers suffering significant right-hemisphere disease, I have encountered a number of patients whose writing performance seems to have remained at or near their pre-morbid level of skill.

Recently, however, some evidence has accumulated to suggest that linguistic capacity may not be mediated entirely by the left hemisphere. Various investigators have taken a much closer look at patients with right-hemisphere injuries and have concluded that they are indeed deficient in certain aspects of linguistic competence. Such individuals have no difficulty in appreciating the literal meanings (denotations) of terms or in responding appropriately to questions. However, they appear lacking in the ability to appreciate the less literal implications or connotations of a question, or the nuances of a familiar metaphor or utterance. For example, asked what is meant by the proverb *Too many cooks spoil the broth,* a right-hemisphere patient may offer the superficially acceptable response, "What you're cooking won't be good if you have too many people cooking it." Further probing, however, may reveal that he is unable to go beyond this very literal, "concrete" interpretation and to acknowledge that the proverb needn't pertain to food or cooks at all. Asked during the course of an interview "how long" he's been here, the patient will likely answer, say, "a few minutes," and express surprise that the length of his hospital stay was the intent of the question. Required to match a word like *lady* with either a straight line or a curved line, he may resist violently and, if pressed, is likely to respond randomly. People and abstract geometric configurations represent two disparate realms to such patients, and they therefore balk at honoring formal or metaphorical links between them.

This avoidance of the metaphorical, this penchant for the concrete particular, stands in striking contrast to the speech of these same patients, which is in fact characterized by certain strange features: a flat, monotonous tone, and a tendency to joke, though with a cutting edge, or to make improbable puns. An individual with right-hemisphere disease will typically call his physician "Doc" and make light of his paralyzed arm: "Oh, I don't need them gills to get around, anyway." Asked for the name of the institution he is in, he may proclaim, "Mount Cyanide Hospital." Although such retorts might superficially seem to indicate a superior sense of humor or irony, they actually signal the patient's unrealistic assessment of his situation—in minimizing the true extent of the injury, or embracing what may appear to be a form of "gallows humor," he demonstrates his unawareness of the full seriousness of his plight.

Indeed, the more one observes the right-hemisphere patient's comprehension of questions (both literal and metaphorical) and his own spontaneous language, the clearer his deficits in linguistic competence become. The patient's command of grammar and of sound structure seem unchanged, but the relationship between his capacity to express himself in language and his knowledge of the world is impaired. He resembles a kind of language machine, a talking computer that decodes literally what is said, and gives the most immediate (but not necessarily the implicitly called for) response, a rote rejoinder insensitive to the ideas behind the questions, the intentions or implications of the questioner. And in his spontaneous speech, the patient again seems to neglect the emotional quality of the present situation or the extent of his impairment in favor of dispensing wisecracks—these, in turn, seem to reflect the operation of a "joke machine" rather than the holistic integration of feelings, situational cues, and interpersonal relations appropriate to a serious interview. Such an individual can provide somewhat amusing "one-liners," but hardly seems likely to produce a balanced, developed work of art. However, to the extent that the patient was merely called upon to adapt or reformulate materials he had penned before (e.g., legal briefs, cooking recipes, letters to friends, bureaucratic memoranda), he might succeed reasonably well.

Precisely because literary competence is likely to be vitiated by aphasia, the aphasic's output may, paradoxically, illuminate the properties of artworks produced by the skilled craftsman. The competent writer is generally able to express himself, and give his characters expression, in a variety of voices, to accompany shifts in tone and feeling with appropriate alteration in the means of expression; beyond this, he will possess an enduring and distinctive personal style, discernible through, and underlying, whatever "voice" he assumes. Aphasic speech and writing, by contrast, feature virtual caricatures of style—extreme forms of a particular way of expression without the modifications and modulations introduced by the master stylist.

The pure Broca's aphasic or agrammatic speaker, for example, may be seen as in effect burlesquing the terse, short-sentence writer—Hemingway, say:

So his mother prayed for him and then they stood up and Krebs kissed his mother and went out of the house. He had tried so to keep his life from being complicated. Still none of it had touched him. He had felt sorry for his mother and she had made him lie. He would go to Kansas City and get a job.

The Broca's aphasic attempting to convey the substance of this passage might come out with: "Ma pray . . . up . . .

Krebs kiss mother . . . go out of . . . house . . . feel sorry
. . . mother . . . Krebs to Kansas City." What works effectively in Hemingway's style—straight, neutral, statements
of fact, the unobtrusive concatenation of momentous feelings and actions—becomes in this aphasic's version an
overly terse recitation of the most important words and
word fragments, a passage rich in meaning, certainly, but
devoid of literary value.

Let us consider now, in sharp contrast, Faulkner's flow-
ing, syntactically complex writing, a style replete with
relative clauses, embedded phrases, prepositional phrases,
relatively impoverished in propositions or substantives:

> . . . the slow outward trickle of food and supplies and equip-
> ment which returned each fall as cotton made and ginned and
> sold (two threads frail as truth and impalpable as equators
> yet cable strong to bind for life them who made the cotton
> to the land their sweat fell on).

Uttered by a Wernicke's or posterior aphasic, this might
resemble a Faulkner parody in somewhat meaningless
doubletalk: "the slow trickling of food and stood and
things you know, what I mean is there's this cotton and
it's made and made and, you know, like, there's these
things and that frailable cotton, that stuff that joins them,
you know where, the land where they are, I think that's
what I said, huh?"

These contrasting styles—one featuring a terse sequence
of nouns, each reflecting a whole proposition; the other
highlighting a lengthy, complex, and interconnected series
of clauses—represent the "two poles of language" posited
by the linguist Roman Jakobson, and respectively epitomized in the modes of expression of the anterior and the
posterior patient. The defining characteristics of other
familiar styles are similarly illuminated by language disturbances. For example, one of our patients, with word-

finding difficulty, resorted to a hypersincere yet rather empty and evasive mode of expression, somewhat reminiscent of an effulgent Richard Nixon. Asked how he liked the hospital, he would answer at great length: "I'm glad you asked that question because I want all of you to know that this is the greatest hospital I've ever seen. And you are the finest doctors, and I want to mention especially Dr. Ishiwara, who's been on my team from the very beginning. And I want to make one thing clear: I'm going to go back to that telephone plant, where I was supervisor for twenty, no thirty, years and I'm going to show all those great guys there, that we're really going to make it. I know I'm going to get better because I have the greatest doctors in the world and I want to thank each and every one of you for making it possible."

Another patient was a twenty-three-year-old veteran suffering from an unusual type of developmental language disorder. Possessed of above-average intelligence, he might, in spontaneous conversation, have appeared completely normal. At worst, he sounded a bit pompous, having a predilection for long words and for lengthy and at times circumlocutory answers. He was admitted for evaluation of a problem in reading, yet we soon confirmed that he had a general language difficulty. When asked to summarize his future plans in writing, he unwittingly produced an almost perfect parody of bureaucratese:

I plan concentrating on improving my special needs for however long necessay, My first measure will be to learn where I may recieve the best qualified guiadance for my difficulties and apply for their consideration. I do recognize that Mr. Johnston is presently organizing a program to inprove some of my difficulities. I will fully cooperate with this progra presently extablished at a one-two month duration. My second measure will be to follow the Aphasia's staff's recommendation of obtaining employment related to my vocational interest. My application will soliciate as a temporary trainee for part-time hours. . . . I shall strongly emphasis that my difficulties have been a contributing factor to the strong development of my special abilities, ie being resourceful and creative. . . . I do recognise and accept that I am the elementary factor to improving my difficultieis, that several of the approahces to improving my difficulities will be experimential, that some phases will be intensive, that all phrases will be demanding upon time and effort for both patient and council.

The treatment we recommended was regular intensive drill in answering questions simply and succinctly; the therapist also required a daily précis of materials read, and taught the student certain elementary rules of speaking and oral expression. Equipping the patient with a normal mode of communicating will not be easy, however; for this amazing style may have evolved, in part, as a defense mechanism, in order to conceal the grave difficulties the patient has in determining precisely what he wants to say, then in transforming these thoughts into clear English. Like the output of classic aphasics, this patient's manner of speaking inflates properties which, when modulated by a writer in control of his material, become the elements of an adequate or at worst stilted style.

Deviations from the norm in ordinary language use are relatively easy to spot. A certain minimum competence can be expected from any high school graduate; in addition, an extensive battery of tests is available to pinpoint strengths and weaknesses. A markedly different situation obtains in the area of music, where extreme variation in capacities is the rule, and where few sensitive measures of ability exist. Interpretation of such results is perilous, but the attempt must be made all the same.

Most schoolchildren have at one time been tested on their appreciation of the elements of music, and in all likelihood, the instrument used was the Seashore tests.

This battery probes the ability to judge which of two pitches is higher, which of two tones is louder; whether two successive rhythmic patterns are identical; which of two tones is longer, whether the tone quality or timbre of two successive tones is identical; and which note in a sequence has been changed during a second playing. These somewhat lifeless and tedious exercises have been used for decades to determine which students possess musical aptitude (and should perhaps croon with the "nightingales"), which are "tone-deaf" (and should instead perch with the "crows" during choral practice).

Psychologist Brenda Milner gave the Seashore tests to matched groups of patients having damage, respectively, in the left temporal lobe (the area of the brain subsuming language activity) and the right temporal lobe (the left's symmetrical counterpart which has very little to do with ordinary language processing). On all Seashore tests, patients with right-temporal-lobe damage performed worse than those with lesions in the left temporal lobe, performance being most severely impaired on comparisons of tonal patterns and tonal quality. On the surgical unit where Milner was working, it was also determined that removal of areas of the right temporal lobe (as a measure to mitigate long-standing epilepsy) causes reductions in the level of performance, whereas comparable removals of left-hemisphere tissues do not have this effect. This research, as well as other studies conducted recently, strongly suggests that the right hemisphere plays a dominant role in musical performance and perception.

Linguistic and musical capacities, then, seem to be at least partially independent of one another. One can be skilled in the verbal realm while musically incompetent or illiterate; and one can be a master with one's fingers while also tongue-tied. Strong right-handed (and left-brained) tendencies generally indicate that an individual will be unusually competent in linguistic activities; precisely the opposite seems to be the case with music. Even though instruments (as generally designed) are difficult for left-handers to use, the proportion of left-handed (and so possibly right-brain-dominant) individuals among musicians is at least equal to that among the population as a whole.

Because of its relatively independent status, musical activity can become quite important in the lives of brain-damaged patients. Severely aphasic individuals who scarcely monitor conversations or watch television, may find music enjoyable and listen attentively to a live performer or to the radio. Even those able to say almost nothing can emit an entire melody; and not infrequently, they can sing words that they are unable to emit in the absence of the melody; moreover, they seem to recognize familiar melodies almost instantaneously (e.g., "Take Me Out to the Ball Game") and can match these to the setting with which they are customarily associated (in this case, a picture of a baseball diamond). Even patients with severe memory disorders, who have not learned their doctor's name after months, can learn a body of information or facts when these are embedded in a melody. On the other hand, patients with right-hemisphere disease, whose mnemonic and linguistic skills are not notably altered, may lose the melody in their voice and thus be unable to sing. (Just as the left-hemisphere patient may speak more easily if he encases the words in music, so right-hemisphere patients seem to hold a tune more accurately if they dub in the words.) Right-hemisphere patients are also more prone to lose interest in their surroundings generally, and this includes a reduction of interest in musical events.

Given lack of information in most cases about the "premorbid" level of musical sophistication, it is difficult to make more precise statements about the effects of brain injury on musical capacity. The greater access (and attraction) to music on the part of individuals suffering from diseases of the left hemisphere has important therapeutic implications to which we will return at the end of this chapter.

Accuracy in determination of the average adult's competence in the visual arts is nearly as elusive as in assessment of his musical flair. Established norms do exist for the capacity of the average person to draw figures, construct patterns, and make fine discriminations among visually presented objects. As regards brain-damaged people, however, the validity of tests in this area is at least partially undermined by the lamentable fact that most persons seen in a neuropsychological laboratory have some paralysis or weakness in the favored hand. Assessment of drawing capacity accordingly requires indirect methods and must rely on the patient's performance with his nonpreferred hand. Needless to say, the picture obtained of the patient's capacities under these far-from-ideal circumstances is considerably blurred.

In evaluating the effects of lesion site on performance in a given field, one must first establish the site independently (through radiological means or from a surgeon's report); then one tests for the symptoms typical of a given pathology. For many years it was believed that the right hemisphere played but a minimal role in higher cortical functions. Eventually, however, this assumption was shown to be erroneous, and the right hemisphere came to be considered dominant for (among other functions) drawing or construction capacity. This conclusion seemed logical, inasmuch as patients with right-hemisphere lesions typically perform poorly at visual and spatial tasks, like distinguishing between two geometrical patterns, or feeling one's way out of a maze. Large-scale studies of patients' drawing productions have since indicated that lesions in either hemisphere will produce a severe diminution in drawing ability—but with qualitative differences in the nature of the difficulty.

Summarizing research on this subject, Elizabeth Warrington of the National Hospital in London portrays each patient group as having its characteristic deficit. The drawings of patients with right-hemisphere lesions display distortion of the general outlines of an object, while frequently preserving quite well the details of its internal structure. A picture of a house will be drawn in a logical fashion and include all necessary elements (window, door, chimney, etc.), perhaps even some additional or redundant features, while the overall shape of the building may be virtually unrecognizable. The spatial relationships among the component parts may also be aberrant. Frequently, because of a tendency—associated with certain unilateral lesions in the right hemisphere—to neglect or ignore the left half of space, the left side of the drawing will be incomplete. The individual with a left-hemisphere lesion, on the other hand, produces simplified versions of an assigned object, sketches which are appropriate and readily recognizable in general shape or configuration, but which may be, rather like drawings by young children, grossly deficient in essential internal details. Their houses are often just a shell, with the bottom rectangle and the trapezoidal roof reliably present and appropriately shaped, but with the less crucial door, windows, and shutters likely to be missing. Acute and obtuse angles are likely to be simplified to right angles, parallelograms to rectangles, oblique lines to straight ones, and lines which change direction into continuous ones. The illustrations reproduced below are typical examples of the contrasting work of right- and left-hemisphere patients.

How to account for these differences? The right-hemisphere patient can perceive adequately, but his overall sense of proportion and of spatial relations is impaired, perhaps owing in part to neglect of, or insensitivity to, half of his phenomenal world. On the other hand, with his language capacities preserved, his knowledge of what should be in, say, a house is adequate. Thus his drawings will be intellectually satisfactory, including the required features placed in logical order, perhaps done in painstaking detail, or even duplicated; yet the overall form or Gestalt of the depicted object, that property difficult to put into words and insusceptible to verbal instruction, will be glaringly deficient. The left-hemisphere patient, on the other hand, may well exhibit in drawing the same general tendency toward simpler classification and less differentiated concepts that is characteristic of his language functioning. The primitiveness of his drawings, the omission of elements, reflects his lack of verbal knowledge about what should be included in a representation and how he should "attack" the task. Yet, because of a relatively intact sense of space, orientation, proportion, and perspective, these facets of his drawings will be unquestionably superior to those of right-hemisphere patients. In brief, the drawings of left-hemisphere patients will, in their oversimplification, suggest production by someone at a lower point in development; whereas one may have to infer, or piece together, the subject of a drawing by a right-hemisphere patient.

It is only fair to note that the picture we have just sketched above is not universally accepted. Those who demur are chiefly our old friends the "generalists" or "holists," who believe that any defect in language necessarily extends to all other cognitive domains. Members of this school predict, as one might expect, that the drawings of aphasic patients will inevitably reflect a deterioration in intellectual level, its extent depending on the degree of language disturbance—whereas our description above is, of course, more closely aligned with the "localizing" or "specifist" view that one set of capacities can be severely impaired without skills of a fundamentally different sort being implicated thereby.

Leading the generalist assault on this front is Eberhard Bay, the German neurologist noted for his skepticism

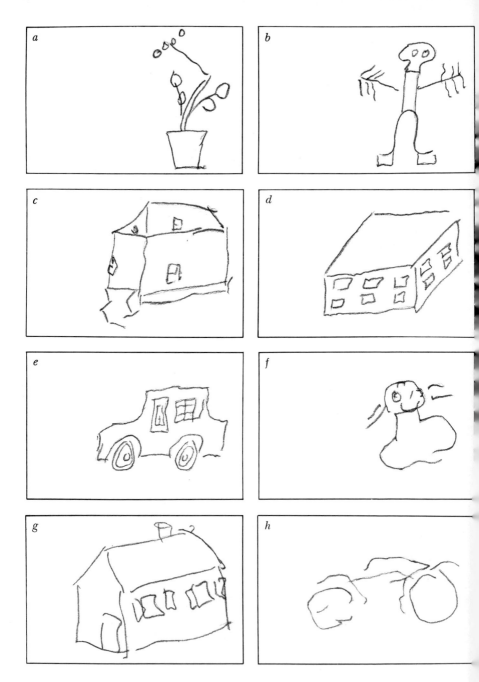

Free-hand drawings of right-handed patients with left-hemisphere lesions: a) flower; b) man; c) and d) house; e) car; f) cat; g) house; h) bicycle. Drawings g and h were done with the non-paralyzed left hand. Note the simplifications and primitivizations and omission of detail, combined with preservation of overall form of model. *(See page 305.)*

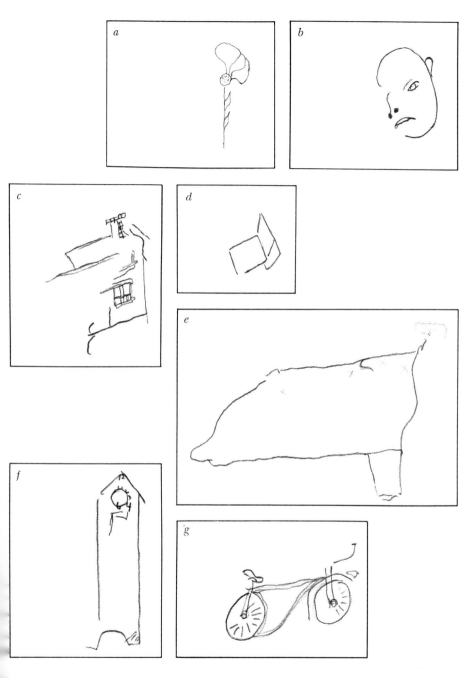

Free-hand drawings by right-handed patients with right-hemisphere lesions: a) flower; b) man's face; c) house; d) cube; e) map of the United States; f) clock; g) bicycle. Note the distortions in contours and in location of detail, omissions on the left side, and difficulty in depicting third dimension. *(See page 305.)*

about visual agnosia. "So far," he claims, "we have never met an aphasic patient who was able to draw a missing part unless he was able to name it as well. . . . if the patient is unable to distinguish in his concepts, he surely cannot make correct use of the respective words." Implicit in this view is a belief in an indissoluble link between the concept of an object (as tapped by the ability to name) and the possibility of giving that object concrete representation in a visual medium.

Bay's argument is certainly parsimonious, and has occasionally won adherents; nonetheless, it is strongly contradicted by my own experience and that of most neuropsychological investigators. Without denying the frequent co-occurrence of the inability to name and the inability to draw, countless instances could be cited where the name is emitted in the absence of the capacity to depict, equally numerous occasions in which the name is inaccessible to the patient but the object can be drawn (or even its name written!).

Documented cases of artists who have become severely aphasic, yet continue to be able to draw with finesse and skill, constitute the strongest evidence against Bay's position. Sometimes, however, Bay has held that severe aphasia of the Broca variety (telegrammatic speech) is not true aphasia, which he then limits to the comprehension difficulties that accompany a posterior, or Wernicke-type aphasia. If one follows him in excluding patients who have primarily motor or Broca's aphasia, then Bay's point of view, though now emasculated, gains in persuasiveness. For it is indeed true that as comprehension becomes severely impaired, drawings suffer as well. The patient with a deficit in comprehension will produce sketches that are greatly simplified, lack crucial elements, fuse features of two different concepts (e.g., a *back* is put on a *table*), omit the third dimension, and so on. His drawings, in short, resemble his speech—featuring confusions between two elements and stray or erroneous components; lacking other parts essential to the designated target; appearing primitive or undifferentiated, like a child's initial efforts. If a certain part of the concept is more fully understood (e.g., the word *sail* in *sailboat*), that portion of the picture will be highlighted. Often, copies are drawn with surprising fidelity, presumably because a set of perceptible components has been presented. In addition, for a patient with communication deficits, performance may improve with repetitive drill; his perceptual-spatial sense being intact, the patient proves able over time to correct deficiencies in his product.

One particularly interesting feature may characterize the drawings of individuals with comprehension defects. When given a model from which to draw, these subjects may copy the model with painstaking accuracy, producing a virtual tracing of the original. Yet on examination, it becomes apparent that the artist has drawn without comprehension: he is slavishly transcribing a graphic configuration which he does not understand, rather than highlighting the defining features of the target in his own style. He bears here a striking resemblance to the patient who does not understand, but who can repeat perfectly. In this regard, patients with comprehension deficits differ strikingly from young children. Whereas in their spontaneous drawings, both groups feature general primitivization, elimination of details, unconcern with perspective, the child tends to employ general schemes which have been adopted by the culture in which he lives (e.g., human stick figures). Furthermore, the child also incorporates into his drawings things that he knows (the pin is shown penetrating the apple) rather than what he perceives (the head of a pin protruding from one side of an apple, the point sticking out the other). The aphasic with comprehension difficulty, however, is more likely to trace what he sees as best he can: rather than using culturally established (and approved) schemes, the patient is likely to evolve his own idiosyncratic ways of depicting a certain element or figure and to employ these throughout his corpus. Even then, however, he may continue to be served by retained technical skill in the use of line.

Even though the view that pictorial and linguistic ability faithfully reflect each other is untenable, bonds do exist between what is understood and what can be drawn. For instance, patients with the so-called Gerstmann syndrome, who have particular difficulty in naming and recognition of individual fingers, may produce drawings in which other parts of the body are well articulated, while the fingers are poorly or incorrectly represented. More compelling support for this association comes from sequential studies of aphasics' drawings during the course of recovery: these reveal a step-by-step return to normal, premorbid levels of competence in drawing, even as there is a strikingly similar advancement in the linguistic competence of the patient. Just as paraphasias, or word confusions, become infrequent, the proportion of appropriate words improves and the overall concept of the sentence is reestablished, so too in drawing, details begin to appear appropriately, inappropriate juxtapositions disappear, skill at deployment of line, shading, color is reestablished. My own guess would be that the improvement in drawing performance reflects a recovery of linguistic abilities; however, the reverse cause and effect—better drawing ability engendering superior language capacity—cannot be excluded.

Our survey of artistic skills in the relatively untrained individual has suggested the following state of affairs: With extensive brain damage, there is usually an across-the-board decrease in the exercise of a wide range of skills; more localized lesions, however, are likely to implicate only particular skills, while leaving others relatively intact. Thus, language and literary ability suffer serious damage with pathology of the major (i.e., the dominant, usually the left) hemisphere; the effects of minor-hemisphere disease on literary activity are not readily apparent, though they may nonetheless be significant. Musical ability presents an essentially complementary picture, with right-hemisphere disease more devastating on most musical capacities, though damage in the major hemisphere may also exact its toll. Finally, difficulties in drawing and painting can be expected from lesions in either hemisphere, with different kinds of impairments, depending on the lesion's location. Drawing capacity may reflect to some extent the type of language disturbance, but this seems true chiefly for those patients with difficulties in comprehension. Those whose motor output is impaired in the face of relatively well-preserved understanding of ordinary language should not suffer significant long-term deficits in skill in the plastic arts (though paralysis may force the patient to relearn techniques using his "spared" limb).

What, however, happens to the individual who has attained a superlatively high level of artistic achievement prior to his suffering brain damage? Is he as impaired as the average person, or does the vast amount of "over-learned" skill and expertise of his pre-morbid days serve as a kind of reserve supply, protecting him against the loss of capacity? Evidence on this question is indeed limited, and is found chiefly in the literature on aphasia, but what has been learned is most suggestive.

The physician who has most intensively studied the effect of brain damage on artistic performance, Théophile Alajouanine, has concluded that aphasia takes its severest toll on the writer. This is hardly surprising, in light of the fact that it is language ability that is most particularly impaired, but such information is nonetheless important. We see that even exquisitely developed skills cannot protect the writer against damage in his language area. Thus, when the poet Charles Baudelaire suffered a stroke—one impairing his language to such an extent that he could only utter the oath "Cré nom"—his literary output was, of course, completely curtailed. There was no magical sparing of the ability to express himself in written symbols, no sudden or spontaneous recovery due to the ascendency of the uninjured portions of the brain. True, Baudelaire *was* able to read the proofs of some of his writings, which suggests that his critical faculty was much better preserved.

While an acute attack of aphasia appears to prevent any kind of creative writing, what of the individual who has recovered from a stroke to the language area? In the relatively rare instances where complete recovery occurs, there is some hope that writing can once again be resumed. The important factor seems to be whether reading and writing were relatively spared by the original lesion, as they are in certain forms of aphasia, or whether these were among the functions most severely impaired. Needless to say, the less impaired reading and writing were initially, the greater the likelihood that the earlier level of competence can once again be reached. I know of no cases in which a writer of fiction has recovered from a significant aphasia and has gone on to create interesting and significant new works; but there are several recorded cases of individuals who were once again able to express themselves effectively through the written word. Noteworthy in this connection are the occasional instances of physicians who became aphasic and were later able to offer descriptive accounts of their aphasia. These accounts, to be reviewed in the final chapter, read well and reveal no latent signs of impairment—though one should not exclude the possibility that these once-aphasic writers benefited from a thorough editing by someone else.

There are also a few cases of aphasic individuals whose general conversational skills were apparently fully restored, but who remained with significant general linguistic impairment. Such patients can produce written communications accurately only with the most painstaking effort. Often the writing of a page will consume an hour or even a day, and the final product may still contain errors. The effort entailed—in searching for words, spelling them and then combining them into meaningful discourse—is so great that these persons write no more than they must. In this they resemble the Broca's aphasic, who, though he has little difficulty with the mechanics of reading, nonetheless desists because of the strain involved.

A case reported by Alajouanine reflects these various aspects. This individual, a major (but unidentified)* French writer who suffered a severe lesion in the anterior portion of his left hemisphere, was left with a Broca's aphasia. At first grossly impaired, he gradually improved to the point where comprehension was good and conversation possible. Nonetheless, a remnant of agrammatism persisted in his speech, such that fully formed sentences were in the minority. The author's writing followed a similar course; it was performed with the nonparalytic hand and exhibited the same difficulty in syntactic construction.

The patient's reading ability eventually returned to a high level. He was able to peruse books in several languages. His literary memory seemed excellent, he was able to edit manuscripts, and he retained a capacity to offer valuable criticism of the artistic output of others. Alajouanine concluded that the "inability of the writer to continue his work" was not related to "a deficiency of memory, reasoning, judgment, or affectivity. Many examples show me that the characteristic trends [sic] of his literary personality have not been modified by the illness."

---

* Just as this book was going to press, I learned that Alajouanine, in a recent book, has identified the writer and presented a detailed description of his course of recovery over a twenty-two-year period. Interested readers with a knowledge of French are referred to *Valéry Larbaud sous divers visages,* published by Gallimard in Paris.

This notwithstanding, the artist of subtlety and nuance had been transformed into an inarticulate speaker and writer who, in the face of preserved skill in other aspects of literary activity, was no longer able to do original creative work in this medium.

It is possible, of course, that a writer with some residual aphasia might be able to effect a shift in style adapted to the limitations imposed by his illness that will yet permit him some restricted measure of creative expression. One such instance may have been the Russian novelist Gleb Ivanovich Uspensky (1840–1902), who suffered from a peculiar speech disorder during his last years, one which might have been due either to schizophrenia or to a lesion in the left hemisphere. (Distinguishing between "word salad" due to a Wernicke's aphasia and that due to a psychotic break may present difficulties even today, and certainly was not reliably done in Russia some seventy-five years ago.) Uspensky nonetheless continued to work, but increasingly embraced a hyperbaroque style. Syntax and detail ran havoc, while the ability to articulate clear propositions and to narrate a sequence of events had atrophied. As Roman Jakobson, who studied the work of Uspensky, maintains, "the reader is crushed by the multiplicity of detail unloaded on him in a limited verbal space, and is physically unable to grasp the whole, so that the portrait is often lost." A typical passage reflects the fate of a literary style when the narrative impulse is relatively attenuated, while powers of vivid, detailed description remain:

From underneath an ancient straw cap with a bleak spot on its shield, there peeked two braids resembling the tusks of a wild boar; a chin grown fat and pendulous definitely spread over the greasy collars of the calico dicky and in thick layer lay on the coarse collar of the canvas coat, firmly buttoned on the neck. From below this coat to the eyes of the observer there protruded massive hands with a ring, which had eaten into the fat finger, a cane with a copper top, a significant bulge of the stomach and the presence of very broad pants, almost of Muslim quality, in the broad ends of which hid the toes of the boots.

Even as some given pathology can exert a powerful destructive influence on a writer's style, however, there may be selected disorders that actually heighten his expressive powers—as witness the case of Uspensky's far greater contemporary, Fyodor Dostoevsky. Dostoevsky clearly suffered from severe epilepsy, which appears to have implicated his temporal lobes. Such a pathology has been known in many instances to exert a dramatic effect on an individual's personality and emotional life. Irrespective of his earlier cosmology (if any), the patient may become deeply concerned about religious issues, highly conscious of good and evil, prone to favor mystical views and to invoke God or Fate as the cause of unusual circumstances, including his own weird behavior. This profound alteration in outlook seems explicable by the fact that, with little prior warning, the patient undergoes a powerful sensory experience (the "aura" of the epileptic fit) which lasts a few moments, immediately thereafter experiences rapid jolting of his musculature and frame, and then goes into convulsions and loses consciousness. This rapid sequence—a brief interval of exquisite rapture, followed by a traumatic fit and a subsequent amnestic period—seems sufficient to convince the individual that he is a "chosen" person; the laws governing the world require reformulation in the light of his experience.

Originally a realistic writer, Dostoevsky turned increasingly into a visionary, one concerned with the religious character, the nature of crime and salvation, the struggle between good and evil, the nature and action of God. He wrote numerous descriptions of his epileptic experiences. Of the aura he exclaimed, "This feeling is so strong and so sweet that for a few seconds of this enjoyment one would readily exchange ten years of one's life—perhaps even his whole life. . . . during these moments as rapid as lightning the impression of the life and the consciousness were in himself ten times more intense . . . his reason was raised up to the understanding of the final cause." Yet the danger and terror of this epiphany are also conceded: "If it were to last more than this five-to-six-second period, the soul would not be able to bear it and would disappear." And the ambivalence of the epileptic toward his condition recurs repeatedly: "God has tortured me throughout my life, meanwhile God sends me at times some moments of entire serenity." Like other tormented artists, Dostoevsky wrestled in his work with his own behavioral and emotional turmoil; he included many descriptions of the ill temper, unmotivated violence, and sudden pangs of remorse common among temporal lobe epileptics; and giving his problems literary expression may well have been of some help to him in confronting his illness. In any event, it seems reasonably safe to say that Dostoevsky's brain disturbance had a significant influence on his artistic development, in terms both of theme and of style.

While the artist dependent upon verbal expression is generally crippled by aphasia, the situation differs dramatically with the painter. True, during the initial days of an aphasic attack, when paralysis is severe, the painter or sculptor is unlikely to be able to do any work. And if the aphasia implicates the areas of comprehension to a significant degree, there may be long-lasting impediments to graphic, as well as verbal, expression. Yet, painting productivity can unquestionably proceed at a high level even in the presence of extensive aphasia. Indeed, it has been maintained on several occasions that a painter's work actually *improved* in quality after the loss of verbal power. Although this extreme claim has yet to be systematically examined—through a critical investigation of an artist's entire *oeuvre*—the mere fact of its reiteration underscores the relative independence of (or even interference between) linguistic and artistic capacities. Two carefully studied cases speak to this question.

A major French painter (not identified in the published literature) who specialized in depictions of marine life and landscapes on the Normandy coast, was stricken at age 52 by a severe case of aphasia. As the lesion was posterior, implicating Wernicke's area, there was no paralysis; however, spoken language was much impaired, word-finding posed difficulties, and understanding was limited to those utterances which could be grasped from the surrounding context. Further intellectual impairment was not found, though previous tendencies toward acidulousness and toward isolation from others were intensified.

According to Alajouanine, who followed him through the course of his illness, the painter's artistic activity remained at its customary high level, even when the aphasia was at its most severe; indeed, there were connoisseurs who maintained that his work had actually gained in intensity and expressiveness. No distortions in form, expression, use of color, or technique were discernible; the painter proceeded at the same rate and developed themes similar to those employed before. This unabated productivity was marvelled at by the painter himself. "There are in me," he explained, "two men, the one who paints, who is normal while he is painting, and the other one who is lost in the mist, who does not stick to life . . . I am saying very poorly what I mean . . . There are inside me the one who grasps reality, life; there is the other one who is lost as regards abstract thinking . . . These are two men, the one who is grasped by reality to paint, the other one, the fool who cannot manage words any more."

Alajouanine's findings are impressively corroborated by K. Zaimov and his colleagues in Sofia, Bulgaria. They describe a major Bulgarian painter, Z.B., who suffered from a severe paralysis and motor aphasia at the age of 48. So debilitating was the paralysis that the painter began to resort to his undamaged left hand. At first, his drawings were very simple in form, utilizing only a few colors and eliminating line configuration; but there was a steady improvement in fluency until the painter, working completely with his left hand, had clearly regained his skill. Yet, unlike the French painter described above, Z.B. embarked on an entirely new style of painting. Earlier his style had been narrative, and he had habitually represented events of the present, past, and future; but now, perhaps from necessity, he ceased to produce these "recitation paintings." He no longer displayed a penchant for stylization, and for the most part avoided using perspective. Instead, he injected into his works many fantastical elements, such as a condensation of images, and an inversion of relations reminiscent of the experiences of a dream. Z.B. also now showed a predilection for clear tones and symmetrical patterns, two preferences which, according to Zaimov, either reflected a change in personality or constituted a defensive ploy to avoid somber colors or unbalanced configurations. The ultimate effect was the emergence of a fresh and direct way of expression which, in the opinion of many critics, signaled "the birth of a new painter." Though now restricted verbally to some seventy or eighty words, capable of understanding only short phrases, unable to read or write (though still able to copy a written text), the painter Z.B. remained at the pinnacle of his art.

Finally, worthy of brief mention is the Spanish painter Daniel Vierge, who was acclaimed as a prodigy during his youth. In 1882, when but 31, he suffered an apoplectic fit which left him with a severe right-sided paralysis, and incapable of emitting anything besides a few meaningless sounds. Undaunted, he taught himself to paint with his left hand and, like Z.B., regained his pre-morbid level of artistic skill. The neurologist G. Bonvicini, who studied Vierge's case in detail, raised the initial possibility that Vierge may originally have been left-handed or ambidextrous, a fact which could account in a simple way for the ability to resume painting. However, Bonvicini subsequently rejected this explanation, on the grounds that, had the painter been left-handed (with speech functions, therefore, governed at least in part by his right hemisphere), language should have improved as well—which it did not.

Although it is highly unlikely that either of the two latter painters we have been discussing was "really" left-handed, another possibility worth considering is that what each had learned to do with his right hand, controlled by the left hemisphere, had simultaneously resulted in the formation of twin "engrams" in the right hemisphere. This could explain the relative ease in resuming painting with the untutored hand (even as it suggests how certain quadriplegics have continued to paint by grasping a brush between their teeth!). However, on further examination this explanation, too, seems less than convincing: if engrams of drawing in the left hemisphere could mysteriously migrate to the right hemisphere, engrams of speech in the left hemisphere should be capable of an analogous journey. The fact that these painters never regained competent linguistic functioning, indicates that the organization of linguistic and of plastic artistic capacities in the brain is different: the re-establishment of drawing competence entails no guarantee that speech will again flourish.

If painters can survive extensive damage to the left hemisphere and still succeed in their artistic endeavors, what of damage to the right hemisphere? Unfortunately, there has been virtually nothing published about this question, perhaps since the dominant role which the right hemisphere may play has been acknowledged only in recent decades. Evidence supplied by the drawings of ordi-

nary individuals stricken by right-hemisphere disease, however, strongly suggests that the capacity to realize form so
essential to the artist is in fact disrupted under such circ-
cumstances. Patients whose cerebral hemispheres have been
surgically split for therapeutic reasons, moreover, display
a remarkable inability to draw adequately when they are
asked to sketch what only the left hemisphere has witnessed—a further indication that a painter might be severely impaired by right hemisphere pathology.

Recently I had the good fortune to speak with Professor
Richard Jung of Freiburg, Germany, who has collected
paintings by four twentieth-century artists who suffered
right-hemisphere disease. Professor Jung is planning to
publish these cases shortly and has kindly made available
to me his findings and allowed me to examine his remarkable collection of slides, which include a number of self-
portraits made before and after the onset of illness. My
interpretation of the works of these four artists is somewhat different from Professor Jung's, however, and he
bears no responsibility for the views expressed here. I
should point out, further, that there were differences
among the works produced by the artists after brain damage, and that not all my generalizations pertain to all four
artists.

In none of the cases in question did a right-hemisphere
lesion lead to a suspension of artistic activity. Indeed, all
of these artists resumed work as soon (more or less) as they
were able to. The most striking feature of drawings and
paintings executed in the weeks immediately following the
illness is a neglect of the left side of the canvas. The
drawing may be executed skillfully on the right side, but
the left side of the face or the landscape has been left out
entirely! At first, it does little or no good to call this to
the artist's attention, as this phenomenon is an intrinsic
reflection of his condition: he simply is unaware of what
occurs on his left side, and presumably he simply mirrors

in his mind's eye the features of the right side of the work. In each case this neglect of the left cleared up within a few months, although residual traces were occasionally discernible either in the overall placement of the subject toward the right side of the canvas or in a somewhat less careful execution of the left side of the work.

The artists' respective styles remain at least recognizable after their brain injury. A before-and-after examination of the texture of their work, of the detailed regularities reflecting in each case the characteristic manner of depositing pigment on canvas, shows a definite continuity. Moreover, the principal visual schemes used—the artist's characteristic way, for example, of drawing his own face—are largely unaffected. Yet, in each instance, the artist's style does seem to change in a number of respects. First of all, although the left of the canvas is no longer "neglected," the picture is often less sharply defined on that side; it appears to "unravel," to become fuzzier and less determinate, with numerous incomplete lines or features. Another trait of the later work is a somewhat lessened inhibition about what aspects of the subject matter are included. It is as if certain previously maintained defenses or notions about what should *not* be included have now evaporated. Perhaps related to this is the fact that overall execution seems to be bolder, more direct, less finely articulated—where formerly an upper lip might have been depicted by a number of delicate lines, there is now perhaps a single thick, even wild stroke.

Such shifts in technique may lead some viewers of these artists' works—and of those of left-hemisphere-diseased artists as well—to speak of a heightened expressiveness or primitiveness in the post-stroke period. Whether these simpler, more direct works are preferred is of course a matter of taste; but it is at least arguable that they possess greater emotional richness, greater passion, and more faithfully capture the essence of the subject. In any event, the question inevitably arises as to the reasons for this development.

Here we must frankly speculate. Perhaps the lowering of inhibitions and the greater directness are simply signs of advancing age, a reaction to the illness-intensified awareness that the time remaining may be limited; there is no time now for subtlety or allusiveness, all must be stated forthrightly. Yet it may also be that such a shift in style is a direct consequence of the brain disease. If, as Norman Geschwind has proposed, the right hemisphere is indeed dominant for emotional behavior, then a lesion there could well lead to a certain change in personality and to a kind of inappropriateness of response which, while perhaps disruptive of the person's social relations, confers a fresh and even exciting cast upon his works. Whatever the reason, it will be instructive to see whether such shifts in style continue to be found among artists with right-hemisphere disease.

In view of the right hemisphere's role in spatial relations and visual forms, it was somewhat surprising to find so little distortion of shape or form, at least on the right side of these painters' works. Perhaps their superior pre-morbid backgrounds placed them in a stronger position than the unskilled painter, either because the skill of form depiction has been overlearned (particularly in the self-portraits studied by Jung), or because spatial abilities are more widely represented in their cortexes. In this regard, painters and other graphic artists seem to differ from artists in other media, who generally become as impaired as non-artists when their brains are injured. In at least some cases that I have seen, however, there does seem to be discernible distortion of form in the works of artistically inclined individuals.

Of the four artists studied by Professor Jung, Lovis Corinth is probably the most renowned. This painter, who lived from 1858 to 1925, was one of the most important and innovative German artists of the period, honored for his bold, expressive portraits and his unsentimental landscapes. In December 1911, Corinth sustained a severe right-hemisphere stroke, one which left him weakened on his left side for many months and also engendered a deep depression. Once he had left his sickbed, however, Corinth resumed painting, and continued to produce highly acclaimed works until his death.

Critics agree that Corinth's works underwent a change of style after his stroke. They are unanimous in attributing this change to purely psychological factors, such as Corinth's depression following his illness, his intensified awareness of the fragility of human life, increasing preoccupation with death, heightened capacity to seize the essence of objects and experience. A typical characterization and interpretation of Corinth's later works appears in the writings of Alfred Kuhn:

When Corinth arose from his sickbed, he was a new person. He had become prescient for the hidden facets of appearance. . . . The contours disappear, the bodies are often as if ript asunder, deformed, disappeared into textures . . . also the faithfulness of portraits had ceased almost entirely . . . all detailed execution came to nothing. With wide stripes the person is captured in essence. Characterization is now exaggerated, indeed, often to caricature. . . . models, no matter who they are, are now just objects to be painted. Indeed, the models must suffer every deprivation. Corinth always seems to be painting a picture behind the picture, one which he alone sees. . . . at this point Corinth shifted from the ranks of the great painters into the circle of the great artists.

Similar sentiments are voiced by Robert Bertrand:

The highest development of Corinth's work came towards the second part of his life, as was the case with Rembrandt. The objects of the world became mere visions. In his paintings they seem to be unreal; dissolved like fog, they travel past the onlooker. Through life he comprehended life and its inner essence was then visible to him in his old age, for he looked at it objectively and serenely. . . . in full possession of his artistic gifts he created his last works.

Perhaps these critics are correct—Corinth's stylistic transformation may indeed have reflected a change in his artistic vision consequent upon his psychological reactions to his illness. And yet, the student of right-hemisphere pathology cannot fail to be struck by the specific features altered in this artist's work: loss of contours, misplacement of details, neglect and obscuring of texture (particularly on the left side of the drawing), alteration of emotional nuance, increased subjectivity, idiosyncrasy, obscurity.

In the case of a single artist, especially one who has not been followed systematically by scientific investigators, no firm conclusions are attainable. Through a judicious accumulation of cases of the sort undertaken by Professor Jung, however, it should prove possible to tease out the effects of neurological and psychological factors on artistic style. If similar changes occur in individuals who are elderly or sickly, independently of the presence or the site of a lesion, then the psychological explanation gains in persuasiveness. If, on the other hand, a multitude of diseases produce diverse symptoms, or no symptoms at all, while painters suffering from right-hemisphere disease typically display the changes found in Corinth's later work, then the organic or neurological interpretation becomes more tenable. At present, our data base is too slender to allow a conclusion, but my own feeling is that at least some of the changes in Corinth's work are best attributed to the lingering effects of damage to his right hemisphere. The reader can form his own tentative conclusions by comparing works produced by Corinth before his illness with later pictures depicting the same subject matter. (See pages

326–9.) And, owing to the kindness of Professor Jung, it has also been possible to include a similar set of works before-and-after by another German painter, Anton Räderscheidt, for whom a similar comparison can be made.

Through the courtesy of my colleague Dr. Harold Good-glass, I have also had an opportunity to examine the drawings of an architect who, as a result of loss of the blood supply to his head for a few moments, suffered significant damage to his right hemisphere (probably with injury in the left hemisphere as well). Dr. Goodglass followed this patient carefully during the weeks in which, presumably because of the reduction of swelling, he was recovering from this major trauma. An examination of the architect's drawings of figures, cubes, and house plans immediately after his admission to the Neurology Service reveals that he was initially reduced to the level of a young child: there appear only the simplest forms of human beings, complete absence of perspective, deficient and oversimplified spatial relations in house plans, maps, and so on. Within two weeks of the initial set of drawings, there are already marked improvements both in left-hemisphere functions (details) and in right-hemisphere components (relations of parts to the whole, general outline) of the picture. A month after his initial testing, the architect was already executing drawings of good quality, as well as plans and diagrams which were at least adequate. The course of recovery can be clearly seen in the accompanying illustrations; these demonstrate, first, how even an individual highly skilled in the graphic arts can be returned to a childish level of capacity by a brain lesion, but second, how a systematically progressive recovery may follow, especially in those cases where the implicated brain tissue has been temporarily incapacitated rather than destroyed.

We have seen above that the symptomatology ensuing upon brain injury in literary artists or in painters follows

Portraits painted by Lovis Corinth before and after he sustained severe right-hemisphere damage in December 1911. *(See pages 322–4.)*

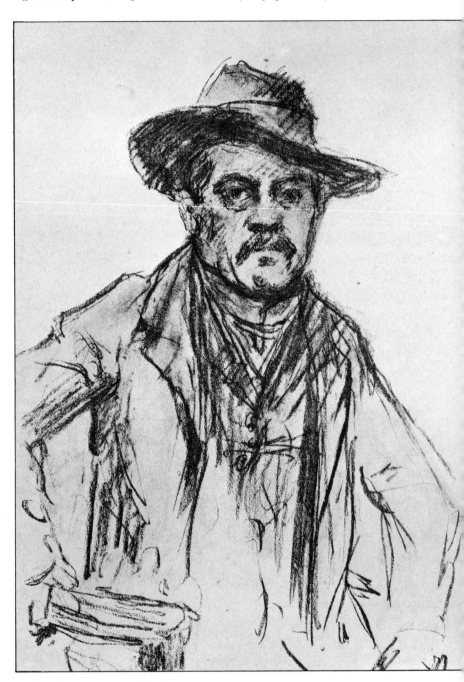

*Self-portrait 1911*

*Self-portrait 1912*

*Self-portrait 1921*

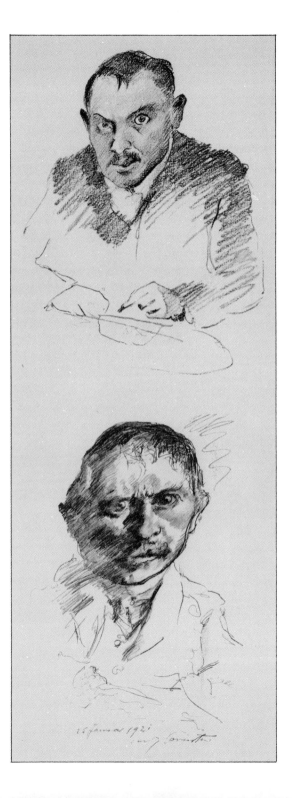

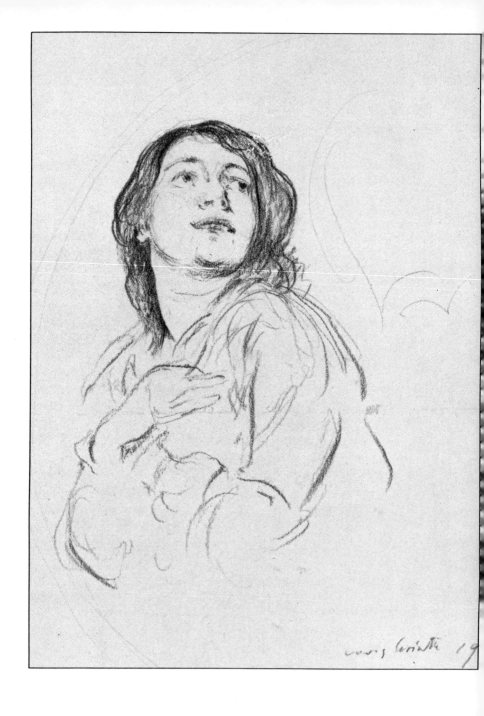

*Corinth's portrait of his wife, Charlotte 1910*

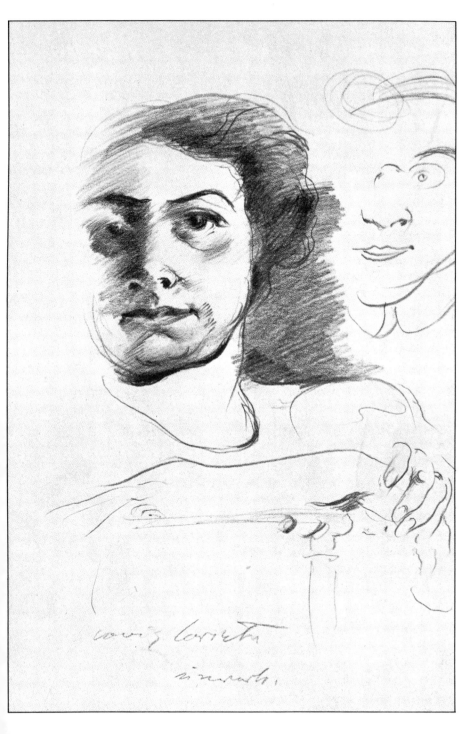

*Portrait of Charlotte 1912*

Self-portraits of the painter Anton Räderscheidt before and after he suffered a right-
hemisphere stroke in October 1967.
a) *Self-portrait of 1965* (two years before).
b) *December 1967* (two months afterward).
First post-stroke attempt at a self-portrait: a
few meager brushstrokes, only right (i.e., "mirrored" left) eye and ear clearly distinguish-
able, left side blank; Räderscheidt quite
unaware of this total neglect of left, though
dissatisfied with picture. c) *March 1968* (five
months). Right side of face now depicted
with some degree of skill, but left side missing
below eyebrow; collar and clothing similarly
depicted only to mid-line. *(See page 325.)*

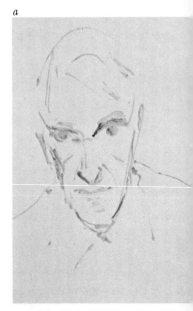

Progressive reduction of neglect of the left in
series of self-portraits by Anton Räderscheidt
from January to June 1968. d) *January* (3½
months after stroke). Neglect of left still
severe, though some improvement observable
over performance of previous month (*b*,
above); colors lively, though crude; outlines distorted even on right, left blank except
for some meaningless brown strokes, perhaps
intended to partially fill this emptiness.
e) *April* (six months). Right side of face now
well delineated; left less so, but notably
improved; color used with greater discretion
and skill, though still with formless brushstrokes at left. f) *June* (eight months). At last
a fairly successful portrait; face depicted with
near-perfect symmetry, though with some
harsh, glaring white brushstrokes on left side.

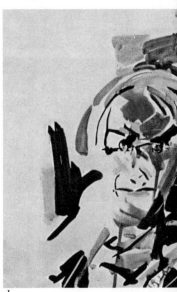

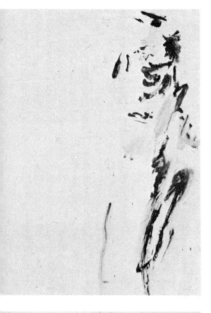

c

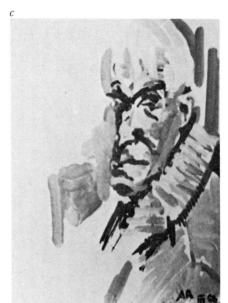

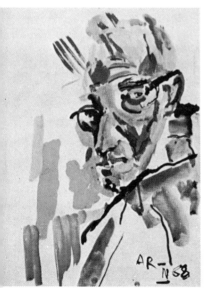

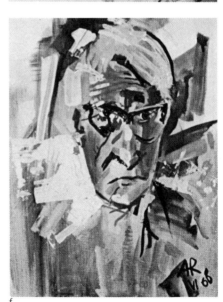

f

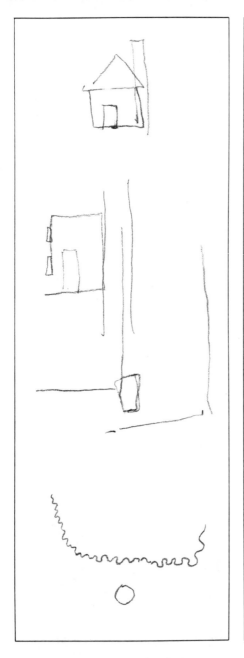

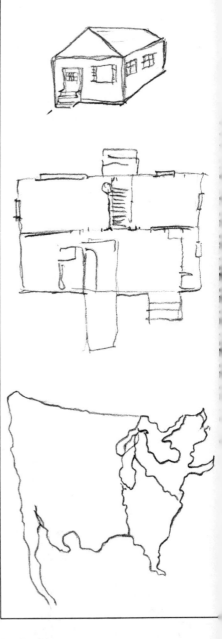

*Session I*
*February 4, 1953*

*Session II*
*February 25, 1953*

Free-hand drawings by architect on two occasions subsequent to brain injury. Depicted at each session were the exterior of a house, the floor plan of the patient's house, and a map of the United States. *(See page 325.)*

certain consistent patterns. When brain damage befalls musicians, however, the picture is far more complex, and far more perplexing. There exist fundamental disagreements about the relationship between aphasia and musical capacity, the localization (if any) of "musical centers" in the brain, the best way to study the dissolution of musical skills, and the overall importance and significance of music as a system of symbolic communication and an area of emotional involvement. Even as the fundamental nature of music has stimulated intensive debate over the centuries, so too the fate of musical ability after brain injury—the precise nature of amusia—continues to challenge neuropsychologists today. If we cannot offer anything like a resolution of the problem here, we can at least essay a coherent summary of the information currently available and describe the various contending positions in this area. Let us begin with a particularly notable case history.

At the height of his powers, the distinguished French composer Maurice Ravel was stricken by a Wernicke's aphasia of moderate intensity. Although he suffered no paralysis, and his memory, judgment, and affectivity seemed unimpaired, he did sustain a diffuse deterioration of his oral and written linguistic capacities. With the help of two musicians, Professor Alajouanine followed Ravel's course carefully for a two-year period and uncovered a fascinating clinical picture.

Ravel was able to recognize melodies and could point out immediately when slight errors were made. Although there was some difficulty in communicating what was wrong, exploration with the help of the examiners invariably enabled him to pinpoint the error. The composer's sense of pitch remained intact, and his general taste and judgment—his ability to criticize performances or to evaluate rhythm and style—seemed impeccable.

In sharp contrast to this preserved discriminating power, however, the composer experienced difficulty in reading notes and in performing from a score. He frequently misplaced notes and encountered extreme difficulty in performing works, including his own. Sometimes phrases and fragments were correctly played, but, just as often, there were transpositions or other confusions of ordering. He was unable to name notes or to sing aloud from a score, and musical writing, though better preserved than language writing, was markedly impaired. Inasmuch as he could neither name notes, write them, nor perform accurately on the piano, Ravel's capacity to compose was effectively annihilated. It is not clear from Alajouanine's report whether the desire to compose—to engage in creative musical expression—was still present. Whether motivation remained or not, however, the potential seemed clearly foreclosed.

The Russian composer V. G. Shebalin suffered from an aphasia which, on clinical description, seems strongly similar to Ravel's. He too had a lesion in the speech zones of the left hemisphere, diagnosed as a sensory or Wernicke's aphasia. His ability to express himself was limited to short phrases, and his command of phoneme production was particularly impaired; understanding of phrases and naming of objects were also significantly limited. Unlike Ravel, however, Shebalin retained the ability to read, and to some extent to write, though "he remained unable to write down long words or a series of words or phrases. When fatigued he would become unable to grasp the meaning of written phrases or paragraphs."

Despite this severe aphasia, Shebalin continued the full range of his musical activities. He worked hard with his pupils, listening to their compositions, analyzing and correcting them. He also devoted a considerable amount of time to composing himself, creating a series of new works that did not differ substantially from those of earlier periods, works that other musicians considered up to his usual standard. The dean of Soviet composers, Dmitri

Shostakovich, described Shebalin's Fifth Symphony as "a brilliant creative work, filled with highest emotions, optimistic and full of life." And T. Khrennikov, another major contemporary Russian composer, commented, "We can only envy the brilliant creative activity of this outstanding man, who, in spite of his illness, created the brilliant Fifth Symphony replete with youthful feelings and wonderful melodies."

We must naturally ponder why Ravel's creative work was abruptly ended by his illness, while Shebalin's output continued unabated in amount and quality. What seems clearly crucial here is the relative degree of preservation of the Russian's ability to express himself in written form, so that he retained a means for communicating his musical ideas; whereas to Ravel, even if he had motifs stored up, ready to be expressed, such channels were simply not accessible. Other, complementary factors may also be involved, however, ranging from differences in personality and motivation to disparities in the extent and nature of the aphasia to contrasts in the organization of musical capacities in the respective nervous systems of these two men. Naturally, given but two cases and limited documentation, it is simply not possible to draw any conclusions regarding the role (if any) of these various factors.*

The variety of ways in which musical capacities can be affected has been illustrated by a number of other case

---

* In his article "Stravinsky in America" in the *New York Review of Books* of August 8, 1974, Robert Craft mentions that the composer Igor Stravinsky suffered a right-hemisphere stroke during his seventy-fifth year. As a result, Stravinsky sustained a permanent partial paralysis on the left side of his body, and an impairment of various "right-hemisphere functions" such as orientation in space. Nonetheless, he remained productive in the years that followed, and, indeed, composed his *Agon* within a matter of months after his stroke. In view of Stravinsky's unique stature, it would be particularly desirable to secure additional information about his clinical picture. Such data might well contribute significantly to our understanding of the cortical organization of musical capacities.

studies. M. I. Botez and N. Wertheim, two Rumanian neurologists, have enlarged our knowledge of amusia by developing a battery of tests for individuals with proven musical competence. Use of this battery has enabled these investigators to identify relatively pure cases of musical difficulty. One patient whom they studied, a right-handed accordion player, had suffered a lesion in the right frontal areas of his brain. A speech difficulty soon cleared up, but the patient remained unable to sing or to play his accordion. His voice was extremely monotonous, and his attempts to play were marked by a distortion in the rhythmic organization of passages, as well as by extensive difficulties in the execution of finger, arm, and bodily movements. He would scramble the order of notes in a sequence, fail to coordinate one hand with the other, and make bizarre substitutions, such as the insertion of a note at an interval of a fourth higher or lower than the intended one.

Surprisingly, the accordionist's "musical sense" and comprehension seemed essentially intact. Although he did have some slight perceptual problems—in recognizing errors in rhythm, for one thing—he remained able to appreciate differences in tone, reproduce individual sounds, recognize intonational faults in a performance, identify the number of sounds in a tune, and discriminate major from minor chords. Somehow, somewhere, there occurred an interruption in the sequence of steps intervening between intended musical ideas and execution by voice or upon a favored instrument. The continued improvement in the patient's speech output suggested that speech capacities were represented in both hemispheres of the patient. Absence of an analogous recovery in his musical expressive capacities may possibly indicate the existence of a unilateral representation of musical expressive functions in the right hemisphere, or at any rate, in the right hemisphere of this particular musician.

At about the same time that they investigated their

hapless accordionist, Botez and Wertheim encountered a patient with a markedly different amusia. This patient, also right-handed, was a former professional violinist, who suffered from a severe aphasia and a right-side paralysis. As in the other case, the patient's speech improved and he became able to write, albeit slowly, with his left hand.

Before his illness, the patient had possessed a well-developed musical sense, including perfect pitch. Testing by Botez and Wertheim following the stroke indicated that the perfect pitch had disappeared, and that there was often a confusion in which a note a fourth higher or lower than the played note was named. Melodies were difficult to recognize: indeed, the patient might play a melody with his left hand without being able to identify it. Intervals were difficult to specify, double and triple meter were confused, rhythms were reproduced with some errors. On the other hand, there was a preserved capacity to name individual notes designated on a clef; this fact, when considered in light of the patient's relatively good linguistic capacity, suggested that his other confusions, such as inability to identify tones, were not merely naming errors, but reflected instead a more fundamental disorder in the *reception* of music. This deduction, that the patient's amusia was primarily of a receptive type, was further reinforced by his impressive performance in singing, transcribing melodies, and playing tunes with his left hand. Like the Wernicke's aphasic, whose ability to express himself is less impaired than his understanding of spoken language, the amusic violinist was disturbed primarily in the accurate perception of musical elements, while only marginally in his ability to execute musical tasks. Botez and Wertheim conclude that in amusia we encounter a situation closely akin to that found in aphasia: the possibility of selective impairment of expressive and of receptive capacities.

To confuse the situation yet further, nearly every reported case of amusia represents a different set of symptoms. A few examples will suffice to indicate the range and
variety of possibilities involved:

• A piano teacher who suffered from Wernicke's aphasia
was able to play the piano quite well after her illness. The
major alteration was a somewhat light, dancelike mood
that came to characterize her playing. She remained able
to execute scales, to detect errors in the performance of
scale, to write music spontaneously or to dictation. In fact,
she was able to sight-read new pieces, even though her
aphasia remained profound for the rest of her life.

• A forty-five-year-old trombonist awakened one day to
discover that he was no longer able to copy music. Though
able to see, read, and sing music perfectly, he suffered
from a "selective agraphia" in the musical realm. One
other accompanying symptom: he was no longer able to
play the trombone, being able to produce only strange
sounds devoid of musical qualities on his instrument.
While hearing the notes perfectly "in his head" and retaining a conception of the entire piece, he was unable to
play it at all.

• A conductor who suffered from a gross jargon (Wernicke's) aphasia due to a malignant tumor in his left hemisphere was nonetheless able to direct his orchestra flawlessly until the day of his admission to the hospital.

• A thirty-four-year-old worker found himself unable to
sing or whistle tunes; he could neither produce them spontaneously nor in accompaniment to an instrument. He
also had difficulty in recognizing noises. Yet, at the same
time, he was able to identify melodies, so long as they had
a distinctive rhythmic configuration. This patient's combination of abilities and disabilities helps to explain how
an individual tone-deaf on clinical examination may nonetheless successfully recognize pieces of music.

• A professional musician who became aphasic remained

able to play musical compositions, both on the cello and the piano. Recognition of instruments and feeling for rhythm and meter remained good. The chief difficulty arose when he attempted to participate in an instrumental ensemble. Although most of the individual elements in his repertoire of musical skills were preserved and his solo performances were adequate, he apparently lacked that keen sensitivity to the details of others' performance which was needed to make him an effective member of the musical group. One possible explanation is that his coordination was sufficiently intact to permit his two hands to work together, when he could set his own pace, but that the split-second timing required for a collaborative effort was now beyond him.

• An amateur musician who suffered a right-hemisphere tumor lost the ability to sing and to play the piano from memory. He remained able to sight-read, but displaced the notes toward the higher end of the piano until he finally ended up off the keyboard. His melody improved when he included the lyrics while singing.

• A patient became tone-deaf and unable to sing along with other people. Although her auditory perception tested by normal methods was adequate, she also failed to recognize melodies when they were sung to her. Yet when shown the title of a song in writing, she was able to sing it perfectly. The engrams of the melodies—the sequence of relations involved in their accurate production—seem to have remained intact. The ability to monitor what she or others were producing was, however, destroyed because of the inability to appreciate pitch values.

In the early 1930's, the neurologist Hans Ustvedt undertook an exhaustive review of the entire neurological literature on amusia. (Since there have been just a handful of additions to the literature since his time—this condition apparently intriguing American and British investigators less than it did the Teutonic research circles devastated by the war—the factual portion of his review requires relatively little revision today.) Ustvedt reached one general conclusion already indicated here: that the literature on amusia is a tangled jungle of claims and counterclaims, difficult to evaluate because of a lack of standardized tests and of sketchy information about the pre-morbid level of patients' musical skills. Nonetheless, on the basis of the insights he managed to glean from this review, and of an intensive examination of fourteen patients whose pre-morbid musical competence had been verified, Ustvedt formulated certain provocative hypotheses.

Most earlier studies had focused on the preservation (or disturbance) of certain elementary musical capacities (e.g., pitch recognition) or of an overall ability to perform or to comprehend music (expressive or receptive competence). This concentration on "cognitive" musical functions had resulted in the neglect of a component crucial to all musical, indeed all aesthetic, experience—its unique potential for arousing and affecting the emotions. Reviewing the effects of brain injury on disparate musical functions, Ustvedt discerned a mixed picture, which we summarize below; but one thing he invariably noted was a change in the individual's emotional relation to music. For the most part, the patients were less involved in their music, and did not perform or listen as fervently as before; their love for music seemed diminished. In an occasional case, there was greater lability in the attitude toward music, wild fluctuations between apparent indifference and a positively maudlin reaction, bordering upon bathos. Ability to evaluate music critically, and to make a finely differentiated musical response, also seemed reduced.

While Ustvedt detected few deficits in the appreciation of tempo, impaired understanding of the unit of the measure was the rule among amusic patients. Comprehension was particularly poor when knowledge was required of the measure in the abstract. The ability to reproduce melodic-rhythmic figures was usually preserved, but duplication of the rhythm alone was impaired; apparently the melody, more tangible in character, is an indispensable factor in accurate reproduction of a musical phrase.

Elementary characteristics of musical perception—sensitivity to pitch, volume, timbre, etc.—seemed intact in these patients, all of whom had left-hemisphere lesions. Yet, with respect to more complex musical elements, there were clear deficits. There was reduction in the capacity to remember old musical elements and to learn new ones; in appreciation of rhythmic and melodic figures; in recognition of melodies. Singing was generally passably accurate, although patients often protested they could no longer sing; there were disturbances in performing instrumental music in most cases, though these could usually be traced to more general disturbances in recognitory or in executive functions.

Singing was also used to explore the relations between speech and melody. Ustvedt found that "the melody facilitates production of the word, whilst the words hamper production of the melody." Overall, he concluded, there was a regression to a more infantile approach to music, with the most primitive elements (rhythm) better preserved than those of moderate complexity (melody) and the most complex functions (speech) being most severely impaired.

It is most disconcerting to find a lack of accord between Ustvedt's conclusions and those reached elsewhere. His study turned up no clear division between receptive and expressive amusia; no evidence of composers or conductors whose musical capacity was selectively destroyed or impaired; no cases of pure tone-deafness, pure instrumental apraxia, or pure arhythmia. Instead, he discerned a general "holistic" decline in music-linguistic sophistication as a result of cortical lesions, more or less irrespective of which part of the left hemisphere was implicated. Even more disturbing, Ustvedt studied three patients with right-hemisphere lesions and found no decline in their musical capacity whatsoever—a finding that indirectly stresses the very connectedness between musical and language functions which other studies have challenged.

The inconclusiveness that emerges overall from our review of the literature on amusia suggests various alternatives. One could, conceivably, dismiss all prior studies as being poorly executed, controlled, or interpreted, and then start from scratch. One could, alternatively, endorse the conclusions of one or another investigator, while dismissing those of his colleagues. It seems more reasonable, however, to assume (as we have elsewhere in this book) that, even if the methods and procedures were not perfectly spelled out, the majority of investigators were describing genuine phenomena as best they could; inconsistencies should be explicable.

In this spirit, we can cherish Ustvedt's individual case studies, and in particular his stress on the emotional component of music—a crucial aspect of musical, and indeed artistic experience in general, but one as yet little understood, in either the normal or the brain-damaged person. At the same time, we need not uncritically embrace Ustvedt's rather strong conclusions about a "general primitivization." The evidence, including his own cases, seems to suggest, instead, that musical functioning, itself far from a unitary capacity, can be disrupted in a great variety of ways, and that it is futile to try to sketch out a single, or even a few, paradigmatic types of amusia. Musical disturbances are not independent of speech disturbances (as disturbances of drawing seem to be), but neither are they closely intertwined with them (as literary deficits seem to be). Nor in most persons can musical capacities be consigned to a single hemisphere. The general preservation of melodic capacity and perception in aphasic—i.e. (usually) left-hemisphere—patients, together with the monotonous quality of voice and song in right-hemisphere patients, indicates a strong right-hemisphere bias for at least the melodic component of music. Ustvedt's own findings point to the left hemisphere as more important for synthetic musical abilities than for elementary perception, thus neatly complementing Milner's demonstration of right-hemisphere involvement in elementary musical functions. Yet recurrent difficulties in perception of fine tone discriminations, and repeated mistakes made in rhythm duplication by patients with injuries in the posterior portion of the left hemisphere, indicate that, at the very least, temporal organization is represented in both cerebral hemispheres.

Comparison among patients and syndromes must also be undertaken with great caution. It may well be that one musician with jargon aphasia can still conduct, while another cannot. One important factor here, of course, is the precise nature of the disease process. If, for example, one conductor has a slow-growing tumor, there is a much greater possibility that his neural organization will adapt sufficiently to allow continuation of a long-established activity than in the case of an abrupt lesion from trauma or stroke. This, however, does not mean that the musical abilities of, say, two composers with lesions in the same brain region—e.g., the posterior portion of the dominant hemisphere—will suffer the identical fate. Whether a composer is left able to read and write seems extremely crucial, for, whatever the status of his "pure" musical capacity, its expression will be effectively thwarted in the absence of command of such a medium of conceptualization and communication. Finally, even assuming that both the premorbid ability and the nature of the lesions are comparable (a situation almost as unlikely as stepping into the same river twice), there remains the question of the patient's "innate" musical proclivities and the way in which musical skills were acquired. For example, just as reading capacities are differently impaired, depending on whether one deals with a phonetic or ideographic written language, musical capacities may also unfold in different ways, depending on the age at which the individual was introduced to formal training, whether he was self-taught or learned to read standard notation, which instruments he plays, and so on. In other words, among the diverse areas of human skill, the realm of music seems to present an especially dizzying mélange of caveats and impediments to its elucidation.

After striking this rather pessimistic note, we can nonetheless point to some promising recent developments. The techniques of dichotic listening (in which different messages are presented simultaneously to the rival hemispheres) and of amytal injection (in which, for diagnostic reasons, one of the hemispheres is temporarily put to sleep) permit us to determine with some authority which hemisphere is dominant for specific musical functions. Such studies have confirmed, with comforting regularity, the dominance of the right hemisphere in most persons for aspects of melodic and timbre recognition and production. Indeed, paralysis of that hemisphere leads to the inability to sustain a melody almost as reliably as paralysis of the left hemisphere produces aphasic difficulties. Other studies indicate that the ability to make "simultaneous judgments" in the musical realm are also strongly lateralized in the right hemisphere. While perception of melodies composed of one tone may be performed equally well by either hemisphere, the right is clearly superior at distinguishing single chords.

One limitation on all these studies, however, is that they have generally been conducted with individuals of average musical ability and a modest degree of training. It remains to be determined whether significant differences obtain with the highly trained musician. It has been observed that there is a high incidence of left-handed musicians, and it has been claimed that a future pianist may be recognized by his superior performance with his left hand. In line with this is a recent study suggesting that, while average individuals have right-hemisphere superiority in musical tasks, for skilled musicians there may exist that left-hemisphere superiority usually associated with language. Thus, we must consider the possibility that musicians have an unusual organization of brain functions. This might be due either to innate predispositions or, possibly, to a shift in cerebral dominance, or at least a progressively wider representation throughout the brain, as musical skills become more developed.

From such experimental investigation, then, comes hope for superior understanding of music's unique status. More sophisticated studies with normal children and adults are sorely needed, and in the wake of the revolution in cognitive psychology wrought by Piaget's research, a similar surge in studies of musical thinking may be forthcoming. And a final source of information about music may well come from the neurological clinic rather than from the research laboratory. For it is becoming increasingly clear that music may make a valuable contribution to the rehabilitation of patients with severe cognitive deficits.

We reported earlier how an individual with a gross memory disorder, one totally unable to assimilate new verbal information, was able to learn a body of facts: the patient first learned a melody, at the same rate as a normal individual, and then was taught lyrics to that melody. Contrary to our expectations, the patient did not find it difficult to sing the melody though it had been originally learned on the piano, or to produce the verbal message apart from the song with which it had been originally associated and entwined. We have noted, too, that even patients who are severely demented, to such an extent that they can hardly speak or recognize objects, may still be able to sing compositions without difficulty and perhaps even to learn simple new melodic fragments.

But perhaps the most promising use of music yet comes from its application in the rehabilitation of severe aphasia. It has been known since the late nineteenth century that anterior aphasics can more readily express themselves and emit words when these are couched in a song. Furthermore, production of melody presents little difficulty for these patients, who can ofttimes hum *"The Star-Spangled Banner"* as flawlessly as any sports stadium enthusiast. However, exploitation of this ability in order to improve speech production *per se* seems to be a new idea, and only recently at our hospital has such an approach been systematically implemented.

A number of patients whose comprehension was reasonably good, yet who had "failed" standard speech therapy, were enrolled in a program called "Melodic Intonation Therapy," or "MIT." Once it had been established that the patients could (and would) sing, they were taught to incorporate familiar utterances like "Good morning, Dr. Albert," "ham and eggs," and "the weather is fine" into simple musical fragments. After these had been mastered, usually without much difficulty, the patients were encouraged to drop the melody while maintaining the stress and articulatory patterns of the prior choral rendition. This procedure generally allowed them to continue making use of these phrases. In case of any regression in the quality of verbal production, use of the melody was resumed and maintained as long as needed. The same or new melodies were also periodically introduced to facilitate the learning of other, more complex phrases, and then similarly phased out gradually as the words themselves were mastered.

From this novel approach, at least two findings seem relatively clear. First of all, since *any* successful verbal communication is extremely important to these aphasics, an effective therapy like MIT bolsters their emotional well-being. Second, and of key importance, music seems to have had a "freeing" or loosening effect on their verbal output. As soon as the patient has mastered the singing of his first one or two phrases, others appear spontaneously: in the space of a few weeks, the patient has at his disposal a fresh vocabulary of words and expressions that have been inaccessible to him since the onset of his illness. In short, from a state of total or near-total inability to communicate, the patient has advanced to the point of at least being able to make his elementary needs known and even sometimes of engaging in extended, if relatively simple, conversation. If the treatment is discontinued, or if the melodies are too soon withdrawn, there may be regression to a more primitive level of language functioning, though the initial spurt or loosening effect is not entirely lost. In such a case, again, reintroduction of the first phases of the training has the desired compensatory effect.

Assuming that this form of treatment continues to be successful (and there is some reason to believe that its success is not wholly transitory), we must ask what is it precisely that is releasing the floodgates of speech. My own guess—and it is just that—is that musical capacities and patterns are very widely diffused in the brain, in both hemispheres. The arousal of these patterns has the same effect as stimulation of wide portions of the brain: it activates a greater proportion of relevant neural connections, hence increasing the probability that the learned patterns critical for production of speech may be aroused. Just as various kinds of verbal cueing help an aphasic patient to produce a word on the tip of his tongue, so melodic cueing may open up blocked pathways leading into the engrams for speech; the melodic patterns must be systematically elicited and drilled, however, since they are less likely to be at the patient's cerebral "fingertips" than such self-stimulating techniques as touching an object, or running through the repertoire of sounds he can emit. Other explanations are also possible, of course—for example, that the patient is speaking completely with his right hemisphere, using engrams laid down there during early childhood—and the issue remains to be resolved.

We have now surveyed an enormous range of disorders of functioning—literary, artistic, and musical. Yet, while a relatively clear division can be made between the capacities crucial in the visual arts and those which figure in the verbal arts, the skills involved in music remain most puzzling. Perhaps this is, in part, because of the varying biological significance of these respective realms: while the survival value or adaptiveness of language and of visual-spatial abilities are evident, with some minimum facility in each characterizing any normal individual, the function of music within the species remains unclear. Whereas the more pronounced uniformity and specialization in the brain for language and for visual constructive processes over the millennia may well be due precisely to the critical importance of these activities for survival, the far less essential character of music allows for a near-stupefying variation among individuals. Some persons exhibit superior gifts from almost the first months of life, often being able to sing before they can talk, to identify and produce pitches perfectly, to achieve virtuoso skills while still in early childhood. Others, often of equal or even superior general intelligence, never display the slightest musical accomplishment, this latter group including many individuals who have received competent formal instruction for years. It is, then, unrealistic to expect a simple pattern of musical organization in the brain, or a compact set of skills which can be compared across individuals; this is especially so, given the presumptive implication in musical capacities not only of the cortex—and both hemispheres at that—but also of the subcortical structures important in rhythmic perception and emotional arousal. Along with each person's unique genetic endowment, background in the field, and customary manner of employing his skills may well come a different neurological pattern, and, hence a different configuration of breakdown in the event of brain damage.

When to these factors is added the incredible assortment of instruments, forms of music, and musical roles—singer, dancer, drummer, pianist, composer, improviser, conductor, and assorted combinations of these—it is hardly surprising that generalizations so handily elude us in this area, that all attempts to find delimited areas involved in all musical competence seem doomed to fail. And yet, the new avenues of research we have described—tests which pit the hemispheres against one another, tests which contrast ordinary individuals and individuals with an extensive musical background and skills, studies of musical thinking in normal adults and in developing children, investigations of therapeutic uses—offer at least some hope that, eventually, sense can be made of music's fascinating status in the mind. In all probability, our ultimate understanding of musical skill, including the mysterious creativity alluded to in the epigraph by Alec Wilder, will depend on our capacity to unravel the riddle of cerebral organization in general and the role of the two cerebral hemispheres in particular. It is to a review of the exciting efforts in this direction that we now turn.

# 9 Contrasting Mirrors

*It was as if that side of the brain had dried up.*
*He was no longer capable of sacrifice, courage,*
*virtue, because he no longer dreamed of them.*

—GRAHAM GREENE,
*The Ministry of Fear*

When the firm gelatinous mass of tissue under the skull is examined by the naked eye, two many-fissured hemispheres of gray matter, mirror-images of one another, are seen. Even when samples of tissue from matching parts of the hemispheres are placed under the histologist's microscope, the differences observable in organization and structure are at best minimal. It is not surprising, therefore, that through most of medical history, clinicians should have assumed that each half of the brain performed the same functions as the other; just like the two eyes or the two ears or the two feet, they were regarded as carbon copies of one another. Yet, during the last hundred years, it has become firmly established that their identical appearance masks radically different functions: the two hemispheres govern significantly different capacities; are, indeed, like two individuals with separate, partially competing identities, each capable of expressing itself and, under appropriate testing circumstances, asserting its importance. The discovery of these different identities, the particular abilities and limitations of each hemisphere, the diverse explanations of the nature and source of each one's distinctiveness—these are the key elements in our review of "lateralization" of function in the human brain.

Recall that each half of the brain controls the movements of the opposite part of the body. When the left foot, the left hand, or fingers of the left hand are moved, impulses have been sent from the right half of the brain; when the individual looks to the left, the impulses (or connections) again go to the right half of the brain; and impulses conveying information from the left ear tend to go to, or "favor," the right half of the brain. This principle of *contralateral* ("opposite-side") representation applies equally well to the right limbs of the body; functioning of the right hand or leg, and other organs on that side, is controlled by the left half of the brain.

If a person is ambidextrous, both brain halves are important in the governance of his movements and actions. Most individuals, of course, are right-handed, and it is therefore the left hemisphere that usually plays a more important role. Thus, an individual with a lesion in his left hemisphere will have to learn anew how to write, eat, or play tennis with his left hand, while the right-hander with injury in his right hemisphere will have lost the use of limbs on which he is much less reliant.

The most fascinating function of the left hemisphere was only recognized a century ago. At that time, sundry hints and clues that had been accruing for many years finally came together into a coherent picture, and scientists first stated publicly that the left hemisphere of the brain played a unique role in (or was "dominant for") human speech and language functions. Lesions in many regions of the left hemisphere would cause difficulty in speaking or in understanding ordinary language; whereas lesions of equal, or even larger size, in the right hemisphere would leave ordinary language unaffected. A different state of affairs prevailed in individuals who were primarily left-handed, perhaps ten percent of the population. In many of these persons, the language function appeared to be represented in both hemispheres, or even primarily in the right hemisphere. Unlike most people, they were "right-brained," with not only the movements of their dominant limbs, but often as well their ability to communicate, dependent upon an intact right hemisphere.

Distinctions between left and right have left an indelible mark on human language and thought. From time immemorial, *right* has been invested with merit and value—we are all familiar with such expressions as *right-hand man,* and with the concept of the right side as the place of honor—whereas *left* has come to designate the worthless or the sinister. (*Sinister,* in fact, means *left* in Latin.) During the Middle Ages, the folds of the left sleeve were thought of as the place to conceal a dagger or other weapon, and it was the left hand, conventionally the instrument of treachery, that might draw it forth. In combat, the right hand, equipped with the chief weapon, did the fighting, but it was the role of the left to administer the fatal blow (the *coup de main gauche*). As recently as a few decades ago, most parents in our society strove to make their naturally left-handed children into "righties" and this practice has by no means died out. Yet, where, thirty-five years ago, only three percent of school-age youngsters wrote with their left hands, this figure is now approximately ten percent. Perhaps the suspicion that there may be disadvantages to being strongly "lateralized" has begun to spread to the general public.

Symmetry is certainly the rule in our natural world and in our bodies. Nonetheless, multiple examples of asymmetry can be found, even in the physical structure of elementary matter. Flatfishes display gross asymmetry in the structure of their bodies; only one-half of the bird's brain and of its vocal system are involved in the production of bird song. In the human, the right arm tends to be longer than the left, the left leg is longer than the right leg, and the left clavicle is longer than the right one. Considering that these measurable differences play little apparent role in human performance, it is indeed striking that an asymmetry so long undetected by scientists can assume critical importance in daily communication.

Once the role of the left hemisphere in speech had been unambiguously established, the general importance of this hemisphere became increasingly apparent. Testing of patients with left-hemisphere lesions revealed deficiencies not only in speech and in right-sided motor functions but also in a range of complex cognitive abilities—in mathematics, in problem-solving, in maze-running, in making drawings and three-dimensional constructions. The left hemisphere became the one to have, if you were having only one. Indeed, neurologists were fond of citing case reports of individuals who had been born without a right hemisphere, or who had lost their entire right hemisphere in an accident or through surgery, who nonetheless coped successfully with the business of living.

It was therefore with some trepidation that a few investigators began to suggest that the right hemisphere might be important too, and not only in the use of the left hand by southpaws. Convincing evidence in this regard came from researchers in England during World War II. Investigators like Oliver Zangwill, Malcolm Piercy, and J. McFie noted that individuals with damage to their right hemispheres would produce bizarre drawings and constructions when asked to copy figures or to draw something "on their own." These patients seemed deficient in their perception of spatial relations; they knew what objects were, they understood what left and right meant, but their drawings were spectacularly disorganized, the relationship among the various elements seriously askew—portions of figures would be omitted (particularly on the left side of the drawing), size relationships would be distorted, sundry aspects of the figure would come unwarrantably to dominate the whole drawing. (See Chapter 8.) Examples of this spatial disorientation could also be observed in such patients' behavior on the ward. They would experience grave difficulties finding their way about, getting from the mess hall back to their beds, remembering the location of the bathroom. Even dressing could pose a major problem for these patients: they would put a shirt or jacket on upside down, insert limbs into the wrong holes, get a garment stuck over the head, or forget to put on a trouser leg (usually the left).

At first, this difficulty appeared explicable in terms of a "neglect" of the left visual field. That is, the patient would readily relate to and interact with individuals or events placed on his right side, controlled by the undamaged left hemisphere; when, however, the "action" took place on his left side, he would appear incognizant of it. Indeed, such neglect can be so strikingly pervasive that the patient will shave only half of his face, brush only one side of his mouth, or eat the contents of only one side of his plate. So bizarre is this behavior that until one has seen it in numerous otherwise intelligent and linguistically intact individuals, one is skeptical of the entire phenomenon.

Sometimes, particularly when the neglect is severe, such a patient may also exhibit "denial"; he will refuse to concede that he has paralysis in his left hand, perhaps seeking to cover over his condition with some feeble joke like "Oh, it's just gone to sleep on me," or "Keep your eyes on it, and you'll see it jump." Such joking, of course, is a "giveaway," bespeaking in itself the patient's awareness that *something* is wrong; yet it is often impossible to get such a person to acknowledge his condition overtly. Alternatively, the patient may invent some sort of bogus explanation for his difficulties; or deny that he is hospitalized altogether; or emit paraphasias only when speaking of his problems (e.g., "My left foot is very sour").

If such patients' bizarre topographical or nosological behavior could in fact be reduced simply to a neglect of elements on the left, however, then one would logically expect left-hemisphere patients to exhibit precisely corresponding deficiencies in behavior. Such proved not to be the case. For individuals with equally large lesions in the left hemisphere, and with equally constricted visual fields, on the right in their case, did *not* similarly deny the existence of their right-side paralysis, nor did they display the kinds of spatial and dressing difficulties almost routinely observed in right-hemisphere patients. Not that left-hemisphere patients performed perfectly on spatial tasks— far from it. Their performances, however, were characterized rather by ignorance of what a figure was (you cannot highlight the appropriate features in a model if you can't identify it), by omission of details, and by simplification of the general configuration of the drawing. Constructions by the left-brain-damaged patient, in other words, might well be primitive, like that of a child, but they would reveal a preserved basic command of spatial relations. Even the most severely afflicted left-hemisphere patient could find his way about the ward and dress himself properly.

A clear inference (among others) from all these observations was that the right hemisphere plays a special distinctive role in the visual and spatial realms—an hypothesis that has received especially strong confirmation in the last two decades. One indirect line of evidence, to be sure, consists in the large number of artists and architects who have been left-handed, including such redoubtable individuals as Michelangelo, Raphael, and Leonardo da Vinci. But the most important measure of support has come from studies of patients who have had brain damage restricted to either one hemisphere or the other, making possible a systematic comparison of their respective performances in a variety of tasks, and accordingly a proper assessment of the domain of "dominance" of each hemisphere.

From these studies, the right hemisphere emerged as playing a crucial role in the processing of visual configurations, particularly those which were unfamiliar, such as random shapes or materials with unusual textures. Whereas familiar shapes could be labeled, and were thus handled routinely, by the left or "verbal" hemisphere, patterns which were not previously known or insusceptible to verbal labels baffled that hemisphere—their detection seemed to depend upon an intact right hemisphere. The right hemisphere was superior at remembering the precise locations of dots in an otherwise empty field and in judging what the whole of a figure (a gestalt) might be like when only parts were exposed.

The once "minor" hemisphere also turned out to play a dominant role in some basic visual skills. For example, the right hemisphere is more important for making fine discriminations among colors (though proper functioning of the more "conceptual" left hemisphere is required for indicating which color or colors are customarily associated with a particular object, like a banana, fireman's hat, or barber pole). The right hemisphere also seems crucial in depth perception, because of its central role in binocular or stereoscopic vision, and as well in the ability to recognize and remember faces. Indeed, cases of prosopagnosia have always entailed significant lesions on the right side of the brain.

Finally, these studies indicated that the right hemisphere is dominant for other than visual functions—notably, for tasks in the tactile or somato-sensory realm. Patients with right-hemisphere lesions displayed difficulty in learning mazes presented to them when they were blindfolded. They also were more impaired than left-hemisphere patients in making subtle discriminations in the tactile modality, such as indicating which of two pressures on the body was sharper, or specifying just where they had been jabbed by a pin. Indeed, whenever fine or subtle pattern discriminations were required, even in the auditory realm, the right hemisphere was found to assume an executive role.

Valuable and revealing as these initial studies were, the vast differences among patients, together with the relative crudeness of the methods employed—they required patient series of as many as one hundred individuals—placed definite limits on their usefulness. With the advent of more sophisticated techniques, and with the reduction in the number of focal brain lesions as the war years receded, other methods for determining hemispheric specialization necessarily came to the fore.

Probably the most exciting and most revealing of these newer methods has been one that allows examination of each hemisphere's performance in total isolation from the other. Such an approach may sound like science fiction, but in fact it became practicable in the early 1960's. At that time, as we have seen, surgeons Philip Vogel, Joseph Bogen, and their associates at California Institute of Technology performed a series of operations in which, as a means of controlling epilepsy, the left hemisphere was surgically separated from the right hemisphere by the cutting of the connections between the two, most particularly the inch-long, quarter-inch-thick bundle of fibers called the corpus callosum. With this operation (usually called a commisurotomy or callosectomy) the patient effectively became "two brains inside one body." Stimulation of the left visual field brought information only into the right hemisphere, since there was now no corpus callosum to transmit the right hemisphere's perceptions to the left. (See the diagram on page 40.) Analogously, information fed into the right visual field, or the right arm, would go directly to the left hemisphere, where it would remain, forever incapable of passing over to the opposite side of the brain. The resulting clinical symptoms in these "commisurotomized" patients resembled those presented by P.K. (see Chapter 7).

Such operations had, it is true, been performed before —for example, by A. J. Akelaitis and his colleagues at Chicago two decades earlier. At that time, it was concluded that this surgery entailed no risks, the corpus callosum then being thought to have no important functions except perhaps, as Warren McCulloch jested, to transmit epileptic fits from one hemisphere to the other. Finding what they expected to find, the psychologists who worked with Akelaitis's patients reported no deficits in them following a commisurotomy. In the 1950's, however, Roger Sperry and his colleagues, also at Cal Tech, began a crucial series of experiments in which they disconnected the two hemispheres in cats. They found that such animals could indeed learn new tasks but that there was no longer any "transfer" between limbs (or hemispheres). If the animal learned a task with his left forelimb, he was unable to perform it with his right. If he had learned to solve a task with one limb before surgery, and then was tested with the opposite limb afterwards, he would again exhibit no retention. This series of studies indicated marked deficits in animals following the surgery *if* one knew how to teach and what to test.

Testing of Vogel and Bogen's first patient produced dramatic results. This patient was a 48-year-old man, a veteran injured during World War II, who had suffered increasingly serious and frequent epileptic seizures in the years thereafter. Nonetheless he had above-average intelligence, keen interest in his surroundings, and normal emotional reactions. After surgery, the patient's seizures were markedly diminished, while his intelligence and personality underwent little or no change. Yet it turned out that he was unable to do many tasks in which cooperation between the cerebral hemispheres was required. For instance, touched on one side of the body while blindfolded, he was unable to point to the matching part of his opposite side, or to use his opposite limb to show where he had been stimulated. Told to point to a certain object in an array (the message reaching his left hemisphere), he would be unable to do so with his left hand (which was connected only with his right hemisphere). This state of affairs sometimes led to amusing consequences: the patient would find himself pulling down his pants with one hand while trying to raise them with his other. Occasionally, however, the consequences were not quite so humorous: the patient once grabbed his wife with his left hand and shook her violently while, with his right hand, he sought to rescue her and bring the violent left hand under control.

Sperry and his co-workers, particularly Michael Gazzaniga and Jerre Levy-Agresti, devised or adapted a number of simple techniques that brought out the unique capacities of each hemisphere. Essentially these techniques involved stimulating each hemisphere separately, then assessing what it could or could not do. Thus, by blindfolding the patient and presenting an object to either one hand or the other, they could ensure that the tactile capacities of each hemisphere were being separately assessed. By asking the subject to fixate on a central point in a visual field and then briefly flashing a target either to the right or to the left of that fixation point, they could ensure that either the right hemisphere (left visual field) or the left hemisphere (right visual field) was being stimulated alone. And by feeding messages auditorily into both ears at the same time—using the dichotic technique of earphone presentation—they could ensure that the left hemisphere heard only what went into the right ear while the right hemisphere perceived only what entered the left ear.

Such techniques enabled the California group to gain unambiguous evidence about the roles assumed by each hemisphere in their patient. With his right hand, the patient could write appropriately, and with his left, he could draw figures accurately. However, he was unable to write with his left hand (because the verbal information in the "linguistic" left hemisphere was inaccessible), and incapable of drawing accurately with his right hand (because the visual-spatial information in the right hemisphere was disconnected from his right hand). Required to copy a three-dimensional model of blocks, the patient was unable to accomplish this with his right hand. While the right hand was fitfully struggling to solve the problem, the left hand, which evidently understood the task, tried like a Good Samaritan to rescue its hapless colleague. It was, however, restrained by the experimenter.

When words were flashed to the patient's right visual field, he reported accurately what he had seen. When the same materials were presented to his left visual field, however, he consistently reported he had seen nothing, or just a flash of light. If, however, instead of asking the agnosic hemisphere what had been seen, the experimenter instructed the patient to use his left hand to point to a matching picture among a collection, the patient could correctly designate the very item that he claimed not to have seen. When verbal information was presented simultaneously to both visual fields, the subject reported orally what he saw in his right visual field, but, at the same time, he was able to draw what he saw in his left visual field. His right hemisphere seemed unable to perceive this inconsistency; the left hemisphere—which could talk—appeared aware of the paradox but remained impotent in the face of it.

Equally striking findings have been manifest in this and other patients in the tactile sphere. Objects placed in the right hand for identification are readily named, while those in the left hand can be cognized and recognized but not named. When, however, after a successful identification by the left hand, patients are asked what has been perceived, they will protest that they cannot feel anything with that hand, or that it is numb. Even when informed that they are successfully recognizing the very objects they claim not to have perceived, they will lamely reply, "Well, I was just guessing" or "Well, I must have done it unconsciously." The left hemisphere is reduced to reporting the information which reaches it and, since discriminations made by the left hand are inaccessible to it, it must plead dumb or "confabulate" a response. A particularly fascinating situation arises when two objects are given to the subject simultaneously, one in each hand, and are then hidden for subsequent retrieval in a large pile. Each hand will then go through the group of objects, searching for the one *it* felt, summarily rejecting the one previously grasped by the other hand.

If a normal person is presented simultaneously with two closely similar auditory messages, for example, *raduct* in his left ear and *poduct* in his right ear, he will fuse the messages, hearing (and reporting) the word *product*. When this test was given to Sperry's first commisurotomized patient, however, he reported only what he had heard in his right ear. Information which had traveled to his right hemisphere from the left ear could not be utilized. In general, the patient completely "extinguished" (failed to report) verbal messages communicated to his left ear, whenever there was a simultaneous input to the right ear. When the patient was presented with "chimerical" stimuli (a face consisting of two disparate halves, or a hybrid portrait composed of two separate objects) and was asked what he had seen, his answer depended on the form of the question. If asked to *point* to what he had seen, he would designate only that part that had been perceived by the right, or minor, hemisphere. If, however, he had to *name* what (or who) had been seen, the patient reported what had been interpreted by the left (or speaking) hemisphere. Indeed, with the perception of faces and nonsense shapes (for which the right hemisphere is specially primed) the patient's verbal performance was scarcely above chance. It took split-brained patients a long time to learn the names for faces, and typically, they had to resort to elaborate verbal strategies, such as the formula *Dick has glasses, Paul has a mustache, and Bob has nothing.* Such a result further confirms the right hemisphere's dominance for the kind of Gestalt perception important in recognizing new configurations: left to its own devices, the major hemisphere performs very poorly in learning new visual configurations.

In another revealing test using chimerical stimuli, patients were asked to point to objects similar to those presented. When the right hemisphere was asked to point, the left hand would select a stimulus that was structurally similar—i.e., related in geometric form—to the perceived chimera; when the left hemisphere (or the right hand) was required to point, "similarity" was reinterpreted, the subject now designating stimuli that belonged to the same conceptual category but bore little structural similarity to the target. Patients asked what they had seen in a chimera routinely chose the left visual field picture; when, however, asked to point to a picture whose name rhymed with that of something seen, they invariably pointed to an object whose name rhymed with that of the picture presented to the right visual field. Where knowledge of auditory-linguistic configurations was required, the left hemisphere took over.

Tests featuring chimerical stimuli not only confirmed that the two hemispheres have different capacities, but also demonstrated a certain rivalry between them. The hemisphere dominant for a given function tends, it was shown, to control the motor performance relative to that function. Thus, in a task for which the right hemisphere is dominant, both right and left hands would point to the left-field stimuli; and, conversely, when the task implicated

a dominant left hemisphere, both hands would point to
what was seen in the right visual field. It is not understood
how the organism "as a whole" decides which visual field,
and which half-brain, should be allowed to "speak for"
both hemispheres and how it then orchestrates the bilateral response.

The California group's early work with split-brained
patients, and particularly with the patient described above,
served to confirm the by now established view that the left
hemisphere is strongly dominant for language: this first
test subject was able to give correct answers to verbal questions only when stimulus information reached his left
hemisphere. Work with subsequent patients, however, undermined this customary view, indicating contrarily a
limited right-brain capacity for language, at least for the
reception of linguistic input. It was found, for instance,
that the minor hemisphere is able to perform simple sums
when presented with numbers in the left visual field or
with block numerals in the left hand. If a word like
*hammer* or *eraser* is flashed in his left visual field, the
patient is often able to select the correct object from a
group. (Yet if the patient is asked afterwards for the name
of his selection, he cannot give it—confirmation that the
left hemisphere has not participated in the patient's correct response.) These patients also seem to have some
capacity for auditory comprehension in their right hemispheres. When an object is named aloud by the examiner,
the patients are able to select the correct object with their
left hands, even if blindfolded. Though both hemispheres
hear the word, the patient cannot tell afterwards what he
has chosen, for only the left hand (and not the left hemisphere) knows what it has selected. The minor hemisphere
can, in certain cases, respond to somewhat more complex
descriptions, such as "shaving instrument" for *razor,* "dirt
remover" for *soap,* or "inserted in slot machines" for
*quarter.* And the most verbally gifted right hemisphere in

the California series endows its owner even with a limited ability to spell with the left hand. Given a few letters in the tactile modality, and asked to form a possible word, this young patient can make an acceptable arrangement, whether or not the word has been spoken by the experimenter.

Such findings—in the face of a massive, century-long accumulation of evidence pointing to exclusively left-hemispheric speech control in right-handed patients—were naturally very surprising. Making them even more so was the fact, as noted above, that the performance of the California researchers' first patient did jibe with established doctrine. Nonetheless, Sperry and his co-workers, pointing to the presence of extra-callosal brain damage in this patient, now claim that the test results they obtained with the others are valid. They conclude that there is in fact some measure of linguistic capacity in the normal individual's right hemisphere, buttressing this assertion with the residual linguistic ability usually displayed even by severely aphasic patients and by the quick recovery of linguistic capacity on the part of young children with severe injury in the left hemisphere.

More critical observers have suggested, however, that it is Sperry's *later* patients who are abnormal. Unlike patient No. 1, who was injured in early adulthood, the others had all had epilepsy from birth or shortly thereafter, and were all operated on in their teens or early twenties. Because of this very early damage, their brain organization naturally would differ drastically from the norm; and because they were operated on while still quite young, the clear-cut dominance found in normal adults would not yet have coalesced. It follows, these critics argue, that the war veteran, a man with a normal brain until early adulthood, who was operated on only in his 40's, more accurately manifests the normal linguistic capacities, or lack thereof, of the right hemisphere.

Neither of these extreme positions seems actually to be warranted, since the varying performances here can be explained quite well simply on the basis of "individual differences." Indeed, there are vast variations within Sperry's series of ten patients, some of whom have remained mute for months, and one for nearly a decade. In addition, and more important, the right-hemisphere linguistic capacity demonstrated in certain patients never really goes beyond very narrow limits. While certain common substantives seem to be comprehended, there is no clear evidence that the right hemisphere can understand verbs. In fact, it even fails on nouns that are either identical in form to verbs (e.g., *fall, hit*) or derived from verbs (*teller* and *trooper*); adjectives derived from verbs (*shiny, leaky, dried,* etc.) are similarly missed, and so for that matter are most adjectives not directly associated with particular nouns. Clearly, messages of any degree of complexity or subtlety elude so taciturn and deaf a hemisphere.* And, despite considerable testing, there is no evidence whatsoever that the right hemisphere can to any extent initiate oral expression. Its meager comprehension, such as it is, can be demonstrated only by pointing; it remains effectively mute.

It is extremely difficult to penetrate into the phenomenal world of a split-brained person, to know just what it is like to have, in effect, two minds within one skull. The two halves of the body can sometimes cooperate, as in tying a shoe, or in making a cat's cradle; but these are precisely the tasks in which two separate individuals can also operate in concert. More complex intermanual tasks, such as playing the piano or knitting, pose grave difficulties. We have seen that sometimes the disconnected

---

* A paper by E. Zaidel presented at the Academy of Aphasia in October 1973 suggests that the right hemisphere in two of Sperry's patients may indeed be able to comprehend more complex messages.

hemispheres interfere with one another, and that there is also a latent competition, depending on whether the given function falls principally into the domain of the left hemisphere or that of the right. Yet the two hemispheres can also cue one another; split-brained patients become increasingly skilled at telling when the other hemisphere has been stimulated, by noting, for example, an eye movement or a shift in bodily orientation.

Investigators have even suggested certain advantages in having a split brain, inasmuch as the hemisphere less skilled or unskilled in given functions does not try to interfere in those realms, and each hemisphere is relieved of the necessity of informing the other of what has been going on as regards its areas of competence. These seem chiefly debating points, however; no one, surely, would recommend such radical surgery, except for those with intractable seizures.

The study of patients with split brains has had a virtually Nobelian effect on the fields of biology, psychology, neurology, and even philosophy (at least upon those philosophers concerned with the unity of mind or the indivisibility of consciousness). No one is yet sure of the precise significance of the findings; nonetheless, everyone agrees that the study of portions of the nervous system in isolation from one another provides an invaluable glimpse into the basic underlying principles of neural organization and behavior. While such radical disconnection, of course, occurs but rarely in humans, surgical experiments *are* possible in animals, permitting an approach to many hitherto inaccessible questions. The principal connections to a specific neural structure can be severed, and the function of the newly isolated structure can be probed, in order to pinpoint what it can accomplish "going it alone." The implications for recovery of function and for rehabilitation are also considerable; for example, evidence on the performance of an isolated zone provides leads about therapeutic methods for those reliant upon that region alone. A certain caution must be employed in drawing conclusions, however: a disconnected region may behave differently than a region still connected to destroyed tissue; in addition, brains whose hemispheres have been disconnected may differ from brains in normally developed individuals, who, unlike the epileptics discussed above, have not had to develop alternative pathways for accomplishing critical functions.

Varying the techniques initially developed with split-brained patients, and drawing on the principles discerned by the California group, a number of other investigators have helped fill out the picture of what each cerebral hemisphere can (and cannot) do. Some of the findings conformed to expectations, others decidedly not. We shall take a look at a few of them in the following pages.

During what we may call the heyday of the left hemisphere, it was widely believed to be dominant not only for speech activity but also for musical expression and comprehension. As we have seen, most of the pertinent evidence now suggests, instead, that the right hemisphere is more important in this area (particularly for singing), that the discrimination of pitch and intensity requires an intact right, but not an intact left, hemisphere. In a neat study, John Bradshaw used delayed auditory feedback— i.e., the playing of speech or music back to a subject a short interval after its original communication—and found that such delayed feedback to the right ear (and the left hemisphere) slows down the speed of oral reading of prose passages, whereas delayed feedback to the left ear (and the right hemisphere) slows down and impairs piano playing. And in a series of important studies using dichotic listening techniques, Doreen Kimura showed that the right hemisphere plays a central role in the discrimination and memory of musical elements, even when those passages are familiar to the listener.

Calculation is another area where the "plaudits" at

one time went exclusively to the left hemisphere. When Sperry's studies revealed a limited calculation capacity in the right hemisphere, Stuart Dimond and his associates were encouraged to take a fresh look. To their astonishment, they found that, when problems requiring equivalent skill were presented respectively to the left and the right visual field, test subjects were better able to solve subtraction problems transmitted to the left field, although there was no difference in speed or accuracy for addition problems. Dimond suggests that what was formerly regarded as the left hemisphere's superiority in this area was merely an artifact reflecting exclusive reliance on verbal responses. When only a manual response, such as pointing, is required, the right hemisphere can then manifest *its* capacities in this respect.

The evidence on whether the right hemisphere plays a role in linguistic function in normal right-handed people is still fragmentary; recent findings increasingly suggest that it is useful, after all, for a speaker to have a right hemisphere. The speech output of patients with injuries in that hemisphere tends to be monotonous and flat, suggesting a loss at least of the melodic component. And patients with exclusively right-hemisphere lesions do make out less well than "normals" on language performance tests. They are often deficient in adopting an abstract attitude, and in performing complex linguistic tasks rapidly. When tested on their sensitivity to the connotations or generalized associations of words—as opposed to their literal meanings—right-hemisphere patients are similarly deficient, suggesting an inability to voluntarily adopt a metaphoric or metalinguistic attitude. And when their diseased condition is the subject of the conversation, such patients are likely to make flagrant naming errors or issue notably inappropriate responses. While this latter defect, being restricted to a particular topic that arouses strong emotions, does not seem at first glance to be really linguistic in nature, it may nonetheless exert considerable influence on these sufferers' language output. If the right hemisphere is able to emit sounds at all, it may well be involuntarily uttered oaths—in fact, such ejaculations have, since the time of Hughlings Jackson, been considered the "speech of the right hemisphere." (This hemisphere is in general perceptually attuned to oaths, gestures, stock responses, and other forms of "automatic speech.") Finally, while the discrimination of consonant sounds is clearly a left-hemisphere function, the ability to detect vowels or make discriminations of pitch or timbre appears to be at least in part a capacity of the right hemisphere. And further confirmation of the right hemisphere's contribution to language is afforded by Macdonald Critchley's report (regrettably undocumented) that creative writers beset by right-hemisphere lesions may suffer impairments in their output.

As we have pointed out in earlier chapters, the presence of a sizable lesion in the brain is naturally reflected in a patient's day-to-day behavior. Individuals with lesions in their frontal lobes may perform adequately on tests of intellectual functioning, but often undergo a more-or-less complete personality change, in which they become flat of affect, slovenly, perhaps giddy or salacious as well. The behavior of a person with injury in the language areas of the left hemisphere will also reflect the locus of injury: if expression is impaired, he will usually exhibit an understandable depression, but will retain an excellent understanding of his condition, and respond appropriately in diverse situations. If the areas of comprehension are disturbed, however, the patient may exhibit a blithe unconcern about his situation, and perhaps appear generally euphoric. His former personality should, nonetheless, still be recognizable.

The unusual personality configuration of those afflicted

with right-hemisphere lesions is just beginning to be recognized. Such patients—as we noted in our study of artists—are usually insensitive in varying degrees to their visual-spatial environment, and tend to neglect objects and, especially, diseased limbs on their left side, while they retain relatively good language capacities; and the behavioral syndrome exhibited by many such individuals is one that follows logically from this combination of abilities and disabilities: The patient will often deny his illness, pretending that there is nothing wrong with him; generally indifferent to what is going on about him, he is likely to spend most of his time just sitting around—he may ask periodically when he can go home, but will usually take no interest otherwise in his surroundings. He has no trouble understanding what is said to him and giving articulate, and at least pertinent, responses; his answers, however, will often be correct in a very strict or narrow sense while betraying an excessive literalness that makes them in normal terms inappropriate. Asked how long he has been "here," a patient will reply, "About five or ten minutes, Doctor. I wasn't looking when I came in." Or, questioned about what floor of the hospital he is on, he will answer, "I'm on this one."

In casual conversation, these individuals will often display a tendency to banter, and may indeed appear quite funny. Closer examination, however, reveals a cutting edge in much of what is said. One recent patient exchanging pleasantries with the attending physician declared that he felt fine, and that he would be "even better at seventy than I am at sixty." Pressed about where he was, he admitted being in a hospital, "though there's nothing wrong with me, as far as I can tell." But he then added, "We're in a dog hospital; they take care of dogs in this hospital." Asked how he liked it in the hospital, he said, "It's O.K., but there are too many ifs, ands, and buts here." This seemed to be a veiled reference to the intensive examination, in-

cluding linguistic evaluation, to which he had been sub-
jected on our Unit. Another patient admitted that he had
been sick because of a fall, but put the matter this way:
"The roof fell in on me . . . this is no Playboy Club, you
know . . . the warden calls me down for dinner." A strange,
forced conviviality—accompanied by tendencies toward
either confabulation or frank invention, or an apparent
gallows humor—seems to be the prevailing mood among
this patient population. At times the inventions will become particularly blatant, as with the patient who insists
that he is in the "Quincy Branch of the Massachusetts
General Hospital," or that his immobile arm was sprained
during a tennis game; and it is then unmistakably clear
even to the casual observer that something is amiss.

Such considerations have led Norman Geschwind to
speculate that the right hemisphere may be dominant for
emotions. A person with a left-hemisphere lesion will usually display normal emotional reactions to situations,
whereas a right-hemisphere patient will most likely be
inappropriately jocular. (The case cited above of some
left-hemisphere patients who appear cheerfully unconcerned about their condition is not really inconsistent with
this comparison, since these individuals' problem derives
from a disturbance of comprehension, not of affect as such.)
Empirical support for Geschwind's speculation has come
from a recent study by Guido Gainotti in which the emotional responses of right-hemisphere patients emerged as
distinctly abnormal.

My own impressions are in accord with this hypothesis
—but with the important qualification that there are actually vast differences among patients, many indeed being
jocose and even euphoric most of the time, yet others
showing themselves extremely hostile, depressed, or taciturn. These variations point to a complex process of interaction between a patient's pre-morbid personality and
the effects of his brain lesion. Whatever a given patient's

emotional "set" may be, however, the key point, again, is that that set is maintained more or less consistently, however inappropriate it may be in various circumstances. The root of the problem seems, as noted above, to lie in the patient's loss of his normal sensitivity to his environment. In many ways, he appears as if cut off from the sensory though not the linguistic world. The literalness already commented on stems from the fact that the patient is responsive chiefly to linguistic input, to the denotations of words and not to their nuances or connotations; he is glaringly insensitive to such factors as tone of voice, the spirit in which a query is put, and other environmental cues that might suggest one as against another response. All this said, it is nonetheless true that most right-hemisphere patients do remain capable of reacting to events of really major significance in their surroundings or in their families. Such reactions are generally only temporary, however; in the absence of continued linguistic reminders, they cannot be sustained, and there follows a rapid return to the status quo. Emotional appropriateness, in sum— being related not only to *what* is said, but to *how* it is said and to what is *not* said, as well—is crucially dependent on right-hemisphere intactness.

On the basis of right-hemisphere patients' reliance on language—particularly in its denotative aspects—and their tendency to neglect information on the left side, Marcel Kinsbourne has developed a more detailed and elaborate, and quite intriguing, interpretation of their behavior. Under normal circumstances, Kinsbourne indicates, the attentional mechanisms located in the mid-portions of the brain will be utilized equally by both cerebral hemispheres. Put differently, each hemisphere controls the capacity to orient to the opposite side—the hemispheres vie with one another for control of the orienting and attention centers of the brain. When some object or element is introduced into either or both of his visual fields, a normal person will be able to attend in either direction. If, however, one hemisphere is injured, it will be more difficult to arouse that hemisphere's attentional capacities and a "super-threshold" stimulus may well be required.

Kinsbourne speculates that when an individual's left hemisphere is activated, for example, during speaking, his orientational mechanism should reflect that arousal and as if by a spill-over effect, his gaze will shift to the right. This surmise was confirmed by requiring normal subjects to locate a gap in a square. When the patients were asked to rehearse a list of words while performing this task, they were less likely to detect a gap on the left side of the square. The act of speech had shifted their attention to the right and so their awareness of gaps on that side had been heightened. On this principle, the patient with right-hemisphere disease should exhibit a persistent inclination to look or orient himself to the right. The usual circumstances of examination involve verbalization by the patient, and orientation to the right is accordingly underscored. This brings about a situation where the right-hemisphere patient is found to be ignorant of that half of the world located on his left.

Why, however, doesn't one find an equivalent degree of neglect of the right side in patients with left-hemisphere damage? At least two factors may be relevant. First of all, the right hemisphere, thought to be more important in visual-spatial behavior, is intact in these patients, and so they may remain more aware of what is going on throughout their surroundings. Second, they still attempt to communicate linguistically, and so they continue to activate their injured left hemisphere. It should be borne in mind, of course, that it is more difficult to assess neglect in left-hemisphere-injured patients, because they do not communicate as well; and it may well be that the degree of neglect exhibited by such patients is for this reason consistently underestimated.

Kinsbourne's model of hemispheres competing for control of attentional mechanisms has generated some imaginative research, both on his part and on that of others. He has found, for example, that skill in balancing a dowel in one hand is enhanced when one is simultaneously speaking, if the dowel is in the left hand, while performance is impaired when one is speaking if the dowel is in the right hand. His explanation is that speaking and balancing are competing activities, which, owing to the "spill-over" effect, interfere with one another when they both occur simultaneously in the same hemisphere; while these same activities become complementary or concurrent when they occur in opposite hemispheres, and they then promote and facilitate one another. Exemplifying the same, complementary side-effect, speaking improves the subject's ability to recognize elements in the right visual field, even when those shapes are nonsensical. In contrast, when the patient rehearses melodies (a right-hemisphere function), a left-visual-field advantage results.

Overall, what emerges from these findings is a more dynamic view of cerebral laterality. Instead of two centers that are alternately clicked on and off, we discern competing fields of forces, which enhance those respective activities in conformity with each field, while impeding and hampering those activities in conflict with the principal preoccupations of each hemisphere. (One fairly common experience exemplifying these conclusions is that of being able to read and write quite easily—or even more easily than usual—when music is being played on the radio, but of finding oneself abruptly distracted when the announcer comes on the air.) The challenge still remains, however, of charting more fully which activities complement, and which conflict with, one another.

One line of investigation presently being pursued in several laboratories tracks eye movement during cerebral activity. If certain functions—for example, language—involve one hemisphere primarily, then the movements of the eyes should reflect this function during linguistic activity. For instance, as one discourses in language, the eyes should shift to the right. Conversely, when a person is using spatial imagery, as in following a route or solving a geometrical problem, his right hemisphere should be activated and his eyes should consequently shift leftwards.

So vigorously is this line of research being pursued that my summary will undoubtedly be passé by the time these lines are printed. Initial studies indicate that eye movements can be a rather fine measure of cerebral activity. Kinsbourne, once again, has provided a paradigmatic study in this regard. In it, both the movements of the eye and those of the head were found to reflect the nature of the thinking required in simple tasks, with verbal reasoning resulting in movements to the right, numerical and spatial reasoning eliciting movement to the left. A separate series of investigations has revealed that people with a rational and objective outlook on life tend to be "right-movers," while individuals whose eyes move to the left are more "subjective" and "intuitive." Stimulated by these findings, Steven Harnad interviewed graduate students and professors in mathematics at Princeton University, classifying them by the direction in which their eyes moved when a series of questions was posed. Those whose eyes moved to the right were found (in the opinion of their peers) to be less creative as mathematicians, displayed less interest in the arts, and utilized a smaller amount of visual imagery in solving problems, than a matched group of mathematicians whose eyes moved to the left, reflecting activity in their nondominant hemisphere. These findings were interpreted as evidence that aesthetic and emotional considerations (presumably mediated by the right hemisphere) are important even for hard-nosed mathematicians.

Such a focus upon the actions and interactions of both hemispheres promises to provide a fuller understanding of what goes on during normal ratiocinative activity. To be sure, brain-injured patients will continue to provide indispensable evidence about what each part of the brain does. Nonetheless, it is almost unthinkable that our "normal" minds should not utilize both halves of the brain during waking activity—any evidence which suggests how these two contrasting "mirrors" interact and modulate one another is most precious. It has already been shown that use of both hemispheres in a task will often increase brain efficiency; for instance, on a visual task in which information was fed independently to each hemisphere (by tachistoscopic presentation) subjects performed better than when information was provided just to one hemisphere. Since the left hemisphere operates primarily by processing elements in sequence, while the right hemisphere treats elements simultaneously ("in parallel"), activities which exploit both forms are particularly enhanced by interhemispheric collaboration. Reaction time is also more rapid in cases of bihemispheric stimulation: even verbal messages are dealt with more efficiently when they are fed to the two hemispheres separately.

Finally, it is worth mentioning that information provided to a single hemisphere may interfere with other information drawing upon that hemisphere. Individuals more efficiently report details of a line drawing when they are asked to describe it verbally than when asked for a spatially monitored output (for example, pointing to the correct items in a column of symbols). Conversely, when individuals are required to recall sentences, a spatially monitored output proves more effective than a linguistic characterization. In each case, it is easier to produce an answer from the hemisphere not involved in rehearsing the information than from a region overlapping the area where the answers are being formulated and rehearsed. The more interhemispheric relations can be based upon cooperative activities, the more probable the organism can achieve an optimal level of productivity.

The distinguished investigators engaged in the monumental task of mapping out the diverse functions of each hemisphere have not been able to resist completely the temptation to engage in "global" speculation, to come up with a single all-encompassing characterization of each hemisphere. The initial such overall characterization— and still the one most popular and most widely espoused —presents the left hemisphere as involved in linguistic activities, the right hemisphere in nonlinguistic activities. This simple explanation is supported by many studies that show the right hemisphere to be superior at dealing with nonsensical or random patterns, irrespective of their modality of presentation, whereas the left hemisphere becomes increasingly more efficient as materials enter the realm of language.

Even should this dichotomy emerge as scientifically impeccable, however, all riddles will by no means have been resolved. Rather, the question then becomes more refined: What is a verbal (or linguistic) element and what is not? What of numbers, punctuation marks, trademarks, flags, musical notation—are these linguistic? What of characters from different alphabets—is English linguistic to a Chinese individual? What of nonsense figures to which one successfully affixes a label—does the same configuration magically become linguistic if the observer is clever (or verbal) enough to make it so? In addition to these as yet unresolved questions about the nature of linguisticality, there is considerable evidence suggesting alternative descriptions of hemispheric specialization. In testing the short-term memory of matched groups of patients, for instance, Nelson Butters and his associates found that patients with right-hemisphere damage had difficulty with visually presented materials whether or not these were verbal, whereas patients with left-hemisphere damage performed poorly with auditorily presented materials, whether or not these were verbal. If these findings can be replicated, they suggest that, at least in the short run, memory is organized on a modality-specific rather than a material-specific basis. In other words, under those circumstances, the left hemisphere seems to be predisposed to deal with auditory materials, the right hemisphere with visual materials. Only when memory is probed over a longer period of time is the traditional characterization upheld—left hemisphere involved with language, right hemisphere with nonlinguistic materials.

The claim of a correlation between the left hemisphere and language function has also been modified by investigators of language perception. Workers at Haskins Laboratory have pointed out that only in the perception and production of phonemes, in particular consonants, is the superiority of the left hemisphere striking. Both hemispheres can receive the auditory parameters of a speech signal, and both can deal efficiently with vowel and tonal sounds. Indeed, the very same acoustic signal will be interpreted (and handled cerebrally) in a different manner depending on whether the individual is "primed" for ordinary language or some kind of nonlinguistic sounds. Only in the former case are left-hemisphere effects encountered. This suggests that the same psychological signal can engage one or the other hemisphere, depending upon whether or not the subject is "set" to perform linguistic operations upon the input.

Yet another way of parceling out the "cerebral pie" has recently emerged. Certain accounts stress the propensity of the right hemisphere for dealing with totalities, gestalten, organized wholes, as, for example, in face or pattern perception, and contrast this with the left hemisphere's mastery of discrete, particularistic elements. A dialectic is thereby proposed between an "elementary" and a "gestaltist" hemisphere—or between a "perceptual" right hemisphere and a "conceptual" left hemisphere. While this approach does not directly contradict the traditional formulation in terms of language-nonlanguage, it does involve rather different functions and, at certain points, cuts across the other characterizations (e.g., language involves both wholes and elements; perception can occur with reference to linguistic or nonlinguistic components).

In an important series of studies, Josephine Semmes and her co-workers have called attention to the surprisingly different ways in which information appears to be stored and handled in each hemisphere. Studies of elementary perception have revealed that tactile perception is represented in a relatively narrow strip of cortex in the left hemisphere (governing the right side of the body) but is represented far more diffusely (throughout large portions of the right hemisphere) for the left side of the body. These findings suggest that information may well be coded and processed differently in the two hemispheres. The left hemisphere, with its focal representation, is better equipped to integrate similar units; accordingly it has gradually been implicated in specialized behaviors requiring fine sensori-motor control, such as manual skills and speech. In contrast, the right hemisphere, with its diffuse representation, is better suited to integrate dissimilar units; this zone therefore specializes in behaviors that require integration of information from diverse sources and modalities. Semmes's model helps explain the right hemisphere's association with spatial functions, for it is preeminently in the individual's sense of space that the unifying of information from disparate loci is most crucial. Indeed, the distinguished neurologist Deryck Denny-Brown has claimed that the major elements of the "right-hemisphere syndrome" are due to a failure to integrate elements of sensation—a condition he called "amorphosynthesis." Spatial disorders found in left-hemisphere-injured patients, on the other hand, are seen as representing a conceptual or linguistic deficit, reflecting not the organization of sensory information *per se* but rather the use to which such information is put.

In addition to challenging the interpretations, it is also possible to question the findings. In a pair of trenchant reviews, the Australian psychologist Murray White has severely criticized the raft of studies of hemispheric specialization, claiming that their techniques are primitive, subject populations poorly controlled, data analysis suspect, and patient groups incommensurable. Without detailing the substance of his attack (which seems to me rather overwrought though not without merit), the kind of ambiguity widespread among findings does seem worth pointing out. It has been found, for example, that when materials are presented simultaneously to both visual fields, materials in the left visual field are more rapidly identified. This is explained by the tendency to begin at the left when one is reading. When the material is presented either to the left or the right, however, then verbal materials are more quickly perceived in the right visual field. This is explained by the dominance of the left hemisphere for verbal processing. Sorting out the contributions of habitual scanning procedures, and those of hemispheric dominance, turns out to be anything but a straightforward task. Indeed, even the use of Hebrew characters, which are scanned from right to left, does not unambiguously resolve such questions. Similar difficulties have arisen in determining laterality effects in the auditory sphere. White concludes that "field effects" depend on the kind of stimulus presentation, the amount, nature, and arrangement of stimuli, the intensity with which information is displayed, the order in which it is reported, the response modality tapped, the viewing condition employed, and the ocular, hand, and speech dominance of subjects. It is not surprising that few, if any, studies meet White's stern requirements; his circumspect conclusions caution those who would unwarily leap from one, two, or even twenty-one studies to a theory of hemispheric dominance.

A final variable in the controversy surrounding cerebral

lateralization is the familiarity of the materials. It has been found, for instance, that unfamiliar shapes tend to be processed by the right hemisphere, whereas shapes capable of verbalization (as well as other linguistic materials) are processed by the left hemisphere. What makes an element "verbalizable" has seldom been considered, but in my view, the familiarity of the item—the frequency with which it is viewed—is probably the crucial factor. We tend to possess, or in lieu of possession, to invent, names for configurations which are frequently perceived; names are much less likely to arise for objects seldom encountered. If we assume that the left hemisphere deals with materials that are familiar and hence readily encoded, while the right hemisphere handles those not readily assimilated into established categories or schemes, we thereby have a ready account of most findings in the neuropsychological literature. Such an account does not invoke any "special" categories of materials, while at the same time it is consistent with the basic assumptions of theories of human learning, according to which a strategy for dealing with unfamiliar materials supplements established ways of dealing with familiar materials.

Even the "familiarity" theory runs into difficulties, however. Why, for instance, should the left hemisphere be predisposed only to deal with consonant sounds, since vowels are presumably as frequent? And why should there be a right-hemisphere effect for the perception of familiar (and presumably easily encoded) musical patterns? It could be argued that it is language *as a whole* that is so familiar and that it is the consonants that are particularly diagnostic of language, vowels being found in nonlinguistic contexts. This argument seems forced, however. It could also be maintained that even familiar music is less familiar than all of language and so remains a right-hemisphere concern. This account will gain in plausibility if a recent finding, alluded to earlier, can be confirmed: Workers at

Columbia University have shown that the strong right-hemisphere effects in musical perception are replaced by left-hemisphere effects when subjects with considerable musical accomplishment are examined. With this skilled population, music appears to involve the left as well as the right hemisphere, and, perhaps because music is so familiar to this group, this realm of experience invades the left hemisphere of the brain.

Overall, we are compelled to say that attempts to reduce hemispheric differences to a simple formula have not encountered striking success; and in view of the long evolutionary history that led to the present cerebral organization, it may, after all, be rather foolish to expect a straightforward solution to this great mystery of the brain. Nonetheless, the question of why hemispheric specialization has occurred is a fascinating and important one, which can be tackled (at least partially) independently of the nature of that division of labor.

Although, as noted earlier, scattered examples of physical asymmetry occur throughout the realm of nature, no other examples as striking as cerebral lateralization have yet been encountered. In a search for precursors of cerebral asymmetry, it is therefore instructive to consider the cousins of man.

Many monkeys do indeed favor particular limbs for most of their activities, though the degree of ambidextrousness and variability is far higher than among *Homo sapiens*. In many activities, of course, all limbs are used. But particularly as regards primitive tool use or the manipulation of disparate elements, monkeys—like humans—will tend to make one hand dominant and the other subordinate. And when their brains are split, the same kind of effects occur, with the hand (and hemisphere) which originally knew the task still master, the hand (and hemisphere) which played a supporting role before, woefully ignorant of how to proceed. The more successfully the task has been mastered, the more likely it is that the subordinate hand will remember how to do it, and easier it is likely to be for that hand to learn the task following callosal surgery. Similar, if somewhat less marked, effects occur with the visual fields of monkeys: tasks which had been more integrally involved with the dominant hemisphere will be retained when its visual field, but not when the contralateral field, is implicated. In the case of primates in general, then, there seems to be an incipient tendency to favor one hand—and this tendency may be innate. Yet across primates, there is little tendency for one hand to be favored over the other. Moreover, the extent to which dominance emerges depends primarily on the amount of environmental activity requiring division of labor and the consistency with which the animal happens to utilize one hand in solving such tasks.

With monkeys, of course, there is no dominance for speech activities—and so no way of determining whether Sarah and Washoe, the two communicating chimpanzees, are favoring one (or the other) hemisphere. Yet the fact that dominance can be observed in the use of tools suggests a comparison with the human infant. It has been proposed that the infant's eventual dominance can be ascertained at birth, for example, by noting the position of the limbs in various reflexes, or the direction in which eyes move during the first hours of infancy. Although these broad claims have not been firmly substantiated, it is generally agreed that an individual's ultimate dominance can be observed by age 1, or at the very latest, by age 2. Few doubt that there are genetic predispositions toward left-handedness in certain families, but again, the centuries-long record of conversion of so-called "natural lefties" into right-handers indicates that this genetic pattern is by no means unmodifiable. Indeed, Thomas Bever has suggested that the left-hander is just that individual with a tendency toward left-handedness who is insensitive to environmental cues and can thereby resist the various "messages" directed toward him by the environment that he, too, should join the legions of right-handers. Modest correlations between left-handedness, thinness, and certain introverted and recalcitrant personality characteristics lend limited support to the imputed relationship between hand dominance and the "kind of person" one is.

Determining which hemisphere controls dominant limb movements is a straightforward process, especially in comparison with determining dominance for speech. It can by no means be assumed that all left-handers have speech dominance in the right hemisphere. If anything, more left-handers are left-brain-dominant for speech; indeed, the ratio may be as high as two left-hemisphere-dominant left-handers to one right-hemisphere-dominant left-hander. One foolproof way of determining speech laterality is by putting one-half of the brain to sleep through the injection of sodium amytal into a carotid artery; this, however, is a rather risky procedure, normally used only when neurosurgery is contemplated. A somewhat less reliable but far more convenient method of assessing hemispheric dominance for speech is simultaneous presentation of verbal inputs into both ears and empirical determination of which inputs are remembered more accurately and more rapidly. On this evidence Doreen Kimura has shown that cerebral lateralization for speech may occur as early as age 4 for girls, and perhaps somewhat later for boys. Since this technique is, at best, a rough measure, it can be assumed that in many persons dominance for speech is established at an even earlier age.

A strong dominance pattern in speech and motor use has generally been regarded as advantageous; indeed, knowing which hand to use and employing it regularly correlates highly with most everything "good": intelligence, mental health, perhaps even a good marriage. Conversely, mixed dominance, an inconsistent lateral pattern, correlates with "bad things"—difficulty in reading, clumsiness in gait and in motor activity, stuttering, behavioral problems. Strangely, the latter dysfunctional pattern is found far more frequently in boys, who for some reason are more prone to have disorganized (or unusually organized) brains. However, the picture is by no means that simple. First of all, even in those individuals (usually girls) with strongly established early dominance, there is still language capacity in the minor hemisphere, as evidenced by the rapid recovery of linguistic capacities in such individuals when they sustain severe injury in the major hemisphere. In addition, early dominance is no more a guarantor of success in school than late dominance a key to failure. Indeed, John Kershner has recently shown that first-graders without firmly established laterality are superior to their more "lateralized" peers in understanding and reproducing spatial relations, perhaps because they are better able to represent space in an "iconic," or more topographically faithful, manner. Any number of individuals who have been "late bloomers" and have originally displayed difficulties in reading, left-right discrimination, speech, or other kinds of "learning disability" have gone on to great accomplishments in their respective fields (Hermann von Helmholtz, Hans Christian Andersen, and Albert Einstein, among others, probably had dominance problems). A somewhat aberrant organization of the brain may well enable one to see things with a fresh perspective (like the left-looking mathematicians), provided that the differences are not so severe as to entail blatant deficiencies.

Sperry's collaborator Michael Gazzaniga has made the provocative proposal that at birth we are all split-brained individuals. This may be literally true, since the corpus callosum which connects the hemispheres appears to be nonfunctional at birth. Thus, in early life, each hemisphere of the brain (or the whole brain, if you like) appears to participate in all of learning. It is only when, for some unknown reason, the left side of the brain takes the lead in manipulating objects, and the child begins to speak, that the first signs of asymmetry are discernible. At this same time, the corpus callosum is gradually beginning to function. For a number of years, learning of diverse sorts appears to occur in both hemispheres, but there is a gradual shift of dominant motor and speech functions to the left hemisphere, while visual-spatial functions are presumably migrating to the right. In those infrequent cases where a corpus callosum fails to develop, the individual develops two independent brains, each of which appears capable of spatial, linguistic, and other functions. But in the normal person, the division of labor grows increasingly marked until, in the post-adolescent period, each hemisphere becomes incapable of executing the activities that the other hemisphere dominates, either because it no longer has access to its early learning, or because early traces have begun to atrophy through disuse.

Still the question remains: Just what is the nature of the relation between the hemispheres? What does it mean to be left-brained or right-handed?—and the question has as yet not begun to be satisfactorily answered. Some observers tend to think of the right-hander as an individual who does everything with his right hand, others speak only of a majority of activities done with that hand, others see one hand taking the leading or master role, the other that of a subordinate in all behavior. Handedness is ascertained in some cases by a lengthy questionnaire, in others by a series of manual tests to be performed, in still others merely by asking the individual, "Are you right- or left-handed?" Indeed, the position has been taken that this phenomenological procedure is in fact the most valid one, since only the individual himself knows which limb he is most comfortable in using, which more readily masters new tasks. Yet it has also been shown that in the learning of a new activity or skill, it is the nondominant limb that often asserts the initial advantage at the outset. The dominant limb demonstrates its prowess only over the long haul, gradually outstripping its minor colleague in efficiency and effectiveness. Clearly answers to questions of dominance and handedness—including the best definitions of each—rest somewhere in the wiring of the nervous system and in the evolutionary saga of its development; but the code in which these answers is inscribed has not yet been broken.

An attractive ploy is to turn these questions around and ask not, why asymmetry, but rather why symmetry? After pondering the visual system of various lower organisms, the noted anatomist J. Z. Young has concluded that a symmetrical version is uniquely equipped to provide information to the organism about its overall orientation in the environment in a speedy, accurate, and useful manner. The visual system allows the organism to build into its brain an accurate representation or topographic "map" of the external world. Elements in their entirety, as well as the relations among these elements, can also be effectively captured by such an "analog" system. Two eyes and two brains are necessary, since a single midline organ would not allow surveillance of a sufficiently wide field, at least not unless it is equipped with complex computing mechanisms. Items of information which don't feed into the map can be ignored; and, if a motor system is added, skills picked up by one side of the body will be simultaneously absorbed by the other side. Thus, both brain halves, without separate learning, are enabled to acquire those "mirror" versions of the behavioral sequences that may prove invaluable in critical situations. One disadvantage of such a symmetrical system—insensitivity to the orientation of elements like alphabetic letters—is considered unimportant. After all, in the natural world with which infrahumans have to deal, there are virtually no instances where absolute knowledge of left and right is important, but

numerous instances in which an internalized map of the
external world is serviceable. (In contrast, only the asym-
metric system in man allows determination of the information necessary for accurate left-right discrimination.)

Young indicates that man has relinquished total reliance
on a topographical map of the world in the course of developing one of his hemispheres for use in the relatively
autonomous realm of language. The left hemisphere is
skilled at a kind of digital computing which involves abstract items and which often proceeds in blithe independence of the external world. Man can master relationships
of position and movement through language as well as
through a faithful map; additional cognitive opportunities
accrue to him through the specialization of each hemisphere. Humans have, in effect, given up bilateral symmetry. Indeed, we are at more of a loss if deprived of the
dominant, less topographical hemisphere. The geometrical
increase in the number of connections in the human brain,
the use of various symbol systems, the associations among
different sensory modalities, all give rise to an elaborate
computer-like mechanism that performs many operations
quite apart from the mundane world of directionality in
space. Yet, Young concludes, "perhaps it is the two together that serve to make the most truly useful representation of the world, partly map-like, partly abstract."

It is through viewing laterality and symmetry in their
biological context—as the gradual outcome of a lengthy
evolutionary course—that some perspective may be gained
on their meaning. Clearly throughout most of evolution,
the advantages of bilateral symmetry and redundancy in
the nervous system were sufficiently apparent that these
features were not seriously challenged. But, when the line
of the primates encountered conditions where manual dex-
terity and tool use were adaptive, some specialization of
each hemisphere became advantageous. Whether the proclivity toward tool use and the initial use of language were

related developments, as Jerome Bruner suggests, or instead reflect two entirely distinctive evolutionary trends, may forever remain a mystery (though the chimpanzees now learning "language" could offer us data relevant to this question). Yet, clearly, the same evolutionary pressures that encouraged a division of labor in the use of hands were also instrumental in creating a division of labor for more general purposes. Under this parceling out of function, which comes to characterize the developing child during the first years of schooling, the left cerebral hemisphere becomes increasingly involved (if not preoccupied) with linguistic and conceptual matters, while the right hemisphere assumes superiority in visual-spatial processing and in the manipulation of unfamiliar, richly patterned information.

Only in the split-brained person does one witness in its most dramatic form the extent to which these systems can operate independently of one another. Presumably in the normal individual the synchrony and support between these systems can be quite productive. The individual deeply involved in conceptual activity, in dealing with familiar elements, may at the same time remain oriented to the spatial world and incorporate the novel information in his environment. Via the corpus callosum these hemispheres transmit information between one another, so that the linguistic centers know what the right hemisphere has seen and attempted to interpret, even as the right hemisphere is told what to look for, and when the left hemisphere reads or hears about something new. Furthermore, what the dominant hemisphere has mastered is not completely withheld from the nondominant hemisphere; most of us can hold a fork or throw a ball passably well with our "minor" hands. With the nondominant hand, moreover, we usually can write in a mirrorlike manner more readily than in the usual left-to-right sequence—a hint that nondominant limbs have been implicitly performing the same movements as the dominant ones, in the mirror-image manner characteristic of a system with bilateral symmetry.

Such convenient adaptability probably explains why humans continue to have at least partial bilateral symmetry. It is very useful for the left hemisphere to partake of what has been learned by the right hemisphere (or for the right hemisphere to be learning at the same time—we do not know which): the right hand need not start anew in mastering a given task. And, of course, we have already seen the great advantages of this symmetry for the young child unfortunate enough to sustain brain damage. Presumably such progress as can be made by the older brain-damaged individual with his contralateral limbs also reflects the degree to which that symmetry is still retained.

Most brain-injured individuals eventually learn to walk again, and if their right hand has been paralyzed, they become able to function with the left. It is curious, therefore, that those individuals who remain aphasic for more than a few months hardly ever learn to communicate again. This outcome was particularly puzzling in view of the brain's apparent anatomical symmetry. In 1968, however, Norman Geschwind and Walter Levitsky introduced the first documented evidence of a clear difference in the neurological organization of the two hemispheres. Specifically, the region of the left temporal lobe involved in language was shown to be larger in sixty-five percent of all individuals, whereas the same region was larger in only eleven percent of the right hemispheres. Geschwind and Levitsky needed no elaborate histological examinations: they simply looked at one hundred brains and found the differences to be highly significant—again a case of the "prepared mind," here perceiving what hundreds of highly serious neuroanatomists had failed to note. Wada has reported the same kind of brain asymmetry even in early infancy. If these findings continue to be confirmed, we will have the first proof that the division of labor in the hemispheres so obvious in behavior also has correlates in the very structure of the brain. It will not be too surprising, then, if more substantive differences are subsequently shown between the molecular structures of brain areas involved in language and those implicated in the computation of spatial information. Indeed, differences in structure of the two hemispheres have already been suggested in the finding that epilepsy and cortical atrophy are more likely to occur in the left hemisphere. This incidence is presumably linked to the kind and amount of activity that occurs there: perhaps increasing specialization comes at the price of increasing risk to the "machinery." However, left-hemisphere injuries may more frequently populate doctors' records because of the greater import of the activities served by this site—the apparent correlation, in other words, may simply be an artifact.

Any well-organized system involves some division of labor. In all organisms there are specialized regions for dealing with digestion, excretion, absorption, and so on. In a highly differentiated organism such as man, this division of labor is naturally at a premium, and should therefore eventually be reflected as well in the physical character of the nervous system. The individual without his left hemisphere is certainly lost, for he cannot communicate with his world in the symbolic coin which it favors. But, in a different way, the individual without his minor hemisphere has also been abandoned, for he can no longer find his way about and cannot make use of the various paralinguistic cues that modulate conversation and dominate nonverbal interaction. The human brain has striven to achieve a fine and productive balance, allowing some redundancy of representation so that brain damage will not completely destroy the individual's chances for survival, yet encouraging much specialization, so as to facilitate efficient execution and skilled mastery in a wide range of activities and functions.

Indeed, it is in its capability for developing a plethora of skills, for achieving excellence in diverse domains, that the human brain has proved an especially stunning achievement of evolution. Just like the gifted mathematicians who look to the left, or the virtuoso musicians who, despite their left-handedness, can superlatively integrate the activities of both hands, unexceptional mortals also have the potential to achieve excellence in language, conception, and the mastery of the familiar, as well as space perception, intuitions, and the mastery of the unknown. Individual proclivities differ drastically, so that some will find left-hemisphere activities easy, while others will inevitably gravitate to those subsumed by the right hemisphere. As matters now stand, education may not foster the full range of these powers, for at least in our society there is a nigh-exclusive emphasis on the verbal and conceptual, and a concomitant deemphasis of the perceptual, the intuitive, and the spatial. As Nelson Goodman's apt quip has it, "Our educational system is half-brained." Yet the very knowledge that the human brain is so constructed as to facilitate the achievement of excellence in competing spheres of knowledge, and that there may be fruitful interaction between theoretically competing systems, should help us to utilize more fully the contrasting mirrors in the mind.

# 10 The Matter of Mind

*Our brain is a democracy of ten thousand million nerve cells yet it provides us with a unified experience.*

—SIR JOHN ECCLES

Psychology fascinates because, perhaps alone among the sciences, it promises to illuminate the fundamental questions that have so relentlessly haunted human beings. First and foremost, perhaps, we seek perspective on ourselves: what we are like, how we became that way, to what extent we can change, what it would be like if we did, whether we are really a unified whole or merely a collection of disparate skills and actions. Interest in self extends to our ideas, our feelings, our personality, our wishes, fears, dreams, anxieties, goals, triumphs and disasters—these multiple facets cry out for clarification and explanation. Hence the throngs who flock to the latest form of analysis, the guru of the week, the "way" (Western, Eastern, or what-have-you) to salvation, happiness, understanding.

Interest in psychology, to be sure, extends beyond purely selfish concerns. We want to know about groups and individuals who differ from ourselves, including ones we can never meet, because they inhabit the past, the future, or the outer reaches of our galaxy. We are captivated about feelings not experienced, drugs not tried, thoughts too perilous to entertain in the night. And, as the twin dragons of science and technology continue their inexorable advance, more cosmic questions arise: Can our minds, bodies, thoughts, and feelings be controlled? If so, who will control them? Can a brain be transplanted, or a new mind constructed? Maybe these questions are not so selfless, for our children will live in 2001, or at least 1984.

During by far the greater part of its long past, psychology has dealt with these issues by drawing upon the wisdom of thoughtful men and women, who contemplated the human condition, and discoursed or wrote on their conclusions. When, something more than a century ago, psychology first wrapped itself in the mantle of empirical science, two new methods of study emerged: systematic introspection by carefully trained observers, and controlled experiments by laboratory researchers. Introspection proved but a short-lived chapter, for agreement among introspectors was too difficult to attain; so, at least in the English-speaking world, serious academic psychology became synonymous with experimentation *à la* physics.

Most of what experimental psychologists have demonstrated in the last decades has added to our understanding of basic perceptual and motor processes; yet, somewhat surprisingly, the bulk of this research fails to clarify the questions that intrigue all of us, including psychologists. Efforts to "know ourselves" continue to rely upon a hodgepodge of sources—experimental findings, self-observation, folk wisdom, the aperçus of artists, philosophers, commentators, not to mention common sense and common nonsense. Much can be learned from the study of normal adults, but there are limits to this source. For one thing, most processes and skills unfold in the ordinary mortal with such rapidity, intricacy, and smoothness that unraveling the relevant components proves a formidable task. It is also more difficult to gain distance from ourselves, or from those like us, than from members of alien cultures. The very ties of social class, cultural heritage, age, education, and moral values that facilitate ready intercourse among Westerners serve to preclude—or at least render elusive— an objective psychology of such persons.

Accordingly, social scientists have looked to individuals and organisms who diverge from normal adult Western men and women in illuminating ways. Clinicians such as Freud turned to the emotionally disturbed individual, highlighting the continuity between the normal and the diseased personality; developmental psychologists such as Piaget examined the young child, discerning the roots of adult reasoning in his conceptions and misconceptions; anthropologists such as Lévi-Strauss voyaged to the home-lands of distant, primitive peoples, in search of the basic elements and variants of human culture; behaviorists such as Skinner and ethologists such as Lorenz have eaves-dropped on the worlds of different species in an effort to pinpoint the evolutionary antecedents of human skills, practices, feelings, and perceptions. While none of these populations has faithfully mirrored ourselves (taking "our-selves" here to be normal adults of Western culture), each has, like a good sketch, captured salient dimensions of those selves. By a judicious assemblage and combination of these sketches, a convincing picture of human nature in general can—perhaps—be limned.

In brief, that we can find glimpses of ourselves in chil-dren, animals, neurotic persons, or primitive peoples is now the conventional wisdom. Yet it is less widely appre-ciated that mentation can be similarly illuminated by a study of the brain-damaged individual. Like the senile or dying person, such an individual has been regarded chiefly as a source of embarrassment or frustration: things would be so much easier if he would either snap out of it or die. We have all been children, we can admit neurotic ele-ments in ourselves, animals and primitive persons are comfortably remote; brain damage, however, can strike anyone at any time, through accident, illness, or the sometimes savage processes of aging. The very immediacy and irrationality of the threat—like sudden death—has caused many to avert their eyes.

Nonetheless, the implications of brain damage, and brain study in general, can hardly be gainsaid. The discovery of centers in the brain which appear to mediate feelings of pleasure, or give rise to violent behaviors, has raised inevitable and disturbing moral questions. The invention of new surgical techniques increases the possibility of altering behavior through physical intervention. And the improvement of bio-feedback techniques raises the spectre of mind control by skillful conditioners. The dramatic results of split-brain research threaten our conventional assumptions about the "whole person" or the "unified self." Efforts to simulate the human mind—through computers, through artificial brains, even through the creation of living matter—underscore the challenge we face in using the 1,300-gram Jello-like mass inside our skulls to explain itself. Our ultimate understanding of the human brain will rely on our discovery of what this organ does—knowledge heavily dependent, in turn, on the study of what this organ can and cannot do subsequent to injury. As a consequence, the existence of brain damage, and the possibility of studying its effects, become major factors in efforts to understand, simulate, or control the human mind.

These will be our concerns in this concluding chapter. We shall ponder what brain damage does to the individual, and the lessons about normal functioning that can be drawn from its study; and shall focus particularly on the implications of this research for the understanding of human consciousness and personhood. How can a small pile of matter, and one that has been damaged at that, continue to give rise to those impressions of consciousness, self, identity, and mind which are so uniquely and deeply human?

Although introspection will never provide a final, scientifically conclusive answer to psychological questions, it is a wise, and perhaps indispensable, point of departure for experimental investigators. But what of the introspections, the subjective impressions, the first-person accounts of individuals whose brains have become damaged? What can be learned from them, how reliable are the lessons, and are different reports at all consistent with one another? Some accounts are of little note; but several remarkable, intensely personal documents, written so far as we know without major help from others, have provided a fascinating glimpse of the world inhabited by the individual suffering from an insult to his brain.

The diagnosis of aphasia had yet to be officially promulgated when Professor Jacques Lordat, Dean of the Faculty of Medicine at Montpellier, discovered in 1825 that he could no longer speak. He had been feverish for two weeks when, as he later recalled: "I noticed that when trying to speak I could not find the expressions that I needed. The thought was completely ready but the sounds were no longer at my disposition. . . . I said to myself: it is true that I can no longer speak!" Within twenty-four hours thereafter, Lordat's condition had worsened. The words he heard had lost their value; the few he could yet produce could not be coordinated into thought.

Carefully observing his own behavior, Lordat was astonished by his lack of control over what he said. He would confuse the order of syllables: instead of *raisin* ("grapes") he would say *sairin,* instead of *musulman* he was likely to utter *sumulman.* He found himself selecting words from spheres entirely alien to the appropriate one—desiring a book, he unaccountably requested a handkerchief. Nor could he console himself by reading: "In losing the memory for the meaning of spoken words, I had also lost the meanings of their visible signs." Only his ability to repeat words was at least partially preserved.

Yet despite his profound difficulties in reading, listening, and expressing himself, Lordat insisted on the unaltered condition of his mind. "Be assured that there was not the least change in the functioning of the innermost intelligence," he declared. "I felt myself entirely the same inside." He admitted that his mental isolation, his sadness, and the stupid air that seemed to surround him, might seem to signify the waning of his intellectual faculties (an event which, he joked, would please some while disturbing others); but he himself discerned no impediments in his ability to think. He found, for instance, that in reflecting on the Holy Trinity, he was able to grasp all of the relevant ideas, though his memory did not reveal a single word to him. Indeed, he claimed that, despite his speech loss, he experienced no difficulty in the exercise of thought. "Accustomed for so many years to literary studies, I congratulated myself on being able to arrange in my head the principal positions of a lecture and on not finding any undue trouble in the alterations which I chose to introduce in the order of my ideas." These experiences convinced Lordat of the importance of separating loss of speech from loss of intelligence. After some weeks of profound sadness and resignation, Lordat underwent a moment of epiphany: in looking over the books on his library shelf, he was suddenly able to make out the title *Works of Hippocrates.* "This discovery made me shed tears of joy. I used the faculty of reading as a means of relearning how to speak and to write. My education was slow but success was noticeable every day."

Lordat's recovery is documented by the clarity of his written presentation. It is a tribute to the keenness of his intellect that, even at this early date in medical history, he was able to describe the principal features of aphasia; problems in relating meanings to sounds; paraphasias of meaning and of sound; the relative ease of repetition; the interrelations between reading, writing, and speaking. Lordat's later career is inspiring: he remained Dean of the Faculty of Medicine until 1831 and pursued an active

writing and scholarly career for many years thereafter. He
died in 1870, in his 98th year, enriched by every title and
honor his colleagues could bestow.

Professor Lordat's memoir exemplifies certain features
found in other accounts by brain-damaged patients. There
is the suddenness of the onset of the difficulty; the initial
disbelief and despair at the difficulty in speaking and understanding; some measure of relief that one's thoughts
and feelings are still accessible to oneself; the months of
loneliness and frustration when recovery proves slow.
Where patients vary, of course, is in the severity of their
condition, which in turn bears on the extent of their recovery. The most impaired patients will die, or never recover appreciably; those with the mildest impairment will
improve with such rapidity that the episode becomes a
brief, if painful nightmare; only a relatively small group
of patients will evolve from a state of relatively severe
damage to a point at which they are sufficiently intact to
share their subjective impressions with a wider audience.

The early history of aphasiology produced two other
reports of distinction. A sixty-five-year-old physician from
Geneva named Saloz composed *Memoirs of an Aphasic
Doctor*. Like Lordat, Dr. Saloz was able to retain his ideas
and conceptions throughout his illness but, unlike his illustrious predecessor, he felt in retrospect that he had
suffered "a more or less strong diminution of intelligence."
For Saloz, everything had become cloudy, as in a dream or
nightmare: his thoughts were like an "uncultivated field,"
on which were sown diverse ideas bereft of connections.
What was relatively unimpaired was his will; through determination and persistence his recovery was facilitated.

Saloz describes a bizarre situation in which meanings entered and escaped his consciousness with unpredictable
speed and force. Thoughts in themselves seemed relatively
intact, but the symbols or vehicles for embodying them
were not, and so the ideas themselves became slippery.
The most familiar names and writings seemed to retain

only a distant echo of their former clarity; it was as if his mind had been "veiled by a kind of woolly gauze." Saloz never knew ahead of time whether a word would come out appropriately; no matter how carefully he planned, the syllable might emerge distorted, or even "incomprehensible, in a baroque way." There seemed to be a desiccation of the glue connecting word and idea.

A number of interesting leads on rehabilitation appear, perhaps for the first time, in Saloz's memoirs. The physician noted that when he sang, the words came out more easily; he had the impression that neural paths were more readily aroused by a musical line. In producing a sequence like the alphabet, it proved helpful to commence with the beginning of a series. The little "grammatical" words posed special difficulty and required special drill. Paradoxically, it was easier to say *Nebuchadnezzar* and *Popocatepetl* than *if* or *since*. Saloz's method of self-rehabilitation entailed a multifaceted attack whereby each language system was used as a control and guide for the others. Thus, to correct speaking, he continually monitored his writing and reading; writing in turn was guided by reading and speaking. He performed many exercises, making himself spectator and actor simultaneously; through this role-playing technique, replete with gestures and other devices, he ultimately attained a high level of recovery. Even as his predecessor Lordat had presciently described the variety of aphasic difficulties, Saloz anticipated several major forms of therapy now utilized with aphasic patients.

The third aphasic of the classic era to pen an introspective account was Auguste Forel, director of an asylum in Zurich. In May 1912, while dictating an article to his secretary, Forel detected a prickling sensation on his arms and, simultaneously, discovered himself unable to find the words for which he was searching. Not even the dictionary could aid him. This first attack soon passed; a week later, however, he developed further sensory and motor difficulty on his right side and an aphasia which affected reading

and writing as well as speech. Forel reports the sort of in-
congruous behavior that today we call *parapraxis*—for example, he buttered his sugar rather than his bread. Such
misplacements and displacements also permeated his symbolic activity: he could not add a column of figures, for
he confused numbers with their neighbors; and sounds
and syllables were confused in both his writing and reading.

As a means of testing his intellectual capacities, and as
a peculiarly apt remembrance of his strange state, Forel
essayed a satirical poem called "The Crazy Scholar."
He printed two versions of this poem—the second a cor-
rection of the first—noting that the first illustrated his
then-inability to maintain the appropriate rhythm and
caesuras, but his preserved capacity to produce rhymes
and meanings. He concluded that, except for the formal
flaws, his imagination and intelligence had not suffered
noticeably; like an earlier stroke victim, Samuel Johnson,
who similarly tested himself by composing verses in Latin,
Forel interpreted his ability to produce verses, no matter
how inferior, as a sign that his mind was still fundamentally sound.

In recent years there has been a spate of accounts by
individuals who have had the misfortune of suffering a
stroke and the good fortune to recover sufficiently to write
about it. In these accounts, as in those reviewed above,
others may have contributed to fluency and readability:
and of course, as the accounts are written at a later time,
they may not accurately reflect conditions at the beginning
of and during the illness. Nonetheless, the surprising similarity across these accounts, often penned in widely distant
locales, lends credence to their major themes and observations.

Of least interest are accounts by individuals who had
only a mild stroke, from which they rapidly recovered.
Nonetheless, an evocative writer can sometimes capture

the bizarre sensations at the onset of even such a transient illness:

> I am a happily married man with a family. . . . About six weeks ago I went to bed one night feeling quite well but I remember I didn't sleep very well and was rather restless. When I woke up I had a bit of a headache and thought I must have been sleeping with my right arm under me because it felt all pins-and-needly and numb and I couldn't make it do what I wanted. I got out of bed but I couldn't stand; as a matter of fact I actually fell on the floor because my right leg was too weak to take my weight. I called out to my wife in the next room and no sound came—I couldn't speak. . . . I was astonished, horrified. I couldn't believe that this was happening to me and I began to feel bewildered and frightened and then I suddenly realized that I must have had a stroke. In a way this rationalization made me feel somewhat relieved but not for long because I had always thought that the effects of a stroke were permanent in every case. . . . I found I could speak a little but even to me the words seemed wrong and not what I meant to say. I felt rather tired by this time and wondered if I was going to die. I seemed to lose interest in my surroundings and I only vaguely remember the doctor coming. . . . I slept a lot and next day was disappointed and depressed to find that I still couldn't speak clearly and sensibly and that my arm was paralyzed. I was a little annoyed when, about three days later, the doctor appeared with a specialist who was obviously very pleased when he found I could move my thumb. This seemed a stupid thing to be so pleased about and I thought, "A fat lot of good that's going to be to me." Of course I realize now how important that little movement was, because it showed the doctors that I was likely to recover quite soon. Next day I could speak what my mind wanted to say and as you know since then I have never looked back.

Such strokes are sufficiently benign that, like President Eisenhower, the victim can resume his normal work and activities, and the aftereffects are negligible.

Of greater interest are accounts by individuals who have been severely aphasic and have recovered some, but not all, of their faculties. Such individuals (at least the writers among them) tend to be highly critical of their output, so much so that they may even refuse to appear in public. They recognize that they have recovered in significant degree but that talking and understanding, instead of being effortless, are now intensely draining experiences.

One such individual was a young Navy enlisted man named Richard Butler, who suffered a severe fall which left him with a permanent language impairment. Looking back at the early months of his malady, he recalls: "I was (to my thinking) an island, a stranger, and afraid, in a world I never made." He became depressed and weary, fearing that the world was unmanageable. Language recovered to the extent that he could, with sufficient time and attention, express himself adequately, but the feeling of loneliness and the absence of self-confidence were never completely overcome. He withdrew into himself:

I must be alone; I'm not good company for others and I don't enjoy much of others' company. . . . Most often feeling unsure of myself, uncomfortable in interpersonal situations, I am either unable or unwilling to communicate.

Butler believes that his thought processes were more seriously disrupted by his illness than were his emotional responses:

I don't think as fast as others around me evidently do. I nevertheless feel the way they feel. The impaired intellect is out of balance with my intact or increased sensitivity.

As a result of this disharmony, Butler has become highly self-conscious. He sees his mind as a revolving card-file of experience which must constantly be spun to select the appropriate word or concept. Because he suffers from "ideational interruption or short-circuitry . . . too often for adequacy, my tabula rasa remains blank." Butler appears to have in much greater degree that difficulty in finding words and expressing oneself cogently that befalls all individuals during moments of strain and stress. While these difficulties are rarely crippling for the normal individual, they are sufficiently pernicious to disable many brain-damaged individuals.

Another, highly illuminating account of aphasic difficulties was penned by a former British radio broadcaster, Douglas Ritchie, who at the age of 50 suffered a major stroke. His recollections of the first days are very hazy: he doesn't remember pain or discomfort and claims not even to have recognized his wife during the first days after his "cerebral vascular accident." He lay in bed, as he puts it, "trying to collect my mind."

Ritchie has since attempted to re-create his mental and emotional state in the weeks after his stroke. "My main desire was to return to work. My mind was all right, I thought, and I was perfectly aware of my name and my environment but I could not think of anything that had happened since my stroke." He found that he could read adequately ("the machinery" was satisfactory) but that he could not handle materials of any complexity. Certain authors—e.g., Graham Greene—were comprehensible; those with more subtle styles, like Ivy Compton-Burnett, were clearly not. "The novels ought to be simple, to be adventurous, and not to be 'who dunnits' because my memory was poor."

Particular difficulties arose when Ritchie tried to express, or even think about, things which were unfamiliar. It is perhaps this difficulty especially which impels brain-damaged persons toward more familiar, functional, and 'concrete' behaviors. Ritchie had special problems in logical deduction: "My brain went around in circles, a simple piece of logic going to the first premise but staying there." As the months passed, fluency in carrying on simple activities improved, but the problems of conceptualizing and then communicating more exotic concepts remained:

> There was, I observed, a wide difference between thinking about words and actually thinking in words and about words. I could daydream. . . . I could think, actively, without words. . . . but . . . . the minute I rehearsed speaking with my tongue, even though I kept silent the words would not come. . . . there was a headline. . . . I understood this. I kept on repeating the words in my brain. But the moment I lowered the words to my mouth and to my tongue, they would not come.

It is not entirely clear from Ritchie's account whether he feels that his difficulty lay primarily in expressing already clear ideas, or in the actual conceptualization of those ideas at a preverbal level. Like other aphasic patients, however, he hints that the difficulty was more "peripheral" than "central":

> My brain could not read very easily and of course it was only half-working. My brain must be made to work. The inside of my brain (I call it that) worked better than the outside—the reacting, the speaking, the calculating, the writing, the humming and the understanding of writing or just speech. And it was the inside of my brain which was the most valuable and that could save me from drowning.

Over many months, with considerable therapy and support from friends, Ritchie recovered his language capacities almost fully. He found, as have other, similarly afflicted writers, that keeping a diary on the course of his illness was a rewarding assignment which may indeed have aided his recovery. Yet the feeling remains that the stroke has left him somehow different:

> I was very egotistical in my normal state, now I am thoroughly "me." But all the same, I am driven inside myself. If I could speak—about politics, music, books, or history—I would be all right.

Accounts of aphasia have also been secured from individuals still recovering and receiving treatment. Generally such patients are interviewed by their physicians or therapists. These reports have the advantage that, in contrast to autobiographical accounts, they are obtained when patients' difficulties are still readily apparent and are reported accurately by trained observers. Having asked several such patients to introspect about their condition, M. Rolnick and his associates obtained the following picture.

At the beginning of the stroke, patients are aghast at their linguistic failings. They think they are talking, only to discover that their words are making no sense; they believe they are understanding others, only to realize subsequently that words have become meaningless sounds. The effort and the will to communicate may be as strong as ever, but the requisite skills are mysteriously suspended; it is as if there are "just bubbles and lots of little marbles" in the patient's mouth.

Sometimes aware of their errors, patients are usually uncertain about the precise nature of a flaw and, in any case, lack the insight and the equipment to correct it; as one phrased it, "I know when I say something it's wrong but I can't remember the right way." Analogous difficulties emerge in the comprehension of spoken language—the patient senses areas of difficulty but even continuous slow repetition may fail to convey the desired meaning. As comprehension is especially difficult in the face of rival sounds, slowness and clarity of speech and a quiet setting are essential.

Echoing the earliest reports on aphasia, these patients generally concur on the relative clarity in their own minds. One recovering patient put it this way:

First I formulate the idea in my mind and then I try to express that idea in the language and then I have the problem. I can get the idea real quickly but to make it into

language or to express it as language . . . I just couldn't do it.
I just lost them . . . I can see them in my mind but I can't
see the words.

The patient apparently possesses a general picture of what
he wants to say, but gaps and lacunae emerge when he
seeks to translate the idea into words. For the normal person, the choice of words appears an almost automatic process, with the appropriate one effortlessly bubbling out of
the mouth; but for the aphasic the words "don't pop up"
—he must "pull them out" and sometimes they just aren't
there at all. These deficits are especially frustrating because
the desired lexical units are at once so close and so elusive.

The patients interviewed by Rolnick raise other revealing, and somewhat unexpected, points. Large print seems
to be desired by aphasics trying to read, even when they
have no known visual problems. They can often read to
themselves with little difficulty, but when they try to express the substance of their reading in their own words,
the meaning recedes. Finally, the patients dwell on the
delicacy of their relations with their families. As frustrating as it may be when the family ignores the sufferer, it
can be equally galling if they are too intent on helping
him, and on stuffing words into his mouth. Great sensitivity on the relatives' part seems to be called for, as family
members must be able to assess just when the patient can
benefit from some intervention, and when such help
would engender more psychological harm than communicative benefit.

In considering the testimony of these and other patients,
one seldom if ever has any sense of the aphasic as a genuinely alien creature. True, he finds difficulty in those very
behaviors—reading, writing, speaking—which most of us
perform with little or no conscious effort; and even with
the efforts he exerts, his products are often studded with
errors. Nonetheless, the patient still appears an individual

basically like ourselves, with ideas and feelings of which
he is consciously aware and wishes that he seeks to fulfil,
who is prevented from communicating successfully by a
breakdown of one or more essential skills rather than any
fundamental deficit in knowledge or ideation. It is as if
the most basic part, the mainspring, of the human machine
is still operating, but various fine parts are in temporary
disrepair, requiring oiling or replacement of parts. Something is the matter with the materials of the brain, but
the mind itself is still relatively intact.

But, we may ask, how could we possibly tell if and when
the aphasic's thought processes are affected in more fundamental ways? Could a patient, after all, conceivably say,
"Doctor, I don't have the words and also I don't know
what to say; I have lost my ability to form ideas"? How
could a patient be aware that he lacked ideas unless he was
able to formulate the idea that he had no ideas? To paraphrase Descartes, how could he even *be* if he could not
think? The most likely thing to expect of a person in such
a state is incoherent babble, or nothing. And indeed, just
such reports often emerge from patients' recollections
about the first days after a stroke—to the extent that they
can recall this period at all, they speak of it as dreamlike,
difficult to describe in words or even to evoke in imagery.
Naturally, we depend upon reports from those who can
describe their experiences, and to this extent, our synopsis
is limited. Moreover, hardly any introspective accounts
provide details about the locus and type of injury; thus
we can only infer the type and the severity of the aphasia
in a given case. All these considerations caution against
undue reliance on details of the cases described here.

Although the gap between the severely brain-injured
and the normal individual may in the last analysis be
unbridgeable, two recent accounts by highly intelligent
brain-injured persons have seemed to me particularly illu-

minating. In one case, the patient recovered and can be regarded as a therapeutic (or natural) success; in the other, recovery was fragmentary but the patient can hardly be considered a failure—indeed, his tale assumes heroic proportions. We turn first to the patient whose recovery was so impressive.

In 1967, C. Scott Moss was a young and successful clinical psychologist who had just been called to a major professional appointment at the University of Illinois. On the morning of October 30, he had a physical checkup, at the end of which he was pronounced in excellent health by the faculty physician. That afternoon, however, he suffered a severe coughing spell, followed by a disturbance in vision in his right eye, numbness in his right hand, and the inability to read the paper in front of him. A sharp pain occurred at the back of his head; Moss fell down, his right side paralyzed, and discovered to his further consternation that he was utterly unable to speak. Although speech (inexplicably) returned for a brief interval at the hospital, he was completely unable to communicate on the following day. His understanding of others was vague at best, he could neither read nor utter words correctly, and communicated only through gestures.

The first weeks after his stroke are vague in Moss's mind. He felt as if he would have to learn anew to coordinate his functions and to convey his thoughts. He was unable even to engage in simple conversation, let alone deal with the abstractions of his work. He blocked on the most trivial sequences: even asking for a pencil became an enterprise requiring painstaking planning.

Moss readily concedes that the account of his earlier convalescence is sketchy. Fortunately, however, his wife kept her own diary of this period. In Bette Moss's view, the year had been a very hectic and trying one for the family, one of continual tension that, she believes, may well have contributed to her husband's stroke. She reports bewilderment at the onset of the illness, at first thinking her husband was just indulging in some sort of weird joke. Especially perplexing was his ability to converse fluently with an internist when he first arrived at the hospital. Yet, as she recalls, he was able to say nothing at all during the days that followed, except to repeat A, B, C. Instead of saying D, he would return to A.

Scott Moss appeared in a happy mood during the early days of his malady, probably because he was unaware of the severity of his difficulties. He dozed off constantly and was in no pain. But just when Mrs. Moss was despairing of his ever recovering, he gave her reason to think that his "sense of self" had been preserved after all. After one brief "conversation," he patted his wife on her behind: "There was that familiar twinkle in his eye, and I knew that I still had the same Scott I started with."

Even after Moss came home from the hospital, he still displayed relatively little interest in his surroundings, except for eating and sleeping. Yet, very gradually, a desire to learn again and to take up his work once more stirred in him, and he thrust himself with every ounce of his energy into language rehabilitation. It was at this point, about 3½ months after his stroke, that Moss began to keep a journal.

A decisive change occurred when Moss's "inner speech" began to return. During the early part of his illness, he had been unable to "engage in self talk, to think about the future. . . . it was as if without words I could not be concerned about tomorrow." He had carried on basic everyday tasks, such as eating and shaving, without, however, being able to express to himself what he was doing. Now, some months after his CVA, he began to regain at least a rudimentary ability to put into words what he was doing, and to reflect upon the significance of his actions. Once able to describe to himself and others the events of the day, he could relive these experiences at night, and he

recommenced dreaming. "As I recovered my internal ver-
balizations, the memory of the nocturnal mentation began
to recur." Moss now partially resumed scholarly activities,
reading (or having read to him) technical articles, putting
the finishing touches on some papers drafted before his
illness.

In the next stage, attained around six months or so after
the stroke, Moss could express himself with some precision
in words and in writing. During this period, all would
seem to be going well—until suddenly the desired words
would be lacking, refusing to come to mind, and Moss
would panic. It was difficult to retain abstractions; he
would start to formulate a theoretical concept only to find
that, even as he sought to maintain a mental hold upon it,
"it would sort of fade and chances were that I'd end up
giving a simplified version rather than one at the original
level of conception." He found it very difficult to keep in
his mind a verbal outline of what he had to say; as a consequence, thought or reflection on matters beyond his immediate ken—for example, about past or future events—
was exceedingly difficult to entertain.

A year after being stricken, Moss was performing daily
activities at a near-normal level. He could read newsmaga-
zines with ease, but encountered difficulty with the more
abstract and complex discourse of professional articles. He
wrote and spoke with some fluency, but many errors crept
in, and, extremely self-conscious about these lapses, he
would find his performance deteriorating under stress. It
proved especially demanding to deal with several individuals at one time, or to rejoin a comment by another, because at such times a premium was placed on speed and
wit: "The main problem is that I block on words and I
am still shocked into silence by my inability to find appropriate words." Yet Moss did not interpret this word-finding
problem as a symptom of poor thinking: "For the most
part my perception is that I am more capable of thinking

things through than explaining them in words. . . . I like to believe that I appear to have remained largely the same person that I was before. . . . I simply fail to recall highly significant and special words that I would like to use. I know what I want to say but cannot get at the words at that particular moment."

Transcripts of Moss's discourse at a late point in his recovery appear in his book *Recovery with Aphasia*. They were made from tapes that (in pre-Watergate days, it should be stressed) he had secretly made in order subsequently to pore over his verbal interchanges with others. These transcripts reveal no evident difficulty in communication, yet Moss stresses his subjective impression that he was simply not as fluent, as effortlessly verbal and conceptual, as before his illness. The normal person, says Moss, attends almost exclusively to what he wants to say; the recovered aphasic is ever attending to the words which he must painstakingly find in order to convey what is on his mind.

At the book's writing, two years after his stroke, Moss feels he has recovered to within a measurable distance of his pre-morbid ability. "I still have all the words that I ever had," he reports, "but I no longer have the ability to recapture them as quickly as before." Returning to his former teaching position, Moss performed creditably, yet remained ill at ease among highly articulate students and peers, and dissatisfied with his own level of performance. As a result, he took a less-demanding position at a federal penitentiary in California, where he felt he could be of service without feeling "on the spot." And yet, his self-doubts notwithstanding, he has continued his scholarly activities at a notably vigorous pace. In 1970 he published two books, one of which was selected for distribution by a professional book club, and in 1972 he produced his compelling treatise on aphasia. As I write, in late 1973, Moss has just participated in a symposium at the American Psychological Association on "Recovery from Aphasia"; and I learn from a circular in the mail that the man who feared to address a class of graduate students has just produced a tape on "Hypnosymbolic Psychotherapy" for the Behavioral Sciences Tape Library! The story of Moss's recovery, in brief—sensitively recorded and compelling to follow—palpably belies the continuing subjective feelings of inadequacy he reports. To have been able to resume a full professional schedule only two years after being thus heavily struck down is a most impressive achievement. There is every reason to believe that his illness will not exact any long-term crippling effect.

One can only surmise why one patient with a significant stroke should recover so well, while others remain moored to a wheelchair and withdrawn from the world. Perhaps it is a consequence of age, perhaps of motivation, perhaps of skilled therapy, perhaps of unusual brain organization, and, more likely, a combination of these and other factors. But one important clue may be that Moss's occupation, for example, can be practiced without his being continuously on the spot. As a writer and thinker, Moss can withdraw to his study to contemplate what he has done, to criticize, revise, and improve it. True, his work must still pass muster in the eyes of others, but he is not constantly on the firing line, in the way that a virtuoso musician, athlete, politician, or salesman may be.

In contrast, it is instructive to consider the fate of individuals whose career depends upon an instant command of their diverse physical and mental resources. A British actor suffering from right-hemisphere disease was unable to continue in his profession—because of difficulty with spatial orientation, he would often misalign himself on the stage, and even turn his back on the audience. He subsequently became a successful radio announcer: in this position he could read his lines and ignore the spatial layouts. The well-known American actress Patricia Neal also had to suspend her professional activities because of a severe aphasia.

Eventually, however, she was able to return to the lime-light, and has since acted in a number of successful movies. But, particularly at the beginning of her professional come-back, she found performing to be a most frustrating ex-perience, for lines either did not occur to her at all or were misspoken. As a biographer indicates, "Her traitor brain would offer old formula phrases, relics of her illness." In-stead of speaking the line, say, "My mother expects us for dinner tomorrow," she would find herself coming out with "We're meant to go to supper" or "I'm very sorry to tell you." Even when she spoke her lines perfectly, moreover, she would sometimes fail to achieve the precise tonality of voice desired and the performance would be either exces-sively wooden or excessively emotional. There has, how-ever, been a steady improvement in her ability to marshal her resources, and she is once again receiving considerable critical acclaim for her screen roles. Indeed, her empathetic powers and her "stage" personality have remained as im-pressive as before. Nonetheless, Miss Neal's word-finding difficulties remain sufficiently evident that she has felt obliged to keep live appearances on stage or television to a minimum.

The extent of one's recovery from brain damage, de-pends, then, not only on a quantitative improvement in functioning, but also on the demands of one's profession and one's avocation. The individual with a career which allows leisurely contemplation and extensive practice is likely to resume his prior activities; the individual who must be continuously on the spot may now be unsuited to his former work, even though the degree of improvement may be comparable in the two cases. Needless to say, thera-peutic efforts should concentrate on preparing the indi-vidual to approach his earlier pursuits in the most effective way and, whenever possible, devising alternative ways for achieving the demands made upon him.

Our final—and to my mind, most remarkable—brain-injured witness is Zasetsky, a 23-year-old Russian soldier wounded in the battle of Smolensk in 1943. The eminent Russian psychologist A. R. Luria remained in close contact with Zasetsky for twenty-five years, during which period this severely impaired individual assembled thousands of pages of notes describing his condition and his reactions and reflections upon it. In an amazing little book, *The Man with a Shattered World,* Luria presents the hapless soldier's story, often related in the latter's own tortured phrases.

Before the war Zasetsky had been a brilliant young scientist. He had studied at the polytechnical institute, where he had done research in many branches of science and technology. As his mother had sacrificed so much that he might receive an education, his most ardent desire after graduation was to aid her, so that she would finally have a chance to rest. These plans were never to be realized, however, for, as he recalls:

It was the beginning of March, warm and sunny, but damp. . . . all of us were eager to get on with the attack. . . . Suddenly everyone stepped up his pace. . . . the Germans waited silently. . . . Then all at once there was a burst of fire from their side, machine guns whirring in every direction. . . . I jumped up from the ice, pushed on . . . toward the west . . . there . . . and . . .

Zasetsky's memory for the days immediately following the shelling is very dim. He vaguely recalls the doctors hunched over him, holding him down, while blood was running over his body. He remembered that his skull was bursting, that there was a sharp rending pain in his head. His breathing stopped and he was going to die. He overheard fragments of conversation, but could not grasp their import, nor, if he did, could he respond appropriately. "Right after I was wounded, I seemed to be some newborn creature that just looked, listened, observed, repeated but still had no mind of its own. . . . Afterwards when I'd had a chance to hear words that people use again and again in conversation or thinking, various clusters of 'memory fragments' developed, and from these I began to make some sense out of the life around me and remember what words meant." But for the most part, Zasetsky's mind was muddled and confused, and his brain felt limited and feeble: "I'm in a kind of fog all the time, like a heavy half-sleep. . . . Whatever I do remember is scattered, broken down into disconnected bits and pieces. That is why I react so abnormally to every word and idea, every attempt to understand the meaning of words. . . . I was killed March 2, 1943, but because of some vital power of my organism, I miraculously remained alive."

Zasetsky was first seen by Professor Luria about three months after his brush with death. Luria was struck by the extreme youth of the boy, and by his shy manner. His speech was reduced to the simplest, most elementary forms of expression; he was unable to write a single word or read a single letter. He could not perceive in his right visual field; and his ability to distinguish right from left was largely lost. At first, he was unable to indicate what month it was, but with some effort he triumphantly located the right word. Yet he was confused about the order of the seasons, unable to add two simple numbers, or even to describe a picture.

Zasetsky had suffered a penetrating wound in the left parietal-occipital area of his head—an injury that drastically crippled him across the full range of his symbolic and conceptual faculties. What he retained intact, however, were those functions associated with the frontal lobes: his will, his desires, his sensitivity to experience, and the ability to form and sustain intentions, plan actions, and carry them through as effectively as possible under the given circumstances. Zasetsky appreciated from the first the dismal nature of his situation, he was all too

aware of the multifarious difficulties and disabilities be-
setting him; but he remained, as Luria observed, "in the
deepest sense . . . a man, struggling to regain what he had
lost, reconstitute his life, and use the power he once
had had." With an ardent desire to better himself and to
prove to himself and others that he was not a hopeless case,
he resolved to undertake some kind of service to his country. And gradually he came to realize that the most valuable service he could perform would be to portray for
posterity the remarkable fragmented world he now inhabited.

As might be expected, Zasetsky's disabilities were most
severe and extensive during the first years of his illness.
Because of his visual-field defect, he was unable to see
objects in their entirety. Looking at a spoon, he might see
only the tip. Moreover, what parts he saw were unstable
in appearance, seeming to be in a constant state of flux.
Familiar scenes were unrecognizable: he did not even remember his native town upon his return home. The visual
difficulty vitiated his reading; he could not see the closing letters of words clearly; he often had hallucinations;
the right side of any scene was obliterated and even his
comprehension of pictorial materials was limited. He also
lost awareness of the right side of his body: not only did
his sense of particular limbs become impaired, but he
found his subjective sense of his own dimensions suddenly
shifting; sometimes he would seem very tall, at other times
exceedingly small. These strange sensations occurred because of destruction of a region of the brain deemed critical to the construction of the "normal body image."

The ability to carry out actions in space was another
casualty. Zasetsky had forgotten how to enact the simplest
gestures, such as beckoning to another individual, and the
most elementary activities, such as hammering. Given a
needle and a thread, he sat helplessly, ignorant of how to
combine these implements. Handed a pencil, he would sit

at a table, unable to write. He could not undertake the simplest chores at home; indeed, he could not even exercise his body or participate in sports or games. So devastated was his sense of orientation—of knowing right, left, back, and forward, finding his way around home or his neighborhood—that he could scarcely undertake any activity out of doors.

With time, Zasetsky was able to compensate to some degree for these abnormalities. His ability to understand and to communicate what was on his mind also improved somewhat, though he failed whenever linguistic constructions beyond a very simple level were used (for example, he could not understand the phrase *mother's daughter*). Even decades after his injury, he was unable to carry out activities of any complexity; he remained unable to play chess, a game at which he had once excelled, nor could he even follow the action in a movie, for this simple pastime required him to move his eyes at a pace which he could not sustain.

Confronted by this bleak array of disabilities, Zasetsky would have had to be superhuman to avoid completely any feelings of despair; and there were moments, particularly at the beginning, when he believed that he would die, and that he was wholly useless. Yet he never quite lost his faith that things would get better, and that time would heal him. This thought, though unduly optimistic, was probably essential in order to keep him going during the depressing days of slow recuperation. Zasetsky would sometimes remember isolated fragments or words from his earlier life, but he could almost never put them back together into a coherent whole—the areas of the brain which codify and organize such information had been largely destroyed. What memories did return came back from his earliest life, as he put it, "from the wrong end." While names and events from early childhood were relatively vivid, that more specialized knowledge he had acquired in the university was forever lost to him. Particularly in his musings, he found himself returning to the words, ideas, and concerns of early childhood, as these alone seemed accessible.

A major portion of Luria's account depicts Zasetsky's efforts to utilize symbolic language, to read and write. Reading continued to pose a tremendous problem, as his field deficit occluded the right side of all visually presented materials. At first, Zasetsky could not even tell if something had been written in Russian. However, with the help of a therapist, he eventually relearned the Cyrillic alphabet. Each step was arduous, but he gradually succeeded in associating specific sounds to their graphemes. Rather than trying to visualize each letter, he found it easier to recite the alphabet orally and this spared sequence aided him in solidifying his knowledge of it. Finally, after many months of daily exercise, Zasetsky was able to read slowly, letter by letter, and, sometimes, word by word. However, the effort entailed was so great, the rewards at this snail's pace so sparse, that he never enjoyed reading again.

Writing proved a more hopeful story. While at first unable even to use a pencil properly, Zasetsky discovered one day—through the suggestion of a friendly doctor—that he was still able to write automatically. That is, while producing a word letter by letter was an arduous and usually unsuccessful process, writing a word without thinking about it at all proved much simpler. Luria explains that, despite its tremendous complexity, for some adults writing has become, at least in part, an automatic skill, a series of overlearned motor acts akin to reciting the alphabet or playing an arpeggio. This decidedly noncognitive approach enabled Zasetsky to produce many words effortlessly; at least he was able to express some of his ideas in writing. When the word did not come automatically, an arduous syllable-by-syllable construction was necessary, but even here the results were more impressive than in reading.

Zasetsky found that, provided he could remember a word, he could also write it. It was then that he decided to keep a journal describing the world he now inhabited and relating his efforts at adjustment.

Zasetsky worked on his notebooks every day for twenty-five years. Writing never came easily: some days he penned hardly a line, on many more he produced half a page, only on his very best days could he execute upwards of a page. Keeping this journal—whose title was at first "The Story of a Terrible Injury," and later changed to "I'll Fight On" —was terribly exacting work, but the prospect of making a scientific contribution encouraged him to persist:

> It was so hard to write. . . . At last I'd turned up a good idea. So I began to hunt for words to describe it and finally I thought up two. But by the time I got to the third word, I was stuck . . . what a torture it was. I'd always forget what I wanted to write. . . . So before I could go on and write my story, I had to jot down various words for the names of objects, things, phenomena, ideas. Then I'd take the words, sentences, and ideas I'd collected in this way and begin to write my story in a notebook, regrouping the words and sentences, comparing them with others I'd seen in books. Finally I managed to write a sentence expressing an idea I had. . . . Sometimes I'll sit over a page for a week or two. . . . It's been an enormous strain (still is). I work at it like someone with an obsession. . . . But I don't want to give it up. I want to finish what I've begun. So I sit at my desk all day sweating over each word.

These efforts helped Zasetsky to improve his vocabulary and his expressive ability; but he persevered chiefly because he wanted to be able to tell himself, his friends, his doctors, his world, about what it was like to have a damaged brain.

And Zasetsky succeeded, at least as well as anyone has up to this time. Where else can one read: "Words have lost meaning for me or have a meaning that's incomplete and unformed. . . . Every word I hear seems vaguely familiar. . . . As far as my memory's concerned I know a particular word exists, except that it has lost meaning. I don't understand it as I did before I was wounded. This means that if I heard the word 'table' I can't figure out what it is right away, what it is related to. I just have a feeling that the word is somewhat familiar, but that's all. So I have to limit myself to words that 'feel' familiar to me, that have some definite meaning for me." Who else has told us: "I've even forgotten what a dandelion is, a flower I knew when I was a child. When it becomes faded, I remember what it is, but until then I just can't imagine, I have absolutely no idea." And what aphasic has captured his combination of intuitions and uncertainty:

> The doctor asked me to give him any answer I could, so I held up two fingers to show I thought the words mean two people—a mother and a daughter. But then he asked me what daughter's mother meant. I thought for a while but couldn't figure it out, just pointed to the two figures in the picture. The expressions *mother's daughter* and *daughter's mother* sounded just the same to me, so I often told him they were.

The uniqueness of Zasetsky's record seems attributable to three circumstances. First, he was, by all accounts, an extremely intelligent and perceptive individual before trauma befell him. In addition, as a young but permanently disabled individual, he had many years to formulate and record his subjective impressions. Finally, and most importantly, his peculiar lesion destroyed a significant portion of the skills which enable the rest of us to function normally, while at the same time sparing that portion of the brain which allows reflection upon one's own activity, as well as planning and realization of a program, in spite of manifest difficulties.

Zasetsky's injury precluded many forms of understanding and many orders of skill, but he was hardly reduced to a primitive level. His appreciation of his surroundings, both natural and social, remained quite acute; for example, in one lengthy passage, he envisages what it is like to lead lives totally different from one another, such as those of a great engineer, a famous surgeon, a cleaning woman, or an invalid. His imagination is vivid, and his ability to appreciate aesthetic phenomena, such as music and scenery, seems to have remained unimpaired. He comprehended the bizarre event that had crippled him, the devastating impact it had on his future, the invaluable perspective which his journal would provide. In all this, as Luria explains, Zasetsky differed dramatically from the individual with injury to the frontal lobes. This latter injury does not seriously disrupt the person's capacity to learn, perceive, or recall prior knowledge, the capabilities so disrupted in Zasetsky's case. Yet the frontal-lobe patient is devoid of intentions, incapable of laying plans or even regulating his own behavior. Lacking a sense of self, he can neither plan nor correct his actions. He is radically impaired in precisely those aspects of personality that are most crucial to our humanity, and which are spared, as on a lonely island, in the brain of Zasetsky.

The testimony of brain-damaged patients presents a congress of individuals who retain a sense of self, a will if not always the capacity to communicate, at least a tenuous relation to the world of other individuals. It is quite possible that other patients, however, unable to leave a record of their feelings or ideas, because of an inability or a lack of desire to communicate, might present a different world-view. Finding evidence for such a world-view is obviously much more difficult, since we cannot invoke the patient's own testimony. Instead, we must draw inferences from the patient's behavior, and especially from what he does not say, or does not do.

At least three conflicting views can be sketched on the

fate of the brain-damaged patient's sense of self. At one end would be the claim that the patient—indeed any person—is simply a collection of individual skills, each of which can be impaired or spared; on this view, belief in a separate self or sense of identity amounts to a romantic deception on the part of a scientifically obtuse observer. The alternative claim, equally extreme, is that the sense of self, the existence of will, desire, and need to communicate, is inviolate, persisting until death, at least. An intermediate and widely held position does not challenge the existence of a rudimentary sense of self in the brain-damaged patient, but suggests that the victim's coherence and level of functioning are necessarily impaired. We shall examine this intermediate claim more closely.

Perhaps its most articulate exponent was the noted neurologist and psychologist Kurt Goldstein. The chief, almost inevitable consequence of brain damage, Goldstein claimed, was the loss of an "abstract attitude." By this phrase, Goldstein meant the ability of the intact individual to transcend the immediate "givens" in a situation, to consider it from a distance, and to arrive at a decision or action by taking the relevant factors into account. Important for the abstract thinker is, not the specific objects in his realm, but rather his rational and exhaustive way of conceptualizing them. In sharp contrast, the brain-damaged person is characterized by a concrete attitude, in which he or she can deal with objects and elements exclusively in some habitual or rigidly mechanical way. Unable to acquire perspective on his situation, to revise his plans in the light of new information, the "concretely" behaving individual is restricted to the here-and-now, to the perpetual enactment and reenactment of overlearned patterns of behavior. A hook is for hanging, a nail is for joining; the possibility of joining two pieces of wood with a hook, or of hanging a picture on a nail, is foreclosed to the concrete individual.

For Goldstein the distinction between abstract and concrete behavior was a qualitative one. Ordinarily, an individual would not appear abstract at one time, concrete at another, nor would he display an abstract attitude in just some of his activities. If a person is able to shift his mental set voluntarily, to keep in mind several aspects of a situation, to ferret out common properties from diverse situations, to detach his ego from the outer world, such capacities should be manifest in every manner of situation. If, on the other hand, he is governed by his senses, by the customary use of an object, by his routine habits and attitudes, by stereotyped, compulsive behavioral patterns, such concrete manifestations should be ubiquitous.

Much confusion has arisen over Goldstein's definition of "attitude." He would not rely on a single test, or on an individual performance, as documentation of one or another attitude; only the patient's "overall approach" to a range of problems and situations would permit a qualitative judgment. To be sure, Goldstein devised a number of ingenious tests which aided in the judgment. For instance, he introduced blocks of different shapes and sizes and colors and required the patient to make groupings; contrasting two performances, he would stress the abstract patient's ability to arrive at new classifications (first grouping by shape, then by size, etc.), with the concrete patient's perseveration on a single (albeit valid) manner of grouping. Yet, as Goldstein repeatedly pointed out, the clinician might be fooled by a single performance, judged out of context:

[The patient] may be able to count if the examiner begins the series, but he cannot begin himself. . . . He can follow and even take part in a conversation on a familiar topic or the immediate situation, but if the conversation shifts to another topic—in itself equally familiar to the patient—he cannot follow. . . . He may be able to orient himself in a complicated building which has become familiar to him but cannot say

anything about even the simplest relations of rooms and floors
to each other.

Only persistent observation of the patient, over a variety
of situations, could definitively reveal the patient's "attitude."

The thrust of this "organismic" view is that the brain-
damaged patient is different. Though able to deal with
thoughts and ideas, he can do so only in a concrete way;
he may, indeed, successfully exercise almost any skill, but
only if the need for that skill arises in a natural situation.
Where he fails is in drawing voluntarily on his arsenal
of skills, deliberately deciding what should be deployed,
under what circumstances, and in what manner.

Goldstein's highly influential position was extended to
its ultimate (and logical) conclusion by the noted phe-
nomenologist Maurice Merleau-Ponty. Having reviewed
in detail the cases and claims of Goldstein's "organismic
school," Merleau-Ponty went on to a forthright assertion
that the brain-damaged and the normal person were not
comparable:

How are we to coordinate this set of facts and how are we
to discover by means of it what function, found in the normal
person, is absent from the patient? There can be no question
of simply transferring from the normal person what the deficient one lacks and is trying to recover. Illness, like childhood
and "primitive" mentality, is a complete form of existence
and the procedures which it employs to replace normal functions which have been destroyed are equally pathological
phenomena. It is impossible to deduce the normal from the
pathological.

Such a perspective leads to the most pessimistic conclusions
for our inquiry: Goldstein implies, and Merleau-Ponty insists, that no bridge can be constructed between the minds
of the "abstract" analyst and that of the "concrete" patient

—they are as two mutually alien entities that must ever remain asunder.

Certainly Goldstein's claims appear to be inconsistent with, if not in contradiction to, the testimony of the aphasic patients reviewed above. The concrete patient is said to have the requisite skills, but to be unable to deploy them voluntarily and flexibly; the aphasic patient is said to be lacking necessary skills (for example, reading or speaking) but to have retained his will, intentionality, and insight into his own condition. Can we reconcile these apparently divergent characterizations of the mind of the brain-injured person?

The first answer, I think, is that any effort to generalize in this area must be suspect. Brain injury varies enormously in degree, size, and type, in effects on individuals of different ages and backgrounds, in potential for recovery or improvement. What characterizes the demented individual, the person with severe memory disorder, or the individual with a visual-spatial defect, may well be totally irrelevant for the individual with frontal-lobe damage, pure alexia, or the Gerstmann syndrome. It must be understood, too, that within each of these diagnoses, there is a definite sequence of events. The initial, difficult-to-assimilate shock gives way to a period of vague understanding; pleasure at being able to accomplish some function is replaced by despair at the lack of progress; steady efforts in therapy or self-education may be finally crowned by success. No set of antonyms, no simplified framework, can possibly account for all these contingencies.

There is, nonetheless, some prospect for reconciling the divergent views of brain damage introduced here. Goldstein is referring to brain damage in general, without attention to the type of lesion, and his remarks are most applicable to the individual who has suffered from a massive, permanent impairment of function. The patient who is globally aphasic, who has had his frontal lobes removed entirely, who suffers from severe right-hemisphere pathology or is grossly demented, may well be characterized by the rigidity and primitiveness of the "concrete" attitude. On the other hand, the individual with a more focal brain injury, as well as the individual who, despite severe pathology, has retained the crucial frontal-lobe structures, will belie the Goldstein description. Indeed, it might be more accurate to say of Zasetsky, for example, that he failed to exhibit a concrete capacity, while displaying the salient characteristics of the abstract attitude.

While the concrete attitude may characterize certain patients, it definitely cannot be uncritically applied to the patients described in this book, and most especially not to brain-damaged individuals who have themselves described their condition after the initial period of hospitalization. It is precisely by virtue of their overall normality that they are potentially capable of revealing much about the operation of specific skills in the intact individual. But are we being fair in attributing a concrete attitude to those patients who cannot communicate with us, who seem to behave concretely, or to be in a perpetual fog? Might it not be the case that they can also conceive of the world in an abstract way, but that they are locked in by their condition, so that we mistakenly consign them to a concrete world?

One source of information must necessarily be the patient's public behavior. If, for example, in attempting Goldstein's object-sorting task, interacting with his friends and his physicians, making his way about the hospital, and seeking to communicate his needs, he appears to rely on the same small set of habits; and if he does not make any effort to alter these, based on changing conditions or altered demands, then Goldstein's characterization gains in persuasiveness. If, on the other hand, some flexibility is evident in the patient's behavioral patterns, if he accommodates to new events or tackles problems in fresh ways, then "concreteness" seems a less apt description.

This approach, however, presupposes that the patient

plays the game by our rules. We are in the position of anthropologists who have entered an exotic land, administered an intelligence test to a random sampling of denizens, and, noting that they have failed, dare to conclude that they indeed exhibit a more primitive level of intelligence. Standardized Western tests in this situation represent only one choice among a variety of possible alternatives. It might have been more desirable—though admittedly more difficult—if we had come to know intimately the ways of the particular group, and then assessed their intellectual, aesthetic, moral, and political proclivities by posing problems clearly relevant to their own situation.

The brain-damaged individual, while remaining in our society, has suffered a blow that immediately places him on a new footing. Perhaps the least we should do is to meet him halfway, to determine which skills and aspects of symbolization remain, and to assess his competence in these latter areas. If the patient is aphasic, we should give him nonverbal problems; if his memory is impaired, we should pose tests which require no memory or provide him with mnemonic aids; if we want to ascertain his flexibility with objects, we should offer him not triangles and circles, but rather foods, or records, or friends, or other materials more likely to be evocative for his troubled mind. Nor should we be surprised if the patient displays little enthusiasm for discussing Platonic dialogues or the latest senatorial race; his concerns will necessarily center on his own illness and problems, and our assessment of his reasoning powers is more sensibly based on his ability to deal in an abstract manner with this set of issues.

Lamentably, little is known about the ability of brain-damaged patients to reason, to feel, or to wish, when the subject matter extends beyond the tester's traditional armamentarium. It is so much more convenient to administer a test that has already been standardized with college sophomores or Norway rats, that only a few clinicians have taken the trouble to devise tests more suited to given patients' condition and interest. As a consequence we are ignorant of patients' capacities to understand and to utilize visual symbols, artistic objects, works of music, games, plays, gestural languages, jokes, cartoons, metaphors, mathematical modes of reasoning, or puzzles, not to mention numerous other less obvious means of expression and communication. Nor can we even speculate about the extent to which patients would react to therapies or tests couched in these relatively unfamiliar symbolic forms. As with any assessment of individuals from different cultures, the conclusions we draw must be regarded as highly tentative, inviting major revisions.

Bearing this proviso in mind, I will convey my own impressions about the degree of qualitative change customary among brain-damaged individuals. While no two such individuals present exactly the same clinical picture, there are discernible similarities among patients who have lesions in comparable locations, striking contrasts among those whose lesions fall in disparate loci. So long as a lesion is relatively circumscribed, the patient may still carry on a great many activities, and retain a plethora of skills. If avenues are tapped other than the ones especially impaired, much preserved functioning should be evident. The aphasic patient will appear grossly deficient so long as questioning and answering are restricted to the auditory-oral modality. But when the same patient is allowed to look at pictures, to listen to or perform music, to enact roles via gesture or imitation, he will emerge as a somewhat slowed-down normal person, rather than as a bizarre freak. By the same token, the patient with a verbal memory disorder will appear completely demented if asked about events in his recent past. But when queried about the remote past, or when tested in nonlinguistic modalities, or when required to play the piano or win at chess, again, he will appear virtually indistinguishable from a control subject. In the case of the patients on whom we have focused in our study, it is by far more misleading to consider them as a totally alien species than as somewhat impaired normal individuals.

And yet, these impairments can be tremendously instructive. They highlight the importance and the essential nature of the capacity that has been injured, suggest the possibilities of circumventing this disability in brain-injured adults and in children with learning disorders, and in many cases, reveal an unsuspected set of spared and impaired capacities surrounding the injury. Through study of brain-damaged individuals, reading has emerged as primarily a linguistic, rather than a visual function, memory for language has been sharply distinguished from memory for nonlanguage functions, and understanding of certain grammatical words, the ability to orient oneself in space, and the capacity to solve arithmetical problems, have been revealed to reflect the same underlying intellectual operations. Even when the brain-damaged individual is reminiscent of the normal person overall, his aberrations cast fresh light on our own functioning.

There is more to say on this question. While I reject the label of "concrete" for the patient who has suffered a circumscribed stroke, tumor, or wound, such a characterization does seem more applicable for the patient who is grossly demented, or whose brain damage has extended through wide areas of cortex and subcortex. These patients are difficult to reach through any channel, and they do appear to function at a less sophisticated level. It remains difficult to determine, however, whether theirs corresponds to the concrete world described by Goldstein. Different, to be sure, but perhaps just vaguer and emptier, rather than more concrete.

A more instructive way to envision the world of the brain-damaged, it seems to me, is to note the tremendous variation in a patient's performance from day to day. I have never seen a brain-damaged individual, with the possible exception of those either completely demented or virtually recovered, who did not display sizable variations in performance from day to day, if not across hours or minutes. This range is no mere outcome of chance: it is blatantly evident in the early stages of recovery and may be endemic to the condition of the brain-damaged person. No skill seems to be completely destroyed or wholly intact; rather, each seems to be in a partial state of disrepair, and, depending upon such factors as the surrounding conditions, the extent of fatigue, the events of the preceding minutes, motivation at the given moment, the degree of alertness or attentiveness, the patient may succeed strikingly or fail dismally on a given set of tasks. This variability is all-important, because it precludes a ready, foolproof description of the patient—as most consulting physicians soon learn, one must speak of the patient at-a-given-moment-in-time, or in particular circumstances, rather than as a fixed set of mechanized routines, always performing at the same level.

The tremendous perturbations in a patient's performance provide another way of conceptualizing his universe. Rather than being completely able or completely unable to read, the patient will succeed ten, twenty, or fifty percent of the time on a given word, phrase, or task. He differs from the normal in the unpredictibility of his performance and this is, literally speaking, a quantitative difference. Yet, viewed from an insufficiently broad perspective, a string of such failures may well lead the observer to conclude that the patient is an alien creature— bizarrely concrete or at a primitive level of functioning. So long as it is borne in mind that the conclusion derives from a partial sampling of the patient's behavior, and does not take into account the extremes to which it may tend, I find "abstract" and "concrete" acceptable, if not terribly illuminating, figures of speech.

It is here, then, in his incredible variability, that the brain-damaged patient differs most pronouncedly from the young child. The latter acquires language in a regular and orderly fashion and repeatedly makes the same kinds of errors at a given stage: the aphasic patient varies markedly in his linguistic skills and may make diverse kinds of error (or correct utterances) within the space of a few moments. Moreover, one never finds in the six-year-old child a sudden demonstration of the ability to read, to play the violin, or to perform the calculus. Not having learned these skills, there is not even a statistical possibility that the child will exhibit mastery of these tasks—he is indeed qualitatively different from the adolescent or the post-adolescent scientist. No such guarantees can be made in the case of the brain-damaged patient, however, for unless the given skill is completely wiped out, he may well succeed with such tasks at certain times and in certain situations. Since these prove unpredictable, we cannot simply say that he succeeds only in concrete circumstances; rather we must admit that success is both variable and fortuitous.

From these generalizations, I would, for different reasons, except two groups. The individual whose brain is globally affected will never succeed at any but the simplest sensori-motor tasks. His attitude is not merely concrete, however; it is completely reflexive and primitive, virtually devoid of any fragments of mental processing. The second exception is the individual with major frontal-lobe disease. In the latter case, the patient may completely fool the unsuspecting psychologist or the physician, who may conclude on the basis of high scores and appropriate answers that he is dealing with a competent individual. That is because the frontal-lobe patient superficially retains the major cognitive, intellectual, and sensory capacities tapped by psychological tests. His deficiencies inhere in those very judgmental capacities to plan ahead, to assess the consequences of actions, to evaluate alternatives, to conceive of a situation in multiple ways, to detect subtle social and emotional cues, which are the keynotes of the highest human functions, indeed those which, according to Luria, "make a person human." Ironically, however, it is just this patient, who, in his "abhorrence of the hypothetical," typifies Goldstein's concrete attitude, who proves virtually impossible to pick out on the basis of test scores or other standard criteria unless one is especially on the look-out for the "frontal signs." In some ways the most virulent form of brain damage, the frontal syndrome, leaves the fewest objective traces.

Far from reflecting but a diminished and atypical stratum of humanity, the assemblage of brain-damaged persons highlights facets of nearly every human capacity, calling, flair, and failing. In contemplating the range of patients described here, and the many more who have been studied over the years by sensitive clinical observers, one beholds a Balzacian universe. The tragedy and fascination of brain damage is that it throws into boldest relief those traits of individuals usually evident only to satirists and caricaturists. Take, for example, some instances from the recent political past in the United States: the word-finding pauses and circumlocutions which populated Dwight Eisenhower's speech even before he suffered a mild stroke are clearly delineated in the linguistic output of an anomic aphasic; the occasional stutterings, neologisms, and reversals of consonants in Senator Sam Ervin's persiflage form the mainstay of conduction aphasia; the somewhat cliché'd characterization of situations and persons which permeates Richard Nixon's informal discourse is captured in the curious "concrete aphasia" of our patient Mr. MacArthur (see Chapter 2). The memory losses noticeable in entertainers who drink heavily forecast what they may experience if they subsequently suffer from Korsakoff's disease, while the occasional errors which creep into the musical performance of elderly skilled pianists hint at the onset of the benign (or occasionally malignant) processes of senility. The aphasic completely reliant on gestures reminds us of the role played by expressive moments in our own conversation, even as the flat affect of the frontal-lobe patient epitomizes our mood in situations where we do not care.

Particularly fascinating for the light shed on the functioning of non-brain-damaged persons are the somewhat more bizarre behavioral patterns often found in right-hemisphere patients, and in individuals suffering from temporal-lobe epilepsy. With individuals who have disease of the right hemisphere, the abilities to express oneself in language and to understand the spoken and written communication of others are deceptively normal. What is unexpected, almost eerie, is such persons' dependence on channels of language for all their contacts with the world. With sensitivity to visual and auditory nonverbal stimuli minimized as a result of his injury, with neglect of one side of space and denial of illness, these patients are strangely cut off from all but the verbal messages of others. They are able and eager to banter or display sarcasm when hearing another's message; but they are insensitive to facial expressions, the surrounding milieu, and other nonverbal cues which constantly modulate the behavior of the normal individual. As a result, they are reminiscent of language machines, automatons responsive to the literal meaning of messages but appreciative of neither subtle nuances nor the nonlinguistic contexts in which the message was issued. The transcripts of such patients appear normal on a quick reading, but suspicions arise about a person who takes every question literally, so literally in fact that he appears to have never heard a figure of speech. The patient's own conversation may be quite imaginative and unexpected, but it is again somewhat anomalous in the situation—it is as if the individual refused to confront the facts (and the gravity) of his illness.

While this clinical picture appears quite remote from the behavior of the average, well-adjusted individual, it may possess revealing analogues with the world outside brain disease. Consider, for example the propensity of right-hemisphere patients to engage in playful banter. Most of us do this only sparingly, but such persiflage reflects a potential which we usually have. Mindless chatter occurs when we are intoxicated, and, revealingly enough, when we find ourselves in situations where we do not much care about the impression made: we might make snide comments to doctors, ignore the apparent thrust of a question, deny what is manifest to onlookers, almost daring them to confront us with the facts. So, too, the right-hemisphere brain-damaged person, oblivious (because of his condition) to the situation in which he finds himself, issues a steady barrage of free-ranging comments. In some ways, he resembles the individual (or animal) deprived of all external sensory input who must eventually invent his own stimulation.

And what of the stilted way in which those suffering from right-hemisphere disease field inquiries and respond to them in a shotgun, semiautomatic manner? Here the patient exemplifies the behavior which is customarily (though not always justifiably) associated with the brilliant young mathematician or computer scientist. This highly rational individual is ever alert to an inconsistency in what is being said, always seeking to formulate ideas in the most airtight way; but in neither case does he display any humor about his own situation, nor does he take into account the many subtle, intuitive, interpersonal facets which form so central a part of human intercourse. One feels rather that the answers are being typed out at high speed on computer printout paper.

As for the temporal-lobe epileptic, he may again strike the superficial observer as being entirely normal. And, indeed, in talking about the weather, or in describing his work, this individual may pass for a quiet, sober, and intelligent person. Only after discussion over a wide range of topics, and after observation over a period of time, may the highly unusual behavior and personality of this individual come to light. Sudden and inexplicable bursts of temper and outrage occur, often instigated by the most harmless remarks or incidents. There is, in addition, a heightened tendency toward philosophizing and an often melodramatic hyperreligiosity, as the patient ardently embraces new faiths and doctrines, assembles copious notes and diaries, entertains delusions of his own grandeur and his special relation to his God. Unusual sexual practices, such as homosexuality or transvestitism, or, alternately, diminished sexual appetite, are frequent (though by no means universal) concomitants of seizure discharges in the temporal lobes.

Such symptoms vary greatly across individuals. If an individual's violent attacks are infrequent, his religiosity mild, he can easily pass in the periods between seizures for a normal or mildly neurotic member of society. And, of course, there are many individuals of this behavioral pattern for whom no pathology can be demonstrated in the temporal lobes. Conversely, if an individual becomes a religious maniac and if, as is all too often the case, he harms or kills others, then ties to the normal are tenuous at best. Yet, particularly in the earlier stages of temporal-lobe epilepsy, these extremes are seldom seen; locating the patient within the spectrum of normality and disease becomes most difficult.

Some characteristics of temporal-lobe epilepsy seem to be relatively fixed, running off almost like automatic reflexes. These may include auras of smell before the epileptic fit, states of unconsciousness subsequent to the fit, as well as the physical sequence in the attack pattern itself (baring teeth, contorting the face, hurling objects). Other symptoms, however, are individually modulated by the particular social factors affecting each patient. While the patient's diaries may contain characteristic sentiments, they will scarcely feature the same phrases: one patient will speak about his conversations with a god, another about the miraculous warmth of his mother, a third will dwell on attacks by the devil, or by noted political figures. The particular way in which a religious interest is exemplified—joining a church, authoring a religious novel, or defining a personal creed—will also reflect the individual's personal situation, as will the extent to which he displays paranoid ideation. Indeed, it remains an open question whether the religious, ideological, and sexual practices of the temporal-lobe epileptic are part-and-parcel of his brain disease, or the reaction of a more or less intact personality to the bizarre events which are unquestionably symptoms of his disease.

Suppose, for example, that as the consequence of a macabre conditioning procedure, you were suddenly compelled to attack your loved ones on a number of occasions. Not only might you seek psychiatric help; you might well construct a scenario which could help you explain to yourself these uncontrolled fits. And, both unaware of and unable to control these paroxysms, you might posit the existence of a plot, or a hidden enemy, or a god, that was inspiring or compelling these transgressions. In this case, it would not be brain disease *per se,* but rather the construction of a normal mind, which would culminate in a clinical picture of religiosity indistinguishable from that of the verified temporal-lobe epileptic.

Indeed, it is the case of the latter syndrome—as is increasingly recognized—that raises most dramatically two questions: the relation between psychological and organic behavioral disorders; and the way in which society should deal with a diseased brain. Were it proved that a given brain disease produced an unpleasant set of behaviors, and that a certain operation could remove only these unpleasant behaviors, while leaving the rest of the individual intact, then some (though perhaps not all) objections against psychosurgery might be allayed. If, however, the individual's symptoms are seen as inextricably tied to his whole personality, with some of his ideas and thoughts a normal reaction to bizarre conditions, others long-standing attitudes that merely happen to have become involved with bizarre behavior; and if, in addition, some normal non-brain-damaged individuals may present symptoms of temporal-lobe epileptics, then the justification for, and the risks of, corrective brain surgery become much more serious, and the operation correspondingly less defensible.

For even though the brain is clearly the seat of the individual's emotions and personality, it is simplistic to attribute the emotions and personality of a brain-injured person strictly to his disease. To be sure, there are recurrent patterns: the indifference of the frontal-lobe patient, the euphoria of the patient with a severe comprehension disorder, the depression of the patient with isolated problems in expressing himself, are not mere coincidences—they are too reliably present with a given lesion. But who is to say that these patterns, or others which are much less predictable, are a direct consequence of the brain disease, rather than, say, the reaction of a normal brain to a situation where one's own values have ceased to matter, where one's own difficulty with communication is insufficiently appreciated, or one's powers for communicating are mysteriously cut off. To my mind, any discussion of brain damage must include, as a vital component in the equation, the personality of the individual in the days prior to his injury. This personality still exists, at least to some extent; so, too, the same mind, attitude, feelings, and fears remain, if in somewhat subdued or altered form. It is this personality which must come to grips with and comprehend the nature of the brain damage. Barring, however, unusually good communication with the patient's family, we generally learn little about this personality, and so must either speculate about it blindly or deny its relevance altogether. It is thus understandable, however regrettable, that many doctors should take the latter course and insist on talking about, say, "the personality of the frontal patient" as a fixed entity.

Even if brain damage is confirmed, and some emotions or views can be directly traced to it, we are hardly justified —on either moral or intellectual grounds—in discounting the patient as a person. Dostoevsky's novels are no less remarkable, impassioned, moving, or brilliant because we now suspect that they are the productions of a temporal-lobe epileptic; Churchill's decisions in the aftermath of World War II cannot be gainsaid just because he suffered a series of strokes; nor do we fail to make use of Louis Pasteur's brilliant discoveries and insights because he suffered a major stroke when still a young man. Many abilities will remain, many others can be repaired or compensated for, and even those mired at a primitive level need not prevent the individual from communicating and expressing himself, nor from dealing effectively with events in the world and people around him. Through music, pictures, gestures, cards, chess, or love, contacts can and should be maintained with the person. To the extent that his family treats the brain-damaged individual as a functioning individual, he is likely to react as before; to the extent that he is treated as bizarre, unaware, stupid, or half dead, he is all too likely to conform (perhaps literally) to their expectations. The performances of many brain-damaged patients are not only variable for organic reasons; they are also extraordinarily sensitive to the environment which is, after all, under control of individuals with whom he is in constant contact.

Although it seems pointless in most cases to question the essential integrity of the brain-damaged person, delicate issues may nonetheless arise which demand an assessment of the effects of his injury. These include questions about financial decisions, family matters, business concerns, plans for rehabilitation and disposition. All too often, the testimony of the brain-damaged individual is ignored; indeed, so often is the onset of a stroke treated by the family as the occasion for dismissing the patient that left-hemisphere damage may correlate more highly with rejection by the family than with aphasia! Yet sometimes the opposite situation may arise, where perhaps out of misplaced sympathy, the ideas and wishes of the brain-damaged patient are uncritically accepted: this state of affairs may be equally inopportune.

The question arises most stingingly in the case of brain-damaged individuals whose testamentary capacity is wanted. The need (or desire) to change a will, to testify in a case, to make a judgment affecting the fates and fortunes of others in a court of law are sample instances. Should the judgment of the brain-damaged person be sought in this situation and, more controversially, should it be followed even when this involves countermanding previous wishes?

Sometimes this question is easy to resolve. If the brain-damaged patient shows no ability to comprehend or communicate, if his actions are completely bizarre, or if his emotional state has changed drastically, then one will obviously wait for an improvement in the condition before listening seriously to his desires. Such would be the case with President Wilson, President Salazar, or Ambassador Joseph P. Kennedy after their strokes. Alternatively, the completely or almost completely recovered person like President Eisenhower and Prime Minister Churchill should certainly be heard.

In many, perhaps most cases, however, the decision on testamentary competence is less obvious. Such is the case, for instance, where there has been an undeniable diminution in certain functions, without however the patient becoming so disabled that he cannot make his wishes known. Naturally, if it is possible to postpone the decision, this course is preferable, for the patient's condition will probably improve, and in some cases the problem may evaporate for other reasons. When, however, an immediate decision is essential, some personal equation-solving is required. In such cases, the advice of neurologist Macdonald Critchley is sound: Donning the cap of the experimenter, one should try to reduce the problem to its essences and then determine, by a series of pragmatic tests, whether the patient appears to understand the outstanding issues involved. If his comprehension of those issues, and of the factors weighing on a judgment, appears competent, then his verdict should be adhered to; if there is substantial doubt, it may be best to withhold testimony. Critchley cites the case of *Moore* v. *Moore* (1900), in which a will had to be drawn up; the physician gave the patient one pack of cards listing *names,* another pack of cards listing *properties.* The patient then sorted out the cards, placed each bequest with its recipient, and a tally was drawn up. Later, the patient went over the will slowly, clause by clause, with the solicitor and the physician, thereby reducing the margin for error. Such elegant solutions notwithstanding, the question of testamentary capacities is, in the last analysis, as insoluble as most other issues on which lawyers cut their teeth. When Hughlings Jackson was asked about whether an aphasic patient should be allowed to make a will, he answered cryptically, "Can a piece of string stretch across a room?"

Questions about the brain, its normal and injured functioning, involve intrinsic fascination, and yet, for most of us its study possesses special appeal because it promises increased understanding of ourselves, our feelings, and perhaps preeminently, our intellects. There are different avenues to such understanding, ranging from subjective introspections by intensively trained students to behavioral experiments with children or with animals. Yet, as we have argued here, certain, perhaps unique forms of insight can be gleaned from the study of the brain-damaged.

As we withdraw somewhat from the individual syndromes which have occupied us, however, we remain faced with the broader question, the relation between the protoplasm in our head and the mental processes in our mind, that problem of body and mind whose eventual solution was termed by William James "the scientific achievement before which all past achievements would pale." I should like to suggest that a study of brain damage may shed some new light on this venerable problem.

When speaking of the brain and of brain processes, our referent is reasonably clear. We refer to that portion of the nervous system which is housed in our skull, the ten-billion-odd nerve cells and their myriad interconnections and such discrete functional entities as the sensory cortexes, the limbic system, or the subcortical structures subserving attentional mechanisms. The physiologist and the anatomist know their tasks: to tease out the various structures in the brain, to determine what each does, to define their relations. Answers are likely to become increasingly specific; we will know the function of individual cells long before we have unraveled the site of consciousness, the self, or the mind.

It may be futile to search for such sites, of course, but the phenomena for which we are searching need not be equally fictitious. For whatever reasons, individuals seem convinced that they exist as individuals, that they have a unique set of feelings, ideas, and wishes to which they are especially privy, that they experience subjective concomitants of these mental processes, and that these events occur in a special region or part of themselves, called by shorthand the mind, the self, the identity. These three terms are scarcely identical in ordinary usage, but as I will suggest, they allude to a peculiarly human capacity to reflect upon one's own actions and one's own past and future. The "I" or the "mind" may be an invention but *it has been invented,* all the same; a cogent account of its purported existence and development is desirable. And it would be quite interesting if this enigmatic structure could be located somewhere—at least figuratively—in the human brain.

Even though the mind-body problem has often, and perhaps increasingly, been viewed as a pseudo- or insoluble problem, certain facts are agreed upon by nearly everyone with professional or amateur interests in the question—for example, the transmission of electrical impulses along neural circuitry, the migration of chemicals across the cell boundaries, these processes giving rise to the perceptual and motor functions. When the electrical signals—and the concomitant brain waves—cease, thought, behavior, and life cease as well. Within the scientific community, what is called mind is generally related to processes occurring within the brain. However, many investigators would prefer not to speak of mind, either because they remain unconvinced that the term has a meaningful referent, or because they feel it is at present futile to attempt to elucidate this process or entity. Ignoring questions of mind is an acceptable ploy, but this does not mean that the questions will evaporate: they are simply inherited by more brazen investigators.

Those individuals who acknowledge that mind is worth talking about sometimes embrace a form of dualism: they insist on the existence of material processes in the brain, and of mental processes in the mind, but are loath to equate them. Other commentators prefer to think of the mind/body distinction as one embodied in language: according to this view, terms about brain functioning (body) are believed to refer to the very same events as terms about an individual's phenomenal mental experience (mind).

There is but one reality, designated by two different conceptual systems. A related view suggests that the *mental* aspect of an event is that of which we are directly (and personally) aware, while the *bodily* aspect is implicated where we interpret the event as an occurrence in the physical universe. This view intimates that there is something more direct, less mediated about the mind, for it is *from* our mental perceptions that all understandings, including those of science, must flow. There are also more extreme positions which emphasize the body, the mind viewed as a mere epiphenomenon, as well as directly opposite views, according to which the mind is capable of directing the activity of the brain (or body).

Common to these diverse views (as usually formulated) is a focus on the operations of the nervous system at its most microscopic level—the firings of individual nerve cells. When the mental processes of which we are subjectively aware are contrasted with these elementary physical events, the gap is understandably enormous. We can, I feel, achieve fresh insights on the problems of mind by examining the neuropsychological syndromes described here.

Let me exemplify this approach. Once the existence of mind and mental processes has been conceded, the conclusion often follows that the mind is a unified field, a consummate conductor combining into a harmonious chorus the various facets of the individual. The existence of disconnection syndromes (see Chapter 7) sharply challenges this assumption, however. Such patients, it will be recalled, have had the fibers connecting their cerebral hemispheres separated in order to control the spread of severe epileptic seizures. After the disconnection, an individual will appear to perform normally if required to move the right side of the body (or the left side of his brain). He will be able not only to draw, recognize objects with his hand, read and write, but also to describe what he has done accurately. Yet when the same tasks are required of the left hand, the patient fails some (like writing) altogether; and even though he succeeds on others (like recognition of objects), he cannot verbalize what he has done and will produce erroneous answers to linguistic questioning. This bizarre picture apparently results because information transmitted to the right hemisphere of the brain cannot be thence conveyed to the left (or speaking) half. As a result, it makes little sense to speak of the *individual's* mind, if by this is meant a single terminus from which all activities are directed and to which all results are reported. For the "mind" as reflected in the individual's testimony and the behavior of the right side of the body will say one thing, while the "mind" as reflected in the behavior of the left side may indicate something entirely different.

Such macabre clinical pictures have had diverse impacts on those who ponder the mind-body problem. Some commentators have cited these results as further proof that the concept of mind (as customarily used) is outmoded or useless. It makes little sense to speak of *one* mind when the individual's right hemisphere is behaving at cross-purposes to his left; for all we know, there may be as many "minds" as there are schemes of behavior. Others, on the basis of an equally serious review, reach quite a different conclusion. For these scientists, interested in the possibility of a separate consciousness in the right hemisphere, split-brain phenomena confirm the extremely complex nature of mind, raising anew the possibility that perhaps mind cannot be accounted for simply as an accretion of nerve impulses, reflex arcs, and perceptual-motor systems.

Were the tendency to resurrect mind as a non- or supramaterial entity but the efforts of a tiny minority, or of fifth-rate scientists, it could be safely ignored. But, instead, a number of the most distinguished neuroscientists have become agnostic on the question of whether mind can be accounted for in material terms. The distinguished physiologist and Nobel Prize winner Sir John Eccles has declared:

If we follow Jennings, as I do, in his arguments and inferences we come to the religious concept of soul and its special creation by God. I believe that there is a fundamental mystery in my existence, transcending any biological account of the development of my body (including my brain) with its genetic inheritence and its evolutionary origin, and that being so I must believe similarly for . . . every human being.

The renowned British biologist J. B. S. Haldane, perplexed by the paradox that if mind was determined by matter, it would not be determined by truth, concluded:

In order to escape from the necessity of sawing away the branch on which I am sitting, so to speak, I am compelled to believe that the mind is not wholly conditioned by matter.

Writing in a similar though more modest vein, one of the greatest of modern physicists, Sir Arthur Eddington, suggested that:

There is in a human being some portion of the brain, perhaps a mere speck of brain matter, perhaps an extensive region, in which the physical effects of his volitions begin, and from which they are propagated to the nerves and muscles which translate the volition into action. We will call this portion of the brain-matter "conscious matter." . . . it cannot be identical in all respects with inorganic matter for that would reduce the body to an automaton acting independently of consciousness.

And the eminent neurosurgeon Wilder Penfield, unequaled in his experience with brain surgery, has conceded:

It must be said that there is as yet no scientific proof that the brain can control the mind or fully explain the mind.

The assumptions of materialism have never been substantiated. Science throws no light on the nature of the spirit of man or God.

Of course, this reluctance to dismiss "the mind" might only demonstrate anew that scientists should not philosophize. Yet, on the assumption that those who know the brain may have something worthwhile to say on its relation to mental processes, I am reluctant to dismiss these statements altogether. I regard them as sincere declarations by observers perplexed by the realization that the nature of the nervous system is alarmingly remote from all they know about their own minds.

One prescient insight into the physical bases of mind has come from Dr. Penfield's own operations upon severely epileptic patients. So that Penfield could determine what portions of brain could safely be excised, he kept the patients alert and awake during surgery; then he began to stimulate various regions of the cortex with electrical current. When certain areas were stimulated, the patient became aphasic or emitted isolated yelps. If at all possible, these regions were declared off limits for surgical procedure. Many others produced silence—that is, stimulation led to no overt response or discomfort on the patient's part; these could be removed if necessary. When certain parts of the temporal and parietal lobes were stimulated, however, patients began to relate fascinating experiences, leading Penfield eventually to the conclusion that he had tapped into the patient's "stream of consciousness."

These cortical stimulations and evoked impressions have been much written about, and so it is important to determine where facts end and inferences begin. What Penfield found was that stimulation in certain parts of the brain would lead to a report of purely sensory experiences— lights, stars, or colored flashes in the case of the visual cortex, ringing sounds or humming in the case of the auditory cortex. Moving on to adjacent areas of cortex the patient would experience more complete experiences, such as voices, music, composite visual scenes, or familiar persons.

Of greatest significance was the patient's testimony when the "interpretive cortex" was stimulated. Now the patient would describe experiences from his past, happenings from his childhood, emotions he had experienced, hallucinations he was now entertaining. In one case a patient heard a specific popular song being performed by an orchestra. Whenever the electrodes returned to that locus the patient hummed the tune. Once the electrodes were moved, the humming ceased and she reported other experiences, for instance, one of her children speaking. A young boy, when stimulated, reported a telephone conversation with his mother. Later, he reported that his mother was telling his brother that he had his coat on backwards. Patients recurrently related experiences of an individual talking or singing, or someone yelling at them, of people coming in and out, of someone pulling an object, or interacting with another individual.

Often these experiences seemed to be housed in a specific locus in the brain. According to Penfield, repeated stimulation of the same point will repeatedly elicit the performance (or the memory of a performance) of a specific piece of music. Sometimes the experiences are linked by a common feature—for example, otherwise diverse incidents in which something was grabbed or snatched. Indeed, Penfield goes so far as to suggest that the brain may house a "classified file" for grabbing. The patient can usually indicate whether the experience is one which happened many times and hence is familiar, or whether it is strange, exotic, or hallucinatory.

Yet certain experiences seem never to have been elicited in the hundreds of patients and thousands of stimulations reported by Penfield. Patients never indicate that they are in the process of making up their mind; they never describe themselves as carrying out skilled activities, as speaking or talking, as writing messages, adding figures, eating, tasting food, engaging in sexual activities, undergoing painful suffering or tragic experiences. Despite these curious lacunae, however, Penfield reaches the strong conclusion that "the evoked experiential response is a random reproduction of whatever composed the stream of consciousness during some interval of the patient's past life. . . . nothing is lost . . . the record of each man's experience is complete . . . the brain of every man contains an unchanging ganglionic record of successive experience."

Should Penfield's interpretation be correct, these regions of the temporal lobe might be regarded as the permanent repository of the individual's mind. That is, the individual's conscious experiences and thoughts at a given moment in time are experienced in this region and recorded, there available to the individual for reflection or reconsideration at a subsequent point in time. A number of factors call such a view into doubt, however. As Ulric Neisser has pointed out after a careful review of these protocols, the experiences are as likely to be typical *kinds* of events from the person's past as unique memories of specific incidents. As such, they only show the kinds of events which were once salient for the patient or which seem to be significant in retrospect, rather than constituting an exact record of what he perceived and felt. Patients often allude to the dreamlike quality of the experience and, as in a dream, often perceive themselves looking at the scene (as a disinterested observer) rather than as an active participant. Many kinds of experiences are never reported, moreover, thus calling into question Penfield's claim of a random sampling from experience. Indeed, these rivulets seem to be events which have strong auditory or visual components, rather than ones more purely in the realm of thought, records of skilled motor activity, or recreations of deep feelings and passionate experiences. The style of narration is that of the "observer-patient," not of the participating actor, highlighting again the degree to which the memory is a construction by the patient. Finally, the fact that these memories or experiences are elicited by a stimulus in the cortex by no means proves that such experiences are stored there. What may instead be happening is that large portions of the brain are reacting to the stimulus, with speech presumably coming from language areas, interpretation and commentary from the frontal lobes, and so on. Penfield seems to have hooked into the mechanism which mediates one's dreams and one's hazy-to-precise memories of prototypical events in the past—but not necessarily into a faithful cinematic record of what has happened in one life, nor into the area in which thoughts and feelings combine into a person.

Nonetheless, Penfield's remarkable findings do suggest how the brain might give rise to perception of mind. His reports confirm the impression that there may be represented separately in the brain highly developed motor skills, pure sensory sensation, vivid sensory impressions of composite events, deep emotional reactions to occurrences, decision-making and evaluative capacities, story-telling or impression-relating capacity. These are all aspects of mental functioning, but they are scarcely identical to one another; it may be necessary (and, through neuropsychological methods, it becomes possible) to examine each separately before their interaction and possible unification within "consciousness" or "mind" can be explicated.

As I see it, previous commentators have erred in two ways: They have either treated man's diverse skills and capacities as an excuse to reject any talk of a unified mind, or they have quickly passed over these distinctive capacities, lest they undermine the concept of a unified mind. In the second case, they have viewed mind as a static entity, frozen at the present, rather than as a dynamic process with roots extending deep into the past of the individual.

Donning the cap of the science-fiction aficionado, let us speculate about how one might construct a mechanical brain, so indistinguishable from a human one that a blind observer could not tell them apart. Into such a brain one would build the capacity to perform the various perceptual and motor skills of the normal person—to discriminate sizes and shapes and colors, to walk and talk, to make computations, play the fiddle, eat, drink, and be merry. To the extent that a program could be devised for each of these activities, the brain might survive this portion of the "human test."

But those who speak glowingly of mind do not allude solely to such disparate skills. They are more likely to intend the "force" or "power" which appears to deploy these various capacities, to decide when the individual is to perceive or to walk; they posit a homunculus somewhere inside the individual that undertakes purposive activities, abandons them when no longer desirable, evaluates progress or failure, has a sense of awareness ("consciousness") of what the individual has done and will be doing.

Where might this most "mental" of presences arise? Conceivably it has always been present, but that would not reflect the facts of early childhood. Perhaps it arises suddenly in adulthood, but that would not square with what we know about pre-adolescents, nor for that matter, with what we know about later development. Careful examination of human development suggests instead, that the formation of the sense of self, of the feeling of a "mind" in touch with and in command of an individual's behaviors and actions, is a bootstrap operation, one aided by peers, by the language, by the surrounding culture, indeed by the individual's total interaction with the world.

This claim requires amplification. Until the child begins to use various symbols, such as words, pictures, or gestures, he is restricted to concrete action in the physical world.

Once able to employ such symbols, however, he can make reference to all manner of physical, social, and immaterial objects, such as rocks, relatives, and reason. Language is certainly critical in this process, but the capacity to refer to entities can also take place with other forms of symbols; nor can language be considered in a vacuum for it is, after all, a product of the surrounding culture, not an independent invention of the child.

The ability to refer and to represent develops slowly, but, within a few years, a child can use appropriately such words as "I," "me," and "self." At first the meaning of these words is rough, but certainly by the age of 7 or 8, the average child recognizes that a unique self-reference is intended. By this time, there has begun a long, indeed an interminable, process in which the child expresses to himself—generally in language—what has happened to him, reflects on its meaning, and begins to create what we have called here "the metaphor of self": this metaphor represents the child's efforts to make sense of his experience, to keep a record of it, to note where he has been and where he is going. We call such an activity *metaphoric* because, through symbols, the child has constructed an account of a hypothetic individual who happens to be himself. Generally the record of the self entails a strong language component—and for this reason we might consider it a left-hemisphere creature. But it must be stressed that all manner of sensory and emotional concomitants permeate this record and it could be captured in symbolic coin other than natural language. The record may indeed be regarded as complete in one sense, for every experience on which the child reflects, or from which he learns, should exert an effect on the metaphor. Yet precisely because the metaphor is ever-changing, and the child as a consequence is attaining ever-higher levels of understanding, it does not seem possible to freeze past experiences. Instead, such experiences come to be interpreted in terms of the individual's present metaphor (with its level of sophistication); only with regression does the possibility (and it is only a possibility) arise that a child may obtain privileged access to some earlier experience.

By the time the child has become an adult, the metaphor of himself—the record and picture of who and what he is (and who and what he is not)—has attained considerable autonomy. Indeed, it is this record, with its importance to the individual and to his society, which Erik Erikson has termed the person's "sense of identity," a chief product of the adolescent "identity-crisis." The mind, the self, the identity, are literally housed inside the individual's brain; but they appear to have an independent extracorporal existence, because in the course of their formation the self attains increasing autonomy. The individual-as-subject is eventually able to treat the individual-as-object as a separate construction—a poem or a story—of whom he happens to be the author. Paradoxically, the self achieves such autonomy that it can tell what has happened to itself.

Can this sense of self, this consciousness which seems so integral to mind, be localized in any portion of the brain? Ultimately the answer would seem to be no. The highest, most complex order of intellectual activity would seem to draw on every portion of the cortex and may well require the complete intactness of the brain, any kind of damage exerting at least some effect on overall performance. And yet, we can at least hypothesize which brain structures play the most crucial role in the formation and maintenance of the sense of self. They must be ones upon which information about the individual's experiences, feelings, and behaviors can readily converge, they must be areas where it is possible to construct some kind of metaphoric representation of the individual, they must be implicated in planning, deciding, and evaluating, and they are likely to be among the latest-maturing portions of the brain.

The frontal lobes, the proud crowning structures of the

human brain, are likely candidates for this subtle but crucial role. As Walle Nauta, the eminent neuroanatomist, has pointed out, the frontal lobes are the meetingplace *par excellence* for information from the two great functional realms of the brain: the posterior (temporal and parietal) regions involved in the processing of all sensory information; and the limbic system, where the individual's motivational and emotional processes and responses are centered. The frontal lobes function, accordingly, both as a sensory (input) and as an effector (output) mechanism; this cortex is the realm where neural networks representing the individual's internal milieu (his subjective feelings) converge with the systems representing the external milieu (the sights, sounds, tastes, and mores of the world) as reported by all the sensory modalities.

Because of their strategic anatomical location and connections, the frontal lobes thus have the potential to serve as a great integrating station. Their late maturation, in middle childhood, provide further circumstantial evidence of their possible implication in these crucial matters. The most compelling evidence, however, consists in findings from patients who have had their frontal lobes selectively impaired or selectively spared.

We know from our earlier cases (see Chapter 7) that the frontal-lobe patient displays bizarre mood changes (euphoria or irritability), emotional indifference, social inappropriateness and changes in his character. These last manifestations are particularly crucial. The individual with frontal-lobe disease may be intellectually equipped to set out alternative possibilities for action, since his ratiocinative powers *per se* have not been devastated; but he lacks the inclination to exercise those powers. He no longer cares, even if he is aware of the alternatives open to him; he neglects his physical person, overlooks his friends and his conflicts, avoids necessary decisions. He is slovenly, sometimes frankly sexual, careless if not criminal. This indifferent, offensive conduct and incapacity for meaningful decision can be attributed, at least in part, to the particular physiological disturbances in the individual's brain. In view of the disconnection of limbic system information from the centers of motor action, the individual cannot monitor possible future actions by considering their emotional concomitants. Where the normal person can realize that "the mere thought of doing such a thing makes me ill" (because he is contemplating the limbic consequences of a behavior), the frontal-lobe patient cannot. Frontal-lobe impairment also prevents the individual from anticipating the sensory changes which might accompany a motor pattern; as a consequence, the pragmatic effects of a decision fail to be monitored.

Owing to these and other deficiencies, the frontal-lobe patient—even while scoring impressively on objective tests of skills and knowledge—strikes us instantly and intuitively as bereft of a sense of self, unconscious of his life, deprived of a metaphor in which his activities and his worth are recorded, or at least of the ability or the incentive to consult this record. He is, in sum, a mature adult in the range and sophistication of activities in which he can engage; he is like a very young child in respect to his ability, or rather inability, to think about and contemplate the effects of his actions. (The child with frontal damage would seem, however, relatively normal, because those mature behaviors associated with the adult frontal lobe would not yet have developed.)

We have seen, on the other hand, most dramatically in the case of Zasetsky, the consequences of spared frontal lobes. Here a patient is crippled in so many of the sensory and motor capacities which we (and the frontal-lobe patient) normally possess. Nonetheless, his sense of self, his concern about what he can and cannot do, his ability to confront and make decisions, have been diminished little if at all. Indeed, even though his communicative system for representing himself and his world has been impoverished, his left hemisphere severely damaged, he works (often tirelessly) with whatever communicative capacities remain in order to continue to monitor his own "self," to remain an active and vital human being. It is because most aphasic patients retain their pivotal frontal-lobe structures that they, too, even when paralyzed and almost mute, retain the dignity of the sense of self.

Attempts to simulate the human brain must certainly contain the sensory and motor patterns alluded to, but the product would strangely resemble the listless frontal-lobe patient unless it proved possible to construct this sense of self, this terminus of mind. Even were it possible to construct a machine that could "feel" in the sense of undergoing the sensations and emotions of pleasure, pain, thirst, anxiety, or love, the product would be inadequate, unless the elusive "homunculus" could also be simulated. My own hunch is that efforts to simulate the brain are more likely to succeed in the biological laboratory than in the computation center; elaborate computer programs seem less promising than the attempts to construct a brain out of organic matter. This is because, it is my firm conviction, the mind cannot be devised or frozen at a single moment in time. Rather, by its very nature, mind is a slow accumulation of increasingly differentiated representations of the self at different stages of development, affected and altered to some extent by each, but never erasing altogether the traces of itself at a more primitive stage of evolution. When we draw on the processes of mind, we are employing a system with deep historical roots which continue to exert an effect on our contemporary activities.

Our sense of self, in other words, is never wholly adult, never wholly mature, established, and finished. True, our current concerns and skills predominate; but underlying them (and accessible to electrical stimulation or to psychoanalysts' proddings) are reservoirs of earlier experiences and feelings which continue to affect and mold our judgments, to be drawn on as limbic inputs in making decisions, to inform our relation to the past and our aspirations for the future. Simulating these inputs by the creation of a "mental metaphor in computer language" would be extremely difficult, because it is by no means clear how all these inputs (representing many years of development) make their several contributions to a mature sense of self. At some times, as shown in Zasetsky's case, the memories, concerns, and impressions of earlier life dominate; at other times, the current factors, or future considerations, play the most dominant roles. Only if one could somehow simulate the *very processes of learning and of developing,* by the manipulation of protoplasm or hardware, might a convincing artificial brain be constructed. Accomplishing this presupposes not only knowledge of how the mature brain functions (as obtained from brain-damaged patients) but also of how the brain and the person develop—matters unlikely to be resolved in our lifetime. The rock whose fissures were formed by accumulation of debris and of matter over the centuries is easily distinguished from the rock whose fissures were produced by yesterday's skilled sculptor.

Of course, the effort to re-create human brains is but a *Gedanken* experiment, a mental exercise; though one might be able to invent a machine whose answers to questions were indistinguishable from those of one or another specific individual, this would by no means constitute proof of the identity of the brains. For instance, I might know my friend so well that I could anticipate every answer he would give. But our brains would hardly be identical, because his answers (and, so to speak, his brain) would be contained only as a subset of my own—there is no reason to conclude that the other person would be able to simulate my answers with equal fidelity. And even if the relationship were reciprocal, we could never prove that a future question might not be answered differently, or that there were no differences in subjective experiences,

feelings, vulnerabilities, or desires, unascertainable because we do not know what questions to ask, or what
measures to take. Our goal should not be to create perfect
replicas of a given brain or of all brains—a futile enterprise, in any case—but rather to use questions as a spur
to specification of what it is that we do (and do not yet)
know about the brain and the mind.

In this quest, no holds are barred. Information from all
manner of subjects—children, animals, brain-damaged individuals, computer models, metaphoric selves—must be
drawn on as evidence. Attempts to understand the *Weltan-
schauung* of those different from ourselves, as well as those
who would seem highly similar, is also an indispensable
step, even though we can never know the extent to which
we legitimately comprehend the mind of the brain-damaged patient, or, for that matter, our own. Consideration
of the relationship between the neural processes in the
brain and those activities which we exalt as "mental" is
also important, even though definitive answers to the
mind-body question may be as remote in years as they are
plentiful in number. Yet even on this arcane and vexed
question the study of brain damage can be suggestive. We
have seen how a disconnection may challenge the notion
of a single, unitary mind within the cerebral hemispheres.
We can behold the miraculous discoveries of Dr. Penfield
as he stimulates the cortex, then consider dispassionately
whether he has indeed touched the heart of consciousness.
And we may consider whether somewhere in the areas of
the frontal lobe is a metaphor, developed over many years
by virtue of our capacity to represent ourselves in symbols,
nurtured by the surrounding culture and stocked with a
record of what we have done and what we are like—a
mere literary figure which not only represents the mind
or self within the body, but even persistently checks up,
equipped with the tools of the scientist or the riddles of
the philosopher, to make sure that it is really there.

# Notes

# Index

# Notes

CHAPTER 1

p. 3  The epigraph is taken from L. Edson, "The Psyche and the Surgeon," *New York Times Magazine,* September 30, 1973, p. 78. I have been unable to locate the original source of this quotation in Eliot's works.

p. 3  Workers in laboratories: For reviews of some recent research on the brain, see M. Pines, *The Brain Changers* (New York: Harcourt Brace Jovanovich, 1973); M. Ferguson, *The Brain Revolution* (New York: Taplinger, 1973).

p. 4  "bio-feedback" loops: See G. Jonas, *Visceral Learning: Toward the Science of Self-Control* (New York: Viking, 1973).

p. 4  "lesion" studies: See P. Milner, *Physiological Psychology* (New York: Holt, Rinehart, and Winston, 1970) Chap. 4.

p. 11  On stroke, see J. E. Sarno and M. T. Sarno, *Stroke: The Condition and the Patient* (New York: McGraw-Hill, 1969); C. McBride, *Silent Victory* (Chicago: Nelson-Hall, 1969); A. Carter, *All About Strokes* (London: Thomas Nelson, 1968). A more technical account appears in R. Bannister, *Brain's Clinical Neurology* (London: Oxford University Press, 1969), Chap. 13.

p. 12  individuals sustaining moderate strokes: See "Stroke Rehabilitation: Report of the Joint Committee for Stroke Facilities," *Stroke,* 1972, *3*, 375–407.

p. 16  Pure alexia: See Chapter 3.

p. 17  lesion in the parietal lobe of the "dominant" hemisphere: See Chapter 6.

p. 17  lesion in the angular gyrus region: See A. R. Luria, *The Higher Cortical Functions in Man* (New York: Basic Books, 1966), pp. 154–8.

p. 19   The outlook for [Mr. Franklin]: For a full discussion of the prognosis of stroke, see M. Ullman, *Behavioral Changes in Patients Following Strokes* (Springfield, Ill.: Charles C. Thomas, 1962); and H. Rusk and E. J. Taylor, *Rehabilitation Medicine* (St. Louis: C. V. Mosby Co., 1964).

p. 20   a brief historical review: There are no comprehensive histories of neuropsychology. Useful information is contained in A. R. Luria, *The Higher Cortical Functions in Man* (New York: Basic Books, 1966); H. Head, *Aphasia and Kindred Disorders of Speech* (New York: Hafner, 1963); T. Weisenburg and K. E. McBride, *Aphasia: A Clinical and Psychological Study* (New York: The Commonwealth Fund, 1935); L. Stevens, *Explorers of the Brain* (New York: Knopf, 1971).

p. 20   A classic work on phrenology is F. J. Gall and J. Spurzheim, *Anatomie et physiologie du système nerveux en général et du cerveau en particulier* (Paris: Schoell, 1810–1818).

p. 21   P. Broca, "Remarques sur le siège de la faculté du langage articulé," *Bulletin de la Société d'anthropologie,* Paris, 1861, 6.

p. 23   G. Fritsch and E. Hitzig, "Über die elektrische Erregbarkeit des Grosshirns," *Arch. Anat. Physiol. u. Wisse. Med.,* 1870, 37.

p. 23   Munk ablated . . . : H. Munk, *Über die Funktionen der Grosshirnrinde* (Berlin: Hirschwald, 1881).

p. 24   Pierre Marie, "Révision de la question de l'aphasie," *Semaine Medicale,* 1906, 21, 241–7.

p. 25   the "holists": H. Head, *Aphasia and Kindred Disorders of Speech* (New York: Hafner, 1963); K. Goldstein, *Language and Language Disturbances* (New York: Grune and Stratton, 1948).

p. 25   The provocative findings of Karl Lashley: K. Lashley, *Brain Mechanisms and Intelligence* (Chicago: University of Chicago Press, 1929).

p. 26   a more moderate, intermediate position: Perhaps the best instance is A. R. Luria, *The Higher Cortical Functions in Man* (New York: Basic Books, 1966).

p. 36   Accessible introductions to neuroanatomy are D. P. Kimble, *Physiological Psychology* (Reading, Mass.: Addison-Wesley, 1963); and A. J. Gatz, *Manter's Essentials of Clinical Neuroanatomy and Neurophysiology* (Philadelphia: F. A. Davis, 1970). A classic text is R. C. Truex and M. B. Carpenter, *Strong and Elwyn's Human Neuroanatomy* (Baltimore: Williams and Wilkins, 1964).

p. 41   On dichotic listening, see D. Kimura, "Functional Asymmetry of the Brain in Dichotic Listening." *Cortex,* 1967, 3, 163–78.

p. 42   On left-handedness, see H. Hécaen and J. de Ajuriaguerra, *Les gauchers* (Paris: Presses Universitaires de France, 1963).

CHAPTER 2

p. 52   The epigraph is taken from William James, *Psychology* (New York: Fawcett, 1961), p. 117.

p. 52   The most comprehensive work on aphasia in recent years is A. R. Luria, *Traumatic Aphasia* (The Hague: Mouton, 1970). A helpful history of the study of aphasia is found in W. R. Brain, *Speech Disorders* (London: Butterworths, 1965).

p. 53   The issues raised by aphasia: An excellent review of many of these issues appears in H. Goodglass and N. Geschwind, "Language Disorders (Aphasia)," to appear in E. Carterette and M. Friedman (eds.), *Handbook of Perception* (in press).

p. 54   a neurology service: The standard examination is described in R. N. DeJong, *The Neurologic Examination* (New York: 1958).

p. 55   Our testing of aphasic patients . . . : An excellent test, developed at the Boston Veterans Administration Hospital, is described in H. Goodglass and E. Kaplan, *The Assessment of Aphasia* (Philadelphia: Lea and Fabiger, 1972).

p. 63   Broca's aphasia: For discussions, see Goodglass and Kaplan, *op. cit.;* see also J. Brown, *Aphasia, Apraxia, and Agnosia* (Springfield, Ill.: Charles C Thomas, 1972), Chap. 6.

p. 63   words most easily accessible: Cf. H. Gardner, "The Contribution of Operativity to Naming Capacity in Aphasic Patients," *Neuropsychologia*, 1973, *11*, 213–20.

p. 66   On apraxia, see J. Brown, *op. cit.;* also, H. Liepmann, "Apraxie," *Ergeb. der ges. Med.*, 1920, *1*, 516–43.

p. 67   Wernicke's aphasia: First described in C. Wernicke, *Der aphasische Symptomenkomplex* (Breslau: Cohn and Weigart, 1874). See also the references cited in the note to p. 52.

p. 69   According to this traditional model: This point of view has been propounded in recent years by Norman Geschwind. See "Current Concepts: Aphasia," *New England Journal of Medicine*, 1971, *284*, 654–6.

p. 75   our third patient, Richard MacArthur: Aspects of this case have been reported in A. Yamadori and M. Albert, "Word Category Aphasia," *Cortex*, 1973, *9*, 112–25. I am grateful to Dr. Albert for permission to quote from the patient's protocols.

p. 77   Anomia: See the references cited in the note to p. 52.

p. 80   Kurt Goldstein, who deemed naming . . . : See his *Language and Language Disturbances* (New York: Grune and Stratton, 1948), pp. 61, 246, 249.

p. 82   On naming difficulties, see N. Geschwind, "The Varieties of Naming Errors," *Cortex*, 1967, *3*, 97–112. A different viewpoint is propounded in E. Bay, "The Classification of Disorders of Speech," *Cortex*, 1967, *3*, 26–31.

p. 84   On other forms of aphasia, see H. Goodglass and N. Geschwind, "Language Disorder (Aphasia)," in E. Carterette and M. Friedman (eds.), *Handbook of Perception* (in press). An alternative classificatory scheme appears in A. R. Luria, *Traumatic Aphasia* (The Hague: Mouton, 1970). Summaries of other typologies are found in J. de Ajuriaguerra and H. Hécaen, *Le Cortex Cérébral* (Paris: Masson et Cie, 1964).

p. 85   On isolation of the speech area, see N. Geschwind, F. Quadfasel, and J. Segarra, "Isolation of the Speech Area," *Neuropsychologia*, 1968, *6*, 327–40. The anecdote about "Der Leben" is related by E. Stengel, "Zur Lehre von dem transkortikalen Aphasia," *Z. ges. Neur. Psychiatr.*, 1936, *154*, 779.

p. 86    On repetition defect, see R. Strub and H. Gardner, "Repetition Defect in Conduction Aphasia," in *Brain and Language* (1974, in press).

p. 88    H. Head's strong conclusions are reported in *Aphasia and Kindred Disorders of Speech* (New York: Hafner, 1963). The work was originally published in England in 1926.

p. 89    For early accounts of aphasic disturbances, see A. L. Benton, "Contributions to Aphasia Before Broca," *Cortex*, 1964, *1*, 314–26; A. L. Benton and R. J. Joynt, "Early Descriptions of Aphasia," *Archives of Neurology*, 1960, *3*, 205–22.

p. 89    Marc Dax: See R. J. Joynt and A. L. Benton, "The Memoir of Marc Dax on Aphasia," *Neurology*, 1964, *14*, 851–4.

p. 90    The original references on Broca's and Wernicke's discoveries can be found in the notes to pp. 21 and 67, respectively.

p. 90    H. Bastian, *Aphasia and Other Speech Defects* (London: H. K. Lewis, 1898); and K. Kleist, *Gehirnpathologie* (Leipzig: Barth, 1934).

p. 91    J. Hughlings Jackson, *Selected Writings* (London: Hodder and Stoughton, 1932).

p. 92    Marie's papers appeared in vol. 21, pp. 241–7, 493–500, and 565–71.

p. 92    The debate between Marie and the Déjerines appeared in the *Revue Neurologique*, 1908, *16*, pp. 611 ff. and 974 ff.

p. 93    Henry Head's remarks are found on pages 65 and 67 of his *Aphasia and Kindred Disorders of Speech* (New York: Hafner, 1963).

p. 94    The best summary of Kurt Goldstein's views is found in *Language and Language Disturbance* (New York: Grune and Stratton, 1948).

p. 95    On the views of current schools of aphasiological analysis: N. Geschwind, "Disconnexion Syndromes in Animals and Man," *Brain*, 1965, *88*, 237–94, 585–644; H. Hécaen and R. Angelergues, *Pathologie du Langage* (Paris: Larousse, 1965); H. Goodglass and E. Kaplan, *Assessment of Aphasia* (Philadelphia: Lea and Fabiger, 1972); A. R. Luria, *The Higher Cortical Functions in Man* (New York: Basic Books, 1966).

p. 97    The Head-Jackson-Goldstein school: E. Bay, "Present Concepts of Aphasia," *Geriatrics*, 1964, *19*, 319–31; E. Lenneberg, *Biological Foundations of Language* (New York: Wiley, 1967); M. Critchley, *Aphasiology* (London: Arnold, 1971); J. de Ajuriaguerra and R. Tissot, "The Apraxias" in P. J. Vinken and G. Bruyn (eds.), *Handbook of Clinical Neurology* (Amsterdam: North Holland Publishing Company, 1969), vol. 4.

p. 98    On inner speech, see L. Vygotsky, *Thought and Language* (Cambridge: M.I.T. Press, 1962); A. R. Luria and F. Ia. Yudovich, *Speech and the Development of Mental Processes in the Child* (London: Penguin Books, 1971).

p. 98    J. Piaget, *Biologie et Connaissance* (Paris: Gallimard, 1967); see also H. Gardner, *The Quest for Mind* (New York: Knopf, 1973), Chaps. 3, 5.

p. 98   On the relationship between thought and language, see the discussions in A. V. de Reuck and M. O'Connor (eds.), *Disorders of Language* (Boston: Little Brown, 1964), *passim*.

p. 100   On aphasia in children, see J. de Ajuriaguerra and H. Hécaen, *Le Cortex Cérébral* (Paris: Masson et Cie, 1964), Part IV; N. Geschwind, "Disorders of Higher Cortical Functions in Children," *Clinical Proceedings, Children's Hospital National Medical Center*, 1972, *28*, 261–72.

p. 101   On aphasia and left-handers, see H. Hécaen and R. Angelergues, *Pathologie du Langage* (Paris: Larousse, 1965); H. Goodglass and F. Quadfasel, "Language Laterality in Left-handed Aphasics," *Brain*, 1954, *77*, 521–48.

p. 102   On pitch in language, see D. Van Lancker and V. A. Fromkin, "Hemispheric Specialization for Pitch and 'Tone': Evidence from Thai," *Journal of Phonetics*, 1973, *1*, 101–9.

p. 106   On aphasia in polyglots, see M. Critchley, *Aphasiology* (London: Arnold, 1971); M. Minkowski, "On Aphasia in Polyglots," in L. Halpern (ed.), *Problems of Dynamic Neurology* (Jerusalem: Hebrew University, 1963); W. Lambert and S. Fillenbaum, "A Pilot Study of Aphasia Among Bilinguals," *Canadian Journal of Psychology*, 1959, *13*, 28–34.

p. 106   aphasia in individuals with atypical language: R. Meckler, J. Mack, and R. Bennett, "Sign Language Aphasia in a Non-deaf Mute," paper presented at the American Academy of Neurology, 1971; M. Critchley, "Aphasic Disorders of Signalling (Constitutional and Acquired) Occurring in Naval Signalmen," *Journal of Mount Sinai Hospital*, 1942, *9*, 363–75; H. Hécaen and R. Angelergues, *Pathologie du Langage* (Paris: Larousse, 1965); J. E. Sarno, L. P. Swisher, and M. T. Sarno, "Aphasia in a Congenitally Deaf Man," *Cortex*, 1969, *5*, 398–414.

CHAPTER 3

p. 114   The epigraph is taken from E. B. Huey, *The Psychology and Pedagogy of Reading* (Cambridge, Mass.: M.I.T. Press, 1968), p. 203.

p. 114   The case of Monsieur C. appears in J. Déjerine, "Contribution à l'étude anatomo-pathologique et clinique des differents variétés de cécité verbale," *Comp. rend. Scean. soc. biol.*, 1892, *9(4)*, 61–90. My attention was called to this case by N. Geschwind. Cf. his "The Anatomy of Acquired Disorders of Reading," in J. Money (ed.), *Reading Disability* (Baltimore: Johns Hopkins University Press, 1962).

p. 118   The two syndromes exhibited by C. . . . : A comprehensive review of the alexias can be found in D. F. Benson and N. Geschwind, "The Alexias," in P. J. Vinken and G. W. Bruyn (eds.), *Handbook of Clinical*

*Neurology* vol. 4 (Amsterdam: North Holland Publishing Company, 1969).

p. 121   Summarizing the accumulated knowledge . . . : J. Hinshelwood, *Congenital Word-Blindness* (London: Lewis, 1917). The quotation appears on p. 57.

p. 124   On the "look-say" and "phonics" methods, see J. Chall, *Learning to Read: The Great Debate* (New York: McGraw-Hill, 1967).

p. 124   As Macdonald Critchley . . . has pointed out: M. Critchley, *Developmental Dyslexia* (London: Heineman, 1964), p. 18.

p. 126   On methods for treating developmental dyslexia, see M. Critchley, *op. cit.*

p. 126   the work of Dr. Samuel T. Orton: S. T. Orton, *Reading, Writing and Speech Problems in Children* (London: Chapman and Hall, 1937).

p. 128   On reading disability and color-naming, see N. Geschwind and M. Fusillo, "Color-naming Defects in Association with Alexia," *Archives of Neurology*, 1966, *15*, 137–46.

p. 129   On effects of lesions on reading of ideographic and phonetic languages, see R. S. Lyman, S. T. Kwan, and W. H. Chao, "Left occipito-parietal tumor with observations on alexia and agraphia in Chinese and English," *Chinese Medical Journal*, 1938, *54*, 491–516; S. Sasanuma and O. Fujimura, "Selective Impairment of Phonetic and Non-phonetic Transcriptions of Words in Japanese Aphasic Patients: Kana vs. Kanji in Visual Recognition and Writing," *Cortex*, 1970, *6*, 1–18.

p. 130   One patient recently seen at the Boston Veterans Administration Hospital: M. Albert, A. Yamadori, H. Gardner, and D. Howes, "Comprehension in Alexia," *Brain*, 1973, *96*, 317–28.

p. 131   On rehabilitation of alexic patients, see A. R. Luria, *Traumatic Aphasia* (The Hague: Mouton, 1970), chap. 16.

p. 131   Aphasic patients with reading difficulties: There has been little published research on this topic. I am relying chiefly on the results of my own research in this area, a portion of which was recently reported at the Academy of Aphasia, Albuquerque, New Mexico, October 1973.

p. 134   On hyperlexia, see K. Voeller, "Hyperlexia in Children with Autistic Features," unpublished paper, 1972; P. R. Huttenlocher and J. Huttenlocher, "A Study of Children with 'Hyperlexia,'" unpublished paper, 1973; C. C. Mehegan and F. E. Dreifuss, "Hyperlexia," *Neurology*, 1972, *22*, 1105–11. The quotation from Dreifuss appears on p. 1107. The quotation from the Huttenlocher paper appears on p. 13 of the unpublished manuscript.

p. 137   Bishop Harmon's advice is quoted on p. 102 of J. Hinshelwood, *Congenital Word-Blindness* (London: Lewis, 1917).

p. 137   Paul Rozin and his associates . . . : See P. Rozin, S. Poritsky, and R. Sotsky, *Science*, 1971, *3977*, 1264–7.

p. 138   J. Isgur, "Letter-sound Associations Established in Reading-disabled People by an Object-Imagery-Projection Method," unpublished paper, 1973.

p. 139   teaching an arbitrary symbolic method: A. Velletri-Glass, M. Gazzaniga, and D. Premack, "Artificial Language Training in Global Aphasics," *Neuropsychologia*, 1973, *11*, 95–104.

CHAPTER 4

p. 142   The epigraph is taken from William James, *Principles of Psychology*, vol. 1 (New York: Henry Holt, 1890), p. 463.

p. 142   On Gestalt psychology, see W. Köhler, *Gestalt Psychology* (New York: Liveright, 1929); K. Koffka, *Principles of Gestalt Psychology* (New York: Harcourt Brace, 1935). Von Ehrenfels reported his discovery in "Über Gestaltqualitäten," *Vierteljahrsch. Wissenschaft und Philosophie*, 1890, *14*, 249–92.

p. 143   The classic text on behaviorism is John Watson, *Behaviorism* (New York: Norton, 1930).

p. 144   Goldstein and Gelb's lengthy case report: K. Goldstein and A. Gelb, "Psychologische analysen hirnpathologischer Fälle auf Grund von Untersuchungen Hirnverletzter," *Z. Ges. Neurol. Psychiatr.*, 1918, *41*, 1–142.

p. 146   Ernst Cassirer met Schn.: See E. Cassirer, *The Philosophy of Symbolic Forms* (New Haven: Yale University Press, 1957), Vol. III, p. 299.

p. 147   "Visual Object Agnosia with Special Reference to Gestalt Theory": In *Brain*, 1941, *64*, 43–62.

p. 148   A Boston physician . . . : See A. Adler, "Disintegration and Restoration of Optic Recognition in Visual Agnosia," *Archives Neurology and Psychiatry*, 1944, *51*, 243–59. A subsequent report appeared some years later: "Course and Outcome of Visual Agnosia," *Journal of Nervous and Mental Disease*, 1950, *III*, 41–5.

p. 149   tracked down the original patient Schn.: See R. Jung, "Über eine Nachuntersuchung des Falles Schn. . . . von Goldstein and Gelb," *Psychiatrie Neurologie und Medizinische Psychologie*, 1949, *1*, 353–62; and E. Bay, O. Laurenstein, and P. Cibis, "Ein Beitrag zur Frage der Seelenblindheit," *Psychiatrie, Neurologie, und Medizinische Psychologie*, 1949, *3*, 73–91.

p. 151   The classic theory of agnosia is described in J. Brown, *Aphasia, Apraxia, and Agnosia* (Springfield, Ill.: Charles C Thomas, 1972); see also J. A. M. Frederiks, "The Agnosias," in P. J. Vinken and G. W. Bruyn (eds.), *Handbook of Clinical Neurology*, vol. 4 (Amsterdam: North Holland Publishing Company, 1969).

p. 152   Sources for this brief sketch of the historical background include: H. Munk, "Erfahrungen zur Gunsten der Localisation," *Verh. Physiol. ges. Berlin; Dtsch. Med. Wschr.*, 1877, *13*, 31; H. Lissauer, "Ein Fall von Seelenblindheit nebst einem Beitrage zur Theorie derselben," *Arch. Psychiatr. Nervenkr.*, 1889, *21*, 2–50; S. Freud, *On Aphasia* (New York: International Universities Press, 1953). Originally published in 1891.

p. 153   three types of agnosia in the tactile realm: J. P. L. Delay, *Les Astéreoagnosies* (Paris: Masson, 1935).

p. 153   prosopagnosia: A good treatment appears in B. Bornstein, "Prosopagnosia," in L. Halpern (ed.), *Problems in Dynamic Neurology* (Jerusalem: Hebrew University, 1963).

p. 155   Support for this hypothesis . . . : R. Yin, "Face Recognition by Brain-Injured Patients: A Dissociable Ability?" *Neuropsychologia*, 1970, *8*, 395–402.

p. 157   On auditory agnosia, see M. Reinhold, "A Case of Auditory Agnosia," *Brain*, 1950, *73*, 203–23; O. Spreen, A. L. Benton, *et al.*, "Auditory Agnosia Without Aphasia," *Arch. Neurology*, 1965, *13*, 84–92.

p. 157   Bay at Badenweiler: An account of this conference is given in M. Critchley, "The Problem of Visual Agnosia," *Journal of Neurological Sciences*, 1964, *1*, 274–90. Bay's argument is detailed in "Disturbances of Visual Perception and Their Examination," *Brain*, 1953, *76*, 515–50.

p. 159   Bender reviewed a large series of cases: See M. B. Bender and M. Feldman, "The 'So-called' Visual Agnosias," *Brain*, 1972, *95*, 173–86.

p. 160   Teuber's views are expressed on p. 294 of B. Milner and H. Teuber, "Alterations of Perception and Memory in Man: Reflection on Methods," in L. Weiskrantz (ed.), *Analysis of Behavioral Change* (New York: Harper and Row, 1968).

p. 161   Critchley's article appeared in the *Journal of Neurological Sciences*, 1964, *1*, 274–90. The statements quoted from patients appear on p. 279.

p. 162   N. Geschwind's views are expressed in "Disconnexion Syndromes in Animals and Man," *Brain*, 1965, *88*, 585–644.

p. 163   G. Ettlinger's results appear in "Sensory Defects in Visual Agnosia," *Journal of Neurology, Neurosurgery and Psychiatry*, 1956, *19*, 297–307.

p. 164   The case of Dr. A. is described in A. B. Rubens and D. F. Benson, "Associative Visual Agnosia," *Archives of Neurology*, 1971, *24*, 305–16.

p. 167   A case recently reported . . . : At the Academy of Aphasia, Albuquerque, New Mexico, in October 1973. See A. B. Rubens, M. G. Johnson, and D. R. Garwick, "Interference with Visual and Tactile Identification by Confabulatory Verbal Responses in a Patient with Associative Visual Agnosia."

p. 167   Mr. S.'s case was reported by D. F. Benson and J. P. Greenberg, "Visual Form Agnosia," *Archives of Neurology*, 1969, *20* 82–9.

p. 168   R. Efron's study of Mr. S. is reported in "What Is Perception?," *Boston Studies in the Philosophy of Science*, IV, 1966–1968 (Reidel Publishing Company, Dordrecht, Netherlands).

p. 171   Excellent treatments of recent research on recognition are found in U. Neisser, *Cognitive Psychology* (New York: Appleton Century, 1967); and L. Uhr (ed.), *Pattern Recognition* (New York: Wiley, 1965).

p. 173   a severely demented patient: This patient's case is described in detail in Chapter 7.

## CHAPTER 5

p. 176   Mr. Sherlock Holmes's views are expressed in A. Conan Doyle, "A Study in Scarlet," in *The Complete Sherlock Holmes* (Garden City, N.Y.: Doubleday, 1927), p. 21.

p. 176   S. S. Korsakoff's original description appeared in "Eine psychische störung, combiniert mit multipler Neuritis," *Allgem. Ztschr. für Psych,* 1890, *46,* 475–85; "Errinerungs-täuschungen (Pseudoremincenzen) bei polyneuritischer Psychose," *Allgem. Zeitschr. fur Psych,* 1891, *47,* 390–410.

p. 188   a group of 245 Korsakoff patients: M. Victor, R. Adams, and G. H. Collins, *The Wernicke-Korsakoff Syndrome* (Philadelphia: F. A. Davis Co., 1971).

p. 191   An excellent review of the various explanations of the Korsakoff syndrome is found in G. Talland, *Deranged Memory* (New York: Academic Press, 1965). In my discussion here, I have relied heavily on Talland's treatment.

p. 195   W. B. Scoville and B. Milner reported their findings in "Loss of Recent Memory after Bilateral Hippocampal Lesions," *Journal of Neurology, Neurosurgery, and Psychiatry,* 1957, *20,* 11–21. The journal issue devoted primarily to the study of H. M. was *Neuropsychologia,* 1965, vol. 3. A recent review by Milner appears in L. Weiskrantz (ed.), *Analysis of Behavioral Change* (New York: Harper and Row, 1968).

p. 198   See A. Starr and L. Phillips, "Verbal and Motor Memory in the Mnestic Syndrome," *Neuropsychologia,* 1970, *8,* 75–88.

p. 198   patient could . . .remember a limited amount of verbal material: Conflicting views will be found in E. K. Warrington, "Neurologic Disorders of Memory," *British Medical Journal,* 1971, *27,* 243–7; N. Butters, R. Lewis, L. Cermak, and H. Goodglass, "Material-specific Memory Deficits in Alcoholic Korsakoff Patients," *Neuropsychologia,* 1973, *11,* 291–300.

p. 203   experimental work . . . conducted at our hospital: Described in N. Butters and L. S. Cermak, "The Role of Cognitive Factors in the Memory Disorders of Alcoholic Korsakoff Patients," unpublished paper, 1973; and L. S. Cermak, N. Butters, and J. Gerrein, "The Extent of the Verbal Encoding Ability of Korsakoff Patients," *Neuropsychologia,* 1973, *11,* 85–94.

p. 203   The bibliographical reference for Talland's book is found in the note to page 191.

p. 210   Luria's account appears in *The Mind of the Mnemonist* (New York: Basic Books, 1968).

p. 213   Penfield's findings are summarized in W. Penfield, "The Permanent Record of the Stream of Consciousness," *Proc., 14th Int. Cong. Psych.,* Montreal Neurological Institute Report, Number 486, 1954.

p. 213   On eidetic imagery, see R. N. Haber and R. B. Haber, "Eidetic Imagery: I. Frequency," *Perceptual and Motor Skills,* 1964, *19,* 131–8.

One way of testing the alternative possibilities is to ask subjects to recite remembered passages backwards; a "reconstructor" will fail at this task. I know of only one documented case of an "eideteker" unequivocally passing such a test—obviously an insufficient basis for drawing conclusions.

p. 214   On transient global amnesia, see E. C. Shuttleworth and C. E. Morris, "The Transient Global Amnesia Syndrome," *Archives of Neurology*, 1966, *15*, 515–20.

p. 216   On reduplication and related disorders, see E. A. Weinstein and R. Kahn, *Denial of Illness* (Springfield, Ill.: Charles C Thomas, 1955).

p. 219   A good review of current research and theory on memory is L. Cermak, *Human Memory* (New York: Ronald Press, 1972).

CHAPTER 6

p. 220   The quotation from Aristotle appears in M. Critchley, *The Parietal Lobes* (New York: Hafner, 1966), p. 203.

p. 222   Josef Gerstmann's original cases were reported in three papers: "Fingeragnosie," *Wiener Klinische Wochenschrift*, 1924, *37*, 1010–12, "Fingeragnosie und Isolierte Agraphie," *Zeitschrift gesamte Neur. Psych.*, 1927, *108*, 152–77; "Zur Symptomatologie der Hirnläsionen im Übergangsgebiet der unteren Parietal und mittleren Occipitalwendung," *Nervenarzt*, 1930, *3*, 691–5.

p. 222   The Critchley article appeared in *Brain*, 1966, *89*, 183–98; the Benton article in *Journal of Neurology, Neurosurgery and Psychiatry*, 1961, *24*, 176–81.

p. 224   The references for Gerstmann's 1927 and 1930 papers are found in the note to p. 222.

p. 227   new explanations or modifications: R. Klein, M. D. Prague, and P. P. Mallie, "A Syndrome Associated with Left-Hand Paralysis of Central Origin," *Journal of Mental Science*, 1945, *91*, 518–22; S. L. Rubins and E. D. Friedman, "Asymbolia for Pain," *Arch. Neurol. and Psychiatr.*, 1948, *60*, 554–73; P. Schilder, "Localization of the Body Image (Postural Model of the Body)," *Assoc. Res. Nerv. Ment. Dis.*, 1932, *13*, 466–84; P. Schilder, "Fingeragnosie, Fingerapraxie, Fingeraphasie," *Der Nervenarzt*, 1931, *4*, 625–9.

p. 228   Gerstmann at the height of the syndrome's "vogue": The quotation appears on p. 398 of "Syndrome of Finger Agnosia, Disorientation for Right and Left, Agraphia, and Acalculia," *Arch. Neurol. Psychiatr.*, 1940, *44*, 398–408.

p. 229   The developmental form of the Gerstmann syndrome: See, for example, M. Critchley, "Aphasic Disorders of Signalling (Constitutional and Acquired) Occurring in Naval Signalmen," *Journal of Mount Sinai Hospital*, 1942, *9*, 363–75; D. F. Benson and N. Geschwind, "Developmental Gerstmann Syndrome," *Neurology*, 1970, *20*, 293–8.

p. 229   Among the psychologists interested in child development were H. Werner and A. Strauss; see their article, "Deficiency in the Finger Schema in Relation to Arithmetic Disability," *American J. Orthopsychiatry*, 1938, *8*, 719–25.

p. 230   The theoretical perspective of Piaget: See J. Piaget and B. Inhelder, *The Psychology of the Child* (New York: Basic Books, 1968).

p. 230   Other scholars also entered the fray: For a discussion of certain aspects of the interdisciplinary controversy surrounding the Gerstmann syndrome, see M. Critchley, *The Parietal Lobes* (New York: Hafner, 1963), pp. 203 ff.

p. 231   who have lost the ability to perform . . . in one sensory modality: Cf. H. Gardner, R. Strub, and M. Albert, "A Unimodal Deficit in Operational Thought," *Brain and Language* (in press).

p. 231   The *idiot savant* L. is described in M. Scheerer, E. Rothmann, and K. Goldstein, "A Case of 'Idiot Savant': An Experimental Study of Personality Organization," *Psych. Mon.*, 1945, *269*, 1–61.

p. 233   The statement by T. Dantzig is taken from *Number, the Language of Science* (Garden City, N.Y.: Doubleday, 1956), p. 37.

p. 234   The remarks by Piaget are taken from "Some Aspects of Operations," in M. W. Piers (ed.), *Play and Development* (New York: Norton, 1973), p. 23.

p. 235   Those of a structuralist bent: See H. Gardner, *The Quest for Mind* (New York: Knopf, 1973).

p. 236   The reference for Benton's chief critique appears in the note below. See also A. L. Benton, *Right-Left Discrimination and Finger Localization* (New York: Hoeber, 1959). I am grateful to Professor Benton for his critical comments on this chapter.

p. 237   "Judged from the standpoint of behavioural analysis": A. L. Benton, "The Fiction of the Gerstmann Syndrome" (originally published in 1961). In M. T. Sarno, *Aphasia: Selected Readings* (New York: Appleton-Century-Crofts, 1972), p. 176.

p. 238   Statistical critiques of the Gerstmann syndrome appear in K. Poeck and B. Orgass, "Gerstmann's Syndrome and Aphasia," *Cortex*, 1966, *2*, 421–37; I. Gloning, K. Gloning, and G. Guttmann; "Eine faktoranalytische Untersuchung der Sogenannten Gerstmanneschen Syndroms," *Wien. Ztsch. für Nervenheilkunde*, 1967, *25*, 182–92; R. F. Heimburger, W. Demyer, and R. M. Reitan, "Implications of Gerstmann's Syndrome," *Journal Neurol. Neuros. Psychiat.*, 1964, *27*, 52–7.

p. 240   The validity of the Gerstmann syndrome: This viewpoint is taken by R. Strub and N. Geschwind, "Gerstmann Syndrome Without Aphasia," *Cortex* (in press); and by M. Kinsbourne and E. K. Warrington, "A Study of Finger Agnosia," *Brain*, 1962, *85*, 47–66.

p. 243   Support of the viability of the Gerstmann syndrome: See for example D. F. Benson and E. B. Tomlinson, "Hemiplegic Syndrome of the Posterior Cerebral Artery," *Stroke*, 1971, *2*, 559–64. N. Geschwind and M. Fusillo, "Color Naming Deficits in Association with Alexia," *Arch. Neurol.*, 1966, *15*, 137–46.

p. 244  Once these special categories . . . : A. L. Benton and R. Meyers, "An Earlier Description of the Gerstmann Syndrome," *Neurology*, 1956, *6*, 841.

p. 244  Gerstmann's last article appeared in Vol. 28, pp. 12–19 of the journal. The epigraph appears on page 12.

CHAPTER 7

p. 253  intelligence testing: Discussion of the role of intelligence testing in neurological diagnostic work is found in L. Small (ed.), *Neuropsychodiagnosis in Psychotherapy* (New York: Brunner/Maizel, 1973). An introduction to Piaget's approach to intellect can be found in H. Gardner, *The Quest for Mind* (New York: Knopf, 1973), Chapter 3.

p. 259  The case of P.K. is reported in N. Geschwind and E. Kaplan, "A Human Cerebral Deconnection Syndrome," *Neurology*, 1962, *12*, 675–85. The quotation from the investigators appears on page 675.

p. 264  On Alzheimer's disease and related disorders, see C. Wells, *Dementia* (Philadelphia: Davis, 1971); *CIBA Symposium on Alzheimer's Disease and Related Conditions* (London, J. A. Churchill, 1970).

p. 265  Klüver-Bucy syndrome: H. Klüver and P. C. Bucy, "An Analysis of Certain Effects of Bilateral Temporal Lobectomy in the Rhesus Monkey with Special Reference to Psychic Blindness," *Journal of Psychology*, 1938, *55*, 33–54.

p. 266  Pick's disease: I. C. Nichols and W. C. Weigner, "Pick's Disease: A Review of the Literature and Presentation of a Case," *Arch. Neurol. Psychiatr.*, 1934, *32*, 241–4.

p. 267  Frontal lobotomies: A description of the popular and medical view toward this procedure is found in L. Edson, "The Psyche and the Surgeon," *New York Times Magazine*, September 30, 1973. See also L. Stevens, *Explorers of the Brain* (New York: Knopf, 1971), pp. 34–5.

p. 267  On frontal lobes and intellect, see D. Hebb, *The Organization of Behavior* (New York: Wiley, 1949); R. M. Hamlin, "Intellectual Function After Frontal Lobe Surgery," *Cortex*, 1970, *6*, 299–307. An exhaustive review of research on the frontal lobes is found in J. M. Warren and K. Akert (eds.), *The Frontal Granular Cortex and Behavior* (New York: McGraw-Hill, 1964).

p. 269  For a fuller description of the case of Zasetsky, see Chapter 10, pp. 414–22.

p. 270  On social behavior of monkeys after lobotomy, see E. A. Franzen and R. Meyers, "Neural Control of Social Behavior: Prefrontal and Anterior Temporal Cortex," *Neuropsychologia*, 1973, *11*, 141–57.

p. 271 Comprehensive reviews of the cognitive effects of aging are found in W. A. Owens, Jr., "Age and Mental Abilities: A Longitudinal Study," *Genetic Psychology Monographs*, 1953, *48*, 3–54; J. Botwinick, *Cognitive Processes in Mature and Old Age* (New York: Springer, 1967); J. Birren, *The Psychology of Aging* (Englewood Cliffs, N.J.: Prentice-Hall, 1964); J. Birren (ed.) *Human Aging: A Biological and Behavioral Study* (N.I.M.H. Publication, 1961).

p. 273 More severe declines are discussed in J. Blum, J. L. Fosshage, and L. F. Jarvik, "Intellectual Changes and Sex Differences in Octogenarians," *Developmental Psychology*, 1972, 7, 178–87.

p. 274 George Talland's remark appears in A. Welford and J. Birren (eds.) *Behavior, Aging, and the Nervous System* (Springfield, Ill.: Charles C Thomas, 1965), p. 558.

p. 275 On disconnection syndromes, see N. Geschwind, "Disconnexion Syndromes in Animals and Man," *Brain*, 1965, *88*, 585–644.

p. 276 Werner's exposition of the developmental process in children is outlined in his book *Comparative Psychology of Mental Development* (New York: Science Books, 1961); Piaget's views are presented in J. Piaget and B. Inhelder, *The Psychology of the Child* (New York: Basic Books, 1968).

p. 277 On figurativity and operativity, see H. Gardner, "Senses, Symbols, and Operations: The Organization of Artistry" in D. Perkins and B. Leondar (eds.), *The Arts and Cognition* (in press).

p. 279 "occasionally on an accidental basis": A. Pick, *Aphasia* (translated by Jason Brown) (Springfield, Ill.: Charles C Thomas, 1973), p. 41.

p. 281 The progression of stages found in normal children . . . is indeed reversed with these patients: Cf. J. de Ajuriaguerra and R. Tissot, "The Apraxias," in P. J. Vinken and G. W. Bruyn (eds.), *Handbook of Clinical Neurology* (Amsterdam: North Holland Publishing Company, 1969), vol. 4.

p. 284 in the infant: J. de Ajuriaguerra, quoted in C. Muller and I. Ciompi, *Senile Dementia* (Baltimore: Williams and Williams, 1968), p. 77.

p. 285 On brain injury in children, see N. Geschwind, "Disorders of Higher Cortical Function in Children," *Clinical Proceedings Children's Hospital National Medical Center*, 1972, *28*, 261–72; E. Guttmann, "Aphasia in Children," *Brain*, 1942, *65*, 205–19; T. Alajouanine and F. Lhermitte, "Acquired Aphasia in Children," *Brain*, 1965, *88*, 653–62.

p. 286 On cerebral dominance, see Chapter 9.

p. 287 children with left-hemisphere lesions: The most recent work on this topic was described at a workshop on "Mechanisms of Functional Sparing After Infant Brain Damage in Mammals Including Man," at the American Psychological Association, Montreal, September, 1973.

p. 288 N. Geschwind's quotation appears on page 267 of the article cited in the note to p. 285.

CHAPTER 8

p. 291    The epigraph is taken from a "Profile" of Alec Wilder by
W. Balliet in *The New Yorker,* July 9, 1973, p. 45.

p. 292    On disturbances in writing, see A. Leischner, "The Agraphias,"
in P. J. Vinken and G. W. Bruyn, *Handbook in Clinical Neurology*
(Amsterdam: North Holland Publishing Co., 1969), vol. 4.

p. 295    On language capacities of right-hemisphere patients, see J. Eis-
enson, in A. De Reuck and M. O'Connor (eds.), *Disorders of Language*
(London: Churchill, 1964); H. Gardner and G. Denes, "Connotative Judgments by Aphasic Patients on a Pictorial Adaptation of the Semantic
Differential," *Cortex,* 1973, *9,* 183–96.

p. 296    On the unusual conversation of patients with right-hemisphere
disease, see E. A. Weinstein and R. L. Kahn, *Denial of Illness* (Springfield, Ill.: Charles C Thomas, 1955).

p. 297    The passage from Hemingway is found in *The Short Stories of
Ernest Hemingway* (New York, 1953), pp. 152–3; that from Faulkner in
"The Bear" in *Go Down Moses* (New York: Modern Library, 1942), pp.
255–6. The contrast between these styles is elaborated on by R. Ohmann,
"Generative Grammars and the Concept of Literary Style" in M. Stein-
mann (ed.), *New Rhetorics* (New York: Scribners, 1967).

p. 301    On the Seashore Tests, see B. Milner, "Laterality Effects in
Audition," in V. B. Mountcastle (ed.), *Interhemispheric Relations and
Cerebral Dominance* (Baltimore: Johns Hopkins Press, 1962).

p. 301    For references on aphasia and musical competence, see the note
to p. 336.

p. 303    Warrington's findings on drawings: E. K. Warrington, M. James,
and M. Kinsbourne, "Drawing Disability in Relation to Laterality of
Cerebral Lesion," *Brain,* 1966, *89,* 53–82; and "Constructional Apraxia,"
in P. J. Vinken and G. W. Bruyn, *op. cit.,* vol. 4.

p. 305    On the generalists and localizers, see my discussion on pp.91–6.

p. 308    The quotation from Bay appears in L. Halpern (ed.), *Problems
in Dynamic Neurology* (Jerusalem, Hebrew University, 1963), p. 95.

p. 308    On patients with comprehension deficit, see R. Ahrens, "Stör-
ungen Zeichnischer Leistungen bei einem Fall Sensorischer Aphasie,"
*Psychiatr. Neurol.* (Basel), 1957, *134,* 322–45.

p. 310    On the Gerstmann syndrome, see Chapter 6.

p. 310    On improvement in aphasic drawings, see G. Engerth and H.
Urban, "Zur Kenntnis der Gestörten Künstlerischen Leistung bei sensorischer Aphasie," *Z. ges. Neurol. Psych.,* 1933, *145,* 753–87.

p. 311    T. Alajouanine, "Aphasia and Artistic Realization," *Brain,* 1948,
*71,* 229–41, reprinted in M. T. Sarno (ed.), *Aphasia: Selected Readings*
(New York: Appleton-Century-Crofts, 1921), pp. 231–9. The quotation
about the writer appears on p. 232.

p. 314 Jakobson's description and translation of the work of Uspensky appears in R. Jakobson and M. Halle, *Fundamentals of Language* (Hague: Mouton, 1956), pp. 80 ff.

p. 315 On Dostoevsky's epilepsy, see N. Geschwind, "Epilepsy in the Life and Writings of Dostoevsky," unpublished manuscript; T. Alajouanine, "Dostoevsky's Epilepsy," *Brain*, 1963, *86*, 209–11. The quotations are taken from the Geschwind manuscript.

p. 316 it has been maintained on several occasions: See, for example, Alajouanine's paper and also that by Zaimov, cited below.

p. 317 The painter described by Alajouanine is quoted on pp. 236–7 of the neurologist's classic paper.

p. 317 K. Zaimov, D. Kitov, and N. Kolev, "Aphasie chez un peintre," *Encephale*, 1969, *68*, 377–417.

p. 319 G. Bonvicini, "Die Aphasie des Malers Vierge," *Wien. Med. Wochen*, 1929, *76*, 88–91.

p. 320 I met with Professor Jung in October 1973, and at that time had the opportunity to view his slides.

p. 322 The characterization of Corinth's later works is by the critic Alfred Kuhn. Cf. his *Lovis Corinth* (Berlin: Im Propyläen-Verlag, 1925), p. 107.

p. 333 Alajouanine's description of Ravel's aphasia is found on pp. 233–4 of his article.

p. 334 V. G. Shebalin: A. R. Luria, L. S. Tsvetkova, and D. S. Futer, "Aphasia in a Composer," *J. Neurol. Sci.*, 1965, *2*, 288–92. The encomiums appear on p. 292 of this article.

p. 336 Botez and Wertheim's pioneering work is summarized in a number of articles. N. Wertheim, "Disturbances of the Musical Functions," in L. Halpern (ed.), *Problems of Dynamic Neurology* (Jerusalem: Hebrew University, 1963; N. Wertheim, "The Amusias," in *Handbook of Clinical Neurology*, vol. 4, op. cit. The case studies appear in N. Wertheim and M. Botez, "Receptive Amusia," *Brain*, 1961, *84*, 19–30; M. I. Botez and N. Wertheim, "Expressive Aphasia and Amusia Following Right Frontal Lesion in a Right-handed Man," *Brain*, 1959, *82*, 186–201.

p. 338 to indicate the range . . .: These cases are drawn mainly from the various reviews cited above. The piano teacher is described in A. Souques and H. Baruk, "Autopsie d'un case d'amusie (avec aphasie) chez un professeur de piano," *Revue Neurologique*, 1930, *1*, 545–56.

p. 339 H. Ustvedt, "Über die Untersuchung der musikalischen Funktionen bei Patienten mit Gehirnleiden, besonders bei Patienten mit Aphasie," *Acta Med. Scand. Suppl.*, 1937, *86*. The quotation is taken from the English summary, p. 727.

p. 344 make simultaneous judgments in the musical realm: H. W. Gordon, "Hemispheric Asymmetries in the Perception of Musical Chords," *Cortex*, 1970, *6*, 387–98.

p. 345 On left-handed musicians, see R. C. Oldfield, *MRC Speech and Communication Unit Progress Report*, 1966–1969, Edinburgh, Scotland.

On laterality in talented musicians, see T. G. Bever and R. Chiarello, "Cerebral Dominance in Musicians and Non-Musicians," unpublished manuscript, 1973.

p. 346   The Melodic Intonation Therapy for aphasia was described in a paper presented by R. W. Sparks, N. A. Helm, and M. L. Albert at the Academy of Aphasia, Albuquerque, New Mexico, October, 1973.

CHAPTER 9

p. 350   The epigraph comes from Graham Greene's *The Ministry of Fear* (New York: Penguin, 1945), p. 71.

p. 350   On anatomy of the nervous system, see my discussion in Chapter 1, pp. 36–41.

p. 351   On left-handers and language, see H. Goodglass and F. Quadfasel, "Language Laterality in Left-handed Aphasics," *Brain*, 1954, *77*, 521–48.

p. 352   For an example of asymmetry, see G. von Bonin, in V. Mountcastle (ed.), *Interhemispheric Relations and Cerebral Dominance* (Baltimore: Johns Hopkins Univ. Press, 1962), pp. 1 ff.

p. 353   The right hemisphere might be important too: See M. Piercy and V. Smyth, "Right Hemispheric Dominance for Certain Non-Verbal Intellectual Skills," *Brain*, 1960, *83*, 775–90; J. McFie, M. F. Piercy, and O. L. Zangwill, "Visual Spatial Agnosia Associated with Lesions of the Right Cerebral Hemisphere," *Brain*, 1950, *73*, 167–90; O. L. Zangwill, *Cerebral Dominance and Its Relation to Psychological Function* (Springfield, Ill.: Charles C Thomas, 1960).

p. 354   On denial and related phenomena, see E. A. Weinstein and R. Kahn, *Denial of Illness* (Springfield, Ill.: Charles C Thomas, 1955); E. A. Weinstein, "Disorder of the Body Schema in Organic Mental Syndromes," in P. J. Vinken and G. W. Bruyn (eds.), *op. cit.*, vol. 4.

p. 355   On constructions and drawings by brain-injured patients, see Chapter 8, pp. 303–10.

p. 356   The right hemisphere played a special role: Summaries of the role of the right hemisphere appear in D. Kimura, "Functional Asymmetry of the Brain in Dichotic Listening," *Cortex*, 1967, *3*, 163–78; D. Kimura, "Spatial Localization in Left and Right Visual Fields," *Canadian Journal of Psychology*, 1969, *23*, 445–57; D. Kimura, "The Asymmetry of the Human Brain," *Scientific American*, 1973, *228*, 70–8; A. Carmon and H. Bechtholdt, "Dominance of the Right Cerebral Hemisphere for Stereopsis," *Neuropsychologia*, 1969, *7*, 29–39; M. Gazzaniga, *The Bisected Brain* (New York: Appleton-Century-Crofts, 1970); N. Butters, M. Barton, and B. A. Brody, "Role of the Right Parietal Lobe in the Mediation of Cross-modal Associations and Reversible Operations in Space," *Cortex*,

1970, *6*, 174–90; J. Semmes, "Hemispheric Specialization: A Possible Clue to Mechanism," *Neuropsychologia*, 1968, *6*, 11–26.

p. 358 The most complete account of Sperry's work is found in M. Gazzaniga, *op. cit.*

p. 358 A. J. Akelaitis: See, for example, "Studies on the Corpus Callosum VII. Study of Language Functions (Tactile and Visual, Lexia, and Graphia) Unilaterally Following Section of the Corpus Callosum," *J. Neuropath. Exp. Neurol.*, 1943, *3*, 226–62. A review of Akelaitis's essentially negative findings appears in R. W. Sperry, M. S. Gazzaniga, and J. E. Bogen, "Interhemispheric Relationships: The Neocortical Commisures: Syndromes of Hemispheric Disconnection," in P. J. Vinken and G. W. Bruyn, *op. cit.*, vol. 4.

p. 359 Levy-Agresti's provocative research is summarized in R. W. Sperry and J. Levy, "Mental Capacities of the Disconnected Minor Hemisphere Following Commisurotomy," paper presented at the American Psychological Association, Miami, September 1970; Gazzaniga's work is described in his book, *op. cit.*

p. 361 On language capacity in commisurotomized patients, see M. S. Gazzaniga and R. W. Sperry, "Language After Section of the Cerebral Commisures," *Brain*, 1967, *90*, 131–48.

p. 365 E. Zaidel, "Laterality Effects with the Token Test Following Commisurotomy," paper presented at the Academy of Aphasia, Albuquerque, October 1973.

p. 367 J. L. Bradshaw, N. C. Nettleton, and G. Geffen, "Ear Differences and Delayed Auditory Feedback: Effects on a Speech and a Music Task," *Journal of Experimental Psychology*, 1971, *91*, 85–92.

p. 367 Doreen Kimura, "Left-Right Differences in the Perception of Melodies," *Quarterly Journal of Experimental Psychology*, 1964, *16*, 355–8.

p. 368 S. J. Dimond and J. G. Beaumont, "A Right-hemisphere Basis for Calculation in the Human Brain," *Psychonomic Science*, 1972, *26*, 137–8.

p. 368 Right-hemisphere language: See E. A. Weinstein, "Affections of Speech with Lesions of the Non-Dominant Hemisphere," in D. Rioch, E. A. Weinstein (eds.), *Disorders of Communication* (Baltimore: Williams and Wilkins, 1964); D. Van Lancker, "Propositional and Automatic Speech: Lateralization Studies," paper presented at the Academy of Aphasia, Albuquerque, New Mexico, October 1973; H. Gardner and G. Denes, "Connotative Judgments by Aphasic Patients on a Pictorial Adaptation of the Semantic Differential," *Cortex*, 1973, *9*, 183–96.

p. 369 Macdonald Critchley, *Aphasiology* (London: Arnold, 1971).

p. 369 On the personality of the right-hemisphere patient, see G. Gainotti, "Emotional Behavior and Hemispheric Side of Lesion," *Cortex*, 1972, *8*, 41–55.

p. 371 N. Geschwind's views on right-hemispheric dominance for emotions were expressed to me in several personal communications in 1973.

p. 372 Kinsbourne's views are expressed in "The Control of Attention by Interaction Between the Cerebral Hemispheres," in *Attention and Performance* (New York: Academic Press, 1973), pp. 239–56. See also M. Kinsbourne and J. Cooke, "Generalized and Lateralized Effects of Concurrent Verbalization on a Unimanual Skill," *Quarterly Journal of Experimental Psychology*, 1971, *23*, 341–5; M. Kinsbourne, "Eye and Head Turning Indicates Cerebral Lateralization," *Science*, 1972, *176*, 539–41.

p. 375   S. Harnad, "Creativity and Brain Asymmetry," unpublished paper, Princeton University, 1971.

p. 376   On hemispheric differences in processing: G. Cohen, "Hemispheric Differences in Serial vs. Parallel Processing," *Journal of Experimental Psychology*, 1973, *97*, 349–56; R. Davis and V. Schmit, "Timing the Transfer of Information Between Hemispheres in Man," *Acta Psychologica*, 1971, *35*, 335–46.

p. 376   individuals more efficiently report details: L. R. Brooks, "Spatial and Verbal Components of the Act of Recall," *Canadian Journal of Psychology*, 1968, *22*, 349–68.

p. 377   On the problem of characterizing the difference between hemispheres, see H. Gardner, "A Psychological Examination of Nelson Goodman's Theory of Symbols," *The Monist*, 1974, *58*, 319–26; H. Gardner, V. Howard, and D. Perkins, "Symbol Systems: A Philosophical, Psychological and Educational Investigation," in the 1974 Yearbook of the National Society for the Study of Education (Chicago: University of Chicago Press, 1974).

p. 377   On short-term memory, see I. Samuels *et al.*, "Short-term Memory Disorders Following Temporal Lobe Removals in Humans," *Cortex*, 1972, *8*, 283–98.

p. 378   Haskins Laboratory: A. M. Liberman, F. S. Cooper, D. P. Shankweiler, and M. Studdert-Kennedy, "Perception of the Speech Code," *Psychological Review*, 1967, *74*, 431–61; D. Shankweiler and M. Studdert-Kennedy, "Identification of Consonants and Vowels Presented to Left and Right Ears," *Quarterly Journal of Experimental Psychology*, 1967, *19*, 59–63.

p. 378   The subject is "set": F. Spellacy and S. Blumstein, "The Influence of Language Set on Ear Preference in Phoneme Recognition," *Cortex*, 1970, *6*, 430–9.

p. 379   Semmes' model is described in a reference given in the note to p. 356.

p. 380   White's reviews: M. J. White, "Laterality Differences in Perception: A Review," *Psychological Bulletin*, 1969, *72*, 387–405; "Hemispheric Asymmetries in Tachistoscopic Information Processing," *British Journal of Psychology*, 1972, *63*, 497–508.

p. 381   workers at Columbia University: T. G. Bever and R. Chiarello, "Cerebral Dominance in Musicians and Non-Musicians," unpublished manuscript, 1973.

p. 382   On laterality in animals, see C. H. M. Beck and R. C. Barton, "Deviations and Laterality of Hand Preferences in Monkeys," *Cortex*, 1972,

*8,* 339–63. See also C. Trevarthen, "Manipulative Strategies of Baboons and the Origins of Cerebral Asymmetry," unpublished paper, Harvard University, 1968.

p. 383  On language in chimpanzees, see D. Premack, "Language in Chimpanzee," *Science,* 1971, *172,* 808–22.

p. 383  Bever's suggestion was made at a Colloquium at Harvard University in 1972.

p. 384  Kimura's discussion of lateralization and dichotic listening appears in her article, "Left-Right Differences in the Perception of Melodies," *Quarterly Journal of Experimental Psychology,* 1964, *16,* 355–8.

p. 384  On mixed dominance: See H. Hécaen and J. Sauguet, "Cerebral Dominance in Left-handed Subjects," *Cortex,* 1971, *7,* 19–48.

p. 385  J. R. Kershner, "Children's Acquisition of Visuo-Spatial Dimensionality," *Developmental Psychology,* 1971, *5,* 454–62.

p. 385  Gazzaniga's suggestion appears in his book *The Bisected Brain* (New York: Appleton-Century-Crofts, 1970).

p. 386  On the definition of handedness, see H. Hécaen and J. de Ajuriaguerra, *Les gauchers* (Paris: P.U.F., 1963); Oldfield, "Handedness in Musicians," *British Journal of Psychology,* 1969, *60,* 91–9; *M.R.C. Speech and Communication Unit: Progress Report, 1966–1969.*

p. 387  J. Z. Young, in V. B. Mountcastle (ed.), *Interhemispheric Relations and Cerebral Dominance* (Baltimore: Johns Hopkins Univ. Press, 1962). The quotation appears on p. 24.

p. 389  Jerome S. Bruner, *Processes of Cognitive Growth in Infancy* (Worcester, Mass.: Clark University Press, 1968).

p. 390  N. Geschwind and W. Levitsky, "Human Brain: Left-Right Asymmetries in Temporal Speech Regions," *Science,* 1968, *161,* 186–7.

CHAPTER 10

p. 393  The epigraph is taken from *The Brain and the Unity of Conscious Experience* (Cambridge: Cambridge University Press, 1965), p. 36.

p. 394  On the history of psychology, see E. G. Boring, *A History of Experimental Psychology* (New York: Appleton-Century-Crofts, 1950).

p. 395  On the different methods used by social scientists, see H. Gardner, *The Quest for Mind* (New York: Knopf, 1973), chaps. 1, 2, 6.

p. 397  Professor Lordat: The descriptions and quotations on the aphasias of Lordat, Saloz, and Forel are all taken from an excellent review by Th. Alajouanine and F. Lhermitte, "Essai d'introspection de l'aphasie (l'aphasie vue par les aphasiques)," *Revue Neurologique,* 1964, *110,* 609–21. The translations are mine.

p. 402  "I am a happily married man . . .": Quoted in A. B. Carter, *All About Strokes* (London: Thomas Nelson and Sons, 1968), p. ix.

p. 403  Butler relates his experiences in L. Sies and R. Butler, "A Personal Account of Dysphasia," *Journal of Speech and Hearing Disorders,* 1963, *28,* 261–6. The quoted passages appear on pp. 263 and 266.

p. 404  Ritchie's account appears in D. Ritchie, *Stroke: A Diary of Recovery* (London: Faber and Faber, 1960). The quotations appear on page 22, 25, 29, 43, 71, 101, and 142.

p. 406  M. Rolnick and H. R. Hoops, "Aphasia as Seen by the Aphasic," *Journal of Speech and Hearing Disorders,* 1969, *34,* 48–53. The quotations appear on pp. 49, 51.

p. 409  C. Scott Moss, *Recovery with Aphasia* (Urbana, Ill.: University of Illinois Press, 1972). The quotations appear on pp. 26, 5, 9, 10, 36, 72.

p. 413  One British actor: This case was cited by Professor Oliver Zangwill in a personal communication to the author, October 1973. Patricia Neal's recovery is described in B. Farrell, *Pat and Roald* (New York: Random House, 1969). See p. 227 for an account of her stage problems.

p. 415  Zasetsky's story is told in A. R. Luria, *The Man with a Shattered World* (New York: Basic Books, 1972). The quotations are on pp. 8, 10, 11, 12, 33, 79, 82, 101, 102, 132.

p. 423  On Goldstein's views on abstract attitude, see K. Goldstein and M. Scheerer, "Abstract and Concrete Behavior: An Experimental Study with Special Tests," *Psychol. Monographs,* 1941, *329* (whole volume).

p. 424  "[The patient] may be able to count": The quotation appears on p. 8 of K. Goldstein, *Language and Language Disturbances* (New York: Grune and Stratton, 1948).

p. 425  M. Merleau-Ponty, *The Phenomenology of Perception* (London: Routledge and Kegan Paul, 1962), p. 107.

p. 433  "make a person human": Luria, *op. cit.,* p. 134.

p. 433  On frontal-lobe patients, see Chapter 7, pp. 266–71.

p. 434  On diseases of the right hemisphere, see Chapter 8, pp. 295–7, and Chapter 9, pp. 369–73. See also G. Gainotti, "Emotional Behavior and Hemispheric Side of Lesion," *Cortex,* 1972, *8,* 41–55.

p. 435  On temporal-lobe epilepsy: V. Mark and F. Ervin, *Violence and the Brain* (New York: Harper and Row, 1970); L. Edson, "The Psyche and the Surgeon," *New York Times Magazine,* September 30, 1973, pp. 15 ff. The personality of a temporal-lobe epileptic is described by Norman Geschwind in a paper cited in the note to page 315.

p. 440  On testamentary capacities, see M. Critchley, *Aphasiology* (London: Arnold, 1971), pp. 288 ff. Hughlings Jackson's remark is cited on p. 295.

p. 442  William James, *Psychology* (New York: Fawcett, 1963), p. 408.

p. 443  On the mind-body problem, see A. Rosenblueth, *Mind and Brain* (Cambridge, Mass.: M.I.T. Press, 1970); see also the essays in S. M. Farber and R. Wilson (eds.), *Control of the Mind* (New York: McGraw Hill, 1961).

p. 444  On disconnection and the mind: R. W. Sperry, "Hemisphere

Deconnections and Unity in Conscious Awareness," *American Psychologist*, 1968, *23*, 123–33; see also N. Geschwind, "Disconnexion Syndromes in Animals and Man," *Brain*, 1965, *88*, 585–644.

p. 446   J.B.S. Haldane is quoted on p. 183 of S. M. Farber and R. Wilson (eds.) *Control of the Mind* (New York: McGraw Hill, 1961); Eddington is quoted on pp. 88–9 of Rosenblueth, *op. cit.;* Penfield on p. 16 of Farber and Wilson (eds.), *op. cit.*

p. 447   Penfield's own operations: See p. 213. W. Penfield and P. Perot, "The Brain's Record of Auditory and Visual Experience," *Brain*, 1963, *86*, 595–696. The quotations come from p. 687 and also from p. 67 of W. Penfield, "The Permanent Record of the Stream of Consciousness," *Proceedings 14th Int. Congress of Psychology*, Montreal Neurological Institute Report, no. 486, 1954.

p. 449   U. Neisser, *Cognitive Psychology* (New York: Appleton-Century-Crofts, 1967), pp. 167–79.

p. 451   A mechanical brain indistinguishable from a human one: See A. M. Turing, "Computing Machinery and Intelligence," *Mind*, 1950, *69*, 433–60.

p. 452   The self: No one has written with greater penetration on this topic than William James. See *Psychology* (New York: Fawcett, 1963), Chap. 12.

p. 453   E. Erikson, "Identity and the Life Cycle," *Psychological Issues*, 1959, *1* (whole).

p. 454   W. Nauta, "The Problem of the Frontal Lobe: A Reinterpretation," *Journal Psychiatr. Res.*, 1971, *8*, 167–87.

# Index

*Note:* The names, initials, or pseudonyms of all brain-damaged patients have been italicized.

A Note on the Type

The text of this book was set on the Linotype in Baskerville. The face is a facsimile reproduction of types cast from molds made for John Baskerville (1706–75) from his designs. The punches for the revived Linotype Baskerville were cut under the supervision of the English printer George W. Jones.

John Baskerville's original face was one of the forerunners of the type style known as "modern face" to printers—a "modern" of the period A.D. 1800.

Composed, printed, and bound
by The Book Press
Brattleboro, Vermont.

Typography and binding based on
a design by Andrea Clark.